AF539872

Electrocardiogram Made Easy

NIPA® GENX ELECTRONIC RESOURCES & SOLUTIONS P. LTD.
New Delhi-110 034

About the Authors

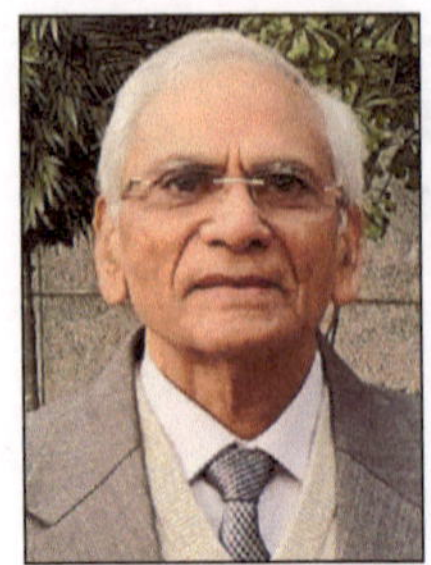

Prof. (Dr.) J.P. Varshney, Former Principal Scientist (Veterinary Medicine, ICAR-IVRI, Izatnagar), with a vast clinical, research and teaching experience of more than 57 years, is still continuing his dedicated yeoman clinical services at Nandini Veterinary Hospital, Surat (Gujarat). His work in animal electrocardiography and cardiology is well recognized and earned him reputation. He has been bestowed with Dr. K.S. Nair Memorial Gold Medal—1990, Dr. C.G. Bhaskar Gold Medal—1996, Ram Lal Agrawal Gold Medal—1997, Award of Merit-2001 (ICAR-IVRI,Izatnagar), Award of Honour-2002 (ICAR-IVRI,Izatnagar), Best Teacher Award 2003-2004 (ICAR-IVRI, Izatnagar), PETCARE Award for Canine Excellence-2005, Dr. C.M. Singh Memorial Lifetime Achievement Award-2020, VIPM Lifetime Achievement Award -2021 and an honour of "Living Legend of Homeopathy-2023" (3rd Homeopathy Vijnana Sammelan, Ahmedabad) besides many other honors and awards. Apart from publications in national/international scientific journals of repute, he is the author of books namely "Equine Parasitic Diseases and Their Management (ICAR-IVRI Izatnagar Publication, 2003), "Research Findings -Homeopathic Bio efficacy and Management of Animal Health (Sintex International Limited, Kalol, Gujarat 2007) , "Electrocardiography in Veterinary Medicine" (Springer Nature, Singapore, 2020), "Handbook of Exotic Pet Medicine" (Brillion Publishing, New Delhi, 2021), "Ultrasound in Veterinary Medicine: Fundamentals and Applications " (NIPA, New Delhi,2022), and "Heart Failure in Animals: Current Concepts" (NIPA, New Delhi,2023)

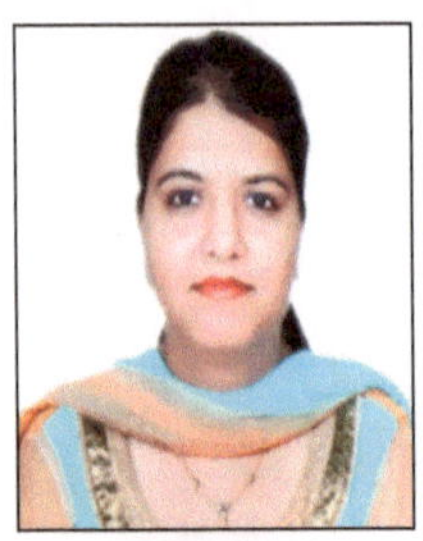

Prof. (Dr.) Neetu Saini, Professor Veterinary Medicine, Guru Angad Dev Veterinary and Animal Sciences University, Ludhiana, Punjab has a vast experience of 20 years in the field of veterinary medicine. She is known for her skill in electrocardiography and echocardiography. She has been bestowed with Young Scientist award besides many other awards. She has publications in national/international scientific journals of repute besides book chapters to her credit

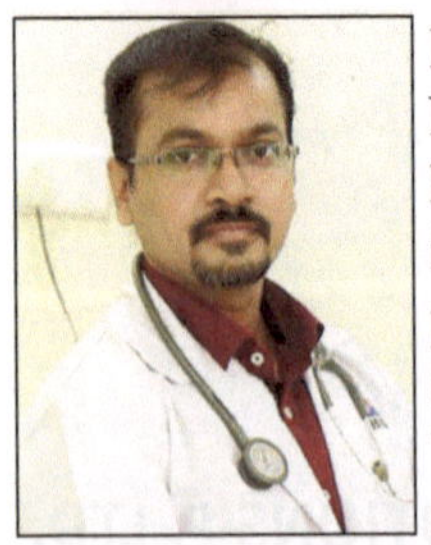

Dr. K. Satish Kumar, Professor and University Head at the PV Narsimha Rao Telangana Veterinary University, Hyderabad, has a vast experience in canine cardiology and diagnostic imaging techniques. He has guided a number of doctoral and post graduate students and has publications in national and international journals. He has been awarded with Fellow of VIPM and Fellow of VASc, Telangana state Best Teacher, and SVVU meritorious Teacher, DC blood Gold medal, PZ Sharma Gold medal, Dr. Rishendra Verma Young Scientist award, and many other prestigious awards.

Electrocardiogram Made Easy
A Fully Illustrated Handbook

J.P. Varshney
B.V.Sc. and A.H.; M.V.Sc. (Vet. Med.); Ph.D. (Vet. Med.)
Ex. Principal Scientist (Veterinary Medicine, IVRI Izatnagar)
Senior Consultant (Veterinary Medicine)
Nandini Veterinary Hospital
Ghod-Dod Road, Surat-395001, Gujarat, India

Neetu Saini
B.V.Sc. and A.H.; M.V.Sc. (Vet. Med.); Ph.D.(Vet.Med.)
Professor (Veterinary medicine)
Department of Veterinary Medicine
Guru Angad Dev Veterinary and Animal Sciences University
Ludhiana - 141004, Punjab, India

K. Satish Kumar
B.V.Sc. and A.H.; M.V.Sc. (Vet. Med.); Ph.D. (Vet. Med.)
Professor and University Head
Department of Veterinary Medicine
College of Veterinary Science
P.V.Narsimha Rao Telangana Veterinary University
Rajendranagar, Hyderabad- 500030, Telangana, India

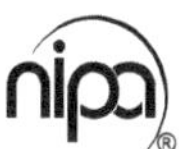

NIPA® GENX ELECTRONIC RESOURCES & SOLUTIONS P. LTD.
New Delhi-110 034

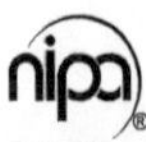

NIPA® GENX ELECTRONIC
RESOURCES & SOLUTIONS P. LTD.
101,103, Vikas Surya Plaza, CU Block
L.S.C. Market, Pitam Pura, New Delhi-110 034
Ph : +91 11 27341616, 27341717, 27341718
E-mail: newindiapublishingagency@gmail.com
Website: www.nipabooks.com
For customer assistance, please contact
Phone: + 91-11-27 34 17 17
Fax: + 91-11-27 34 16 16
E-Mail: feedbacks@nipabooks.com

ISBN: 978-81-19072-01-9

Composed and Designed by NIPA®.

Dedicated to
Parents, Teachers
and
Doyens of Electrocardiography

Acknowledgements

This book would not have seen the light of the day without the support of my family. I am grateful to my better half, Jai Prabha Varshney, for her patience, understanding, unconditional support, and care without any complaint during the long hours of my working on this text. Love, support, and care of my daughters (Pratibha, Ritu and Prabhanshi), sons (Atul, Prabhat and Ajit), and grandchildren (Agrima, Vedaant, Devansh and Anvi) had been a great asset to me in completing the task.

I thank my co-authors Prof Neetu and Prof. Satish for sharing similar vision of the future role of electrocardiogram in assisting diagnosis and prognosis especially in canine and feline practice; for their wisdom, insight and resolute attention in decoding an electrocardiogram in the simplified manner for veterinary students and practitioners.

I would also like to thank Shri Nayan N. Bharatia, Managing Trustee and Board of Trustees, Nandini Veterinary Hospital, Surat for providing me an opportunity to work with them for the greater cause of wellbeing of the animals. Direct or indirect help rendered by colleagues, and staffs is duly acknowledged.

I am indebted to my all animal patients for their unearthly patience in teaching me why this collection of knowledge on electrocardiogram is vital.

(J.P. Varshney)

Preface

Electrocardiogram is a visual record of the electrical activity of the heart recorded at the surface of the body of humans and animals during cardiac systole and diastole. It is one of the simplest and fasted technique employed for evaluating the rhythm, rate, and electrical activity (impulse formation and its conduction) of the heart. Though, Waller initially considered electrocardiography as an experimental method useful to physiologists rather than physicians, it has now become the most useful, handy, non-invasive and cost effective technique with clinicians for evaluating electrical activity of the heart in routine clinical practice.

Arrhythmias and conduction abnormalities are frequently encountered cardiac disturbances not only in canines and felines but also in equines, ruminants and exotic pets. Cardiomyopathy is another heart disease in canines and felines having great clinical importance. Traditional cardiac auscultation remains ineffective in distinguishing the various types of arrhythmias and conduction disturbances; and in recognizing chamber enlargement. The problem of differentiating arrhythmias and conduction disturbances can be easily addressed by adopting the technique of electrocardiography.

The other useful information that can be derived from electrocardiogram is mean electrical axis. It can assist in knowing whether the cardiac axis is normal or deviated. Electrocardiogram is also valuable in medical examination of healthy, geriatric, sport and sniffer dogs; pre-surgical evaluation; differentiating dyspnea of cardiac and respiratory origin; prognostication of dogs with hyperthermia, hypothermia, snake bites; and evaluating dogs with seizures, syncope, coma or trauma

As no technique is cent-percent perfect, electrocardiography has its own limitations. Besides limitations of the technique, patient restrain and positioning; preparation of sites and adequate application of gel; proper electrode clip positioning; and recording of electrocardiogram plays a significant role in interpretation of the electrocardiogram. Any hanky-panky or casual approach in ECG recording may yield erroneous results defeating the purpose of cardiac evaluation.

Majority of veterinary graduates and practicing veterinarians in India are not well versed with the technique of electrocardiography and interpretation of the resultant electrocardiogram because of their poor exposure to the technique. Dearth of a simplified, illustrative and low cost books dealing with all aspects of electrocardiography, right from basics to interpretation of various alterations in an electrocardiogram, also refrain them from using electrocardiography for cardiac evaluation in routine field practice.

The book "Electrocardiogram Made Easy A Fully Illustrated Handbook" has been designed keeping in view the requirements of the novice veterinary graduates and practitioners inclined to do cardiac evaluation of their patients. A chapter on self-exercise has been intended as a study aid to provide reader with an additional opening to assess his own understanding of an electrocardiogram. On one side of the page, ECG strip is given along with a short narration and a question. On the reverse side of the page, same ECG strip is again presented with the answer of the question and detailed analysis of the electrocardiogram.

It is anticipated that the book will achieve its goal of simplifying the technique of electrocardiography and assisting the readers in interpreting electrocardiogram so that the technique is extended to even primary veterinary practices for routine cardiac evaluation.

(J.P. Varshney)

Contents

1

Electrocardiograph, Electrocardiography and Electrocardiogram

Electrocardiograph, electrocardiography and electrocardiogram are the three terms commonly associated with ECG or EKG. Though, these terms are interdependent, there is clear differentiation and demarcation between these terms and should not be used as synonym.

Electrocardiograph

The term "Electrocardiograph" refers to an instrument or machine that records surface potentials associated with the electrical activity of the heart to generate a graphic representation, the electrocardiogram (Fig.1).

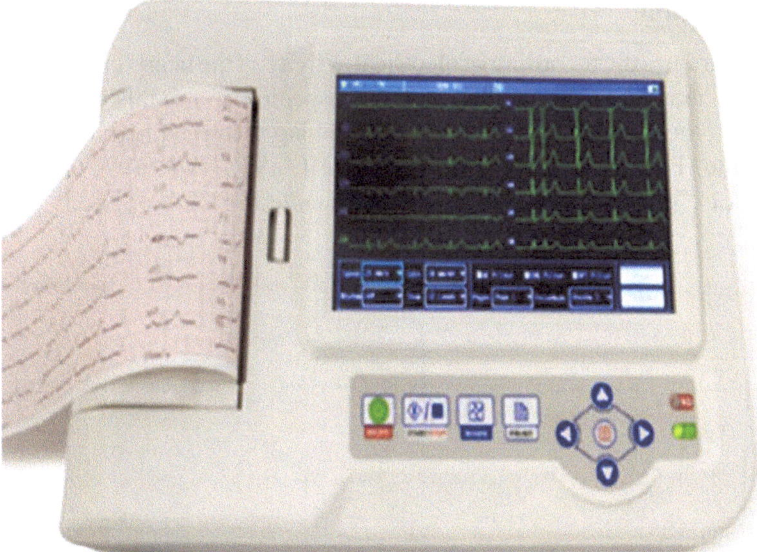

Fig. 1: The Electrocardiograph unit or machine

With the advancement of research, the basic electrocardiograph has taken a revolutionary progress. In the present scenario, a pocket based or smart-phone based electrocardiograph is also available, that is more economical and easier to carry. A Holter electrocardiograph is another type of portable ambulatory devise used to record ECG continuously over a period of time. It is a dynamic mode of recording ECG most commonly used for patients with arrhythmia, if a traditional electrocardiogram doesn't provide enough details (Fig. 2 and 3).

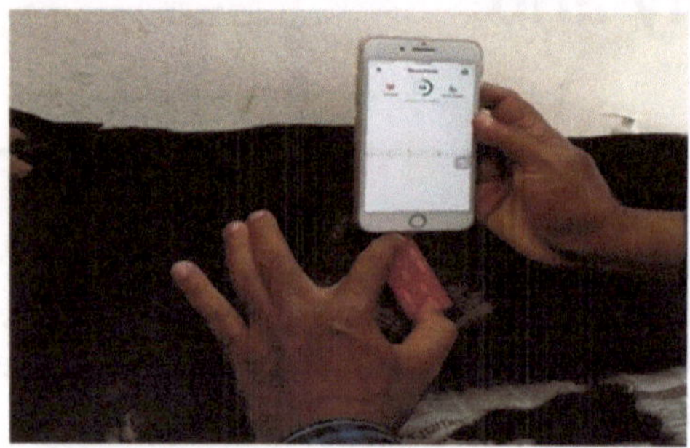

Fig. 2. Smart-phone based ECG device

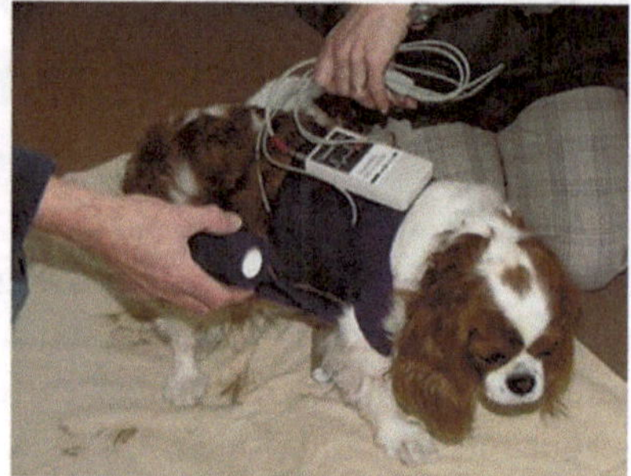

Fig. 3. Holter ECG with attachments

Electrocardiography

Electrocardiography is the process of recording electrical activity of the heart on the surface of the body to produce an electrocardiogram.

Electrocardiogram

Electrocardiogram is the recording of electrical activity of the heart representing voltage on 'Y' axis and time on 'X' axis in all species of animals as well as in humans. In other words, it is a line graph showing electrical activity of the heart over time (Fig.4) in different leads (I, II, III, aVR, aVL, aVF, CV$_5$RL, CV$_6$LL, CV$_6$LU, V$_{10}$). Electrocardiogram is also called as ECG or EKG.

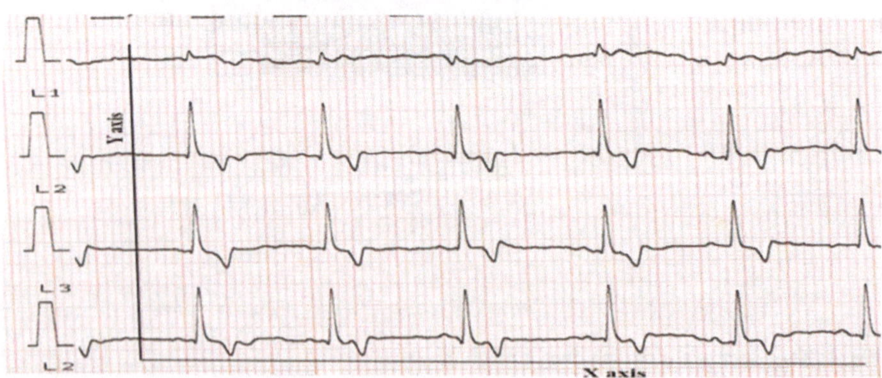

A

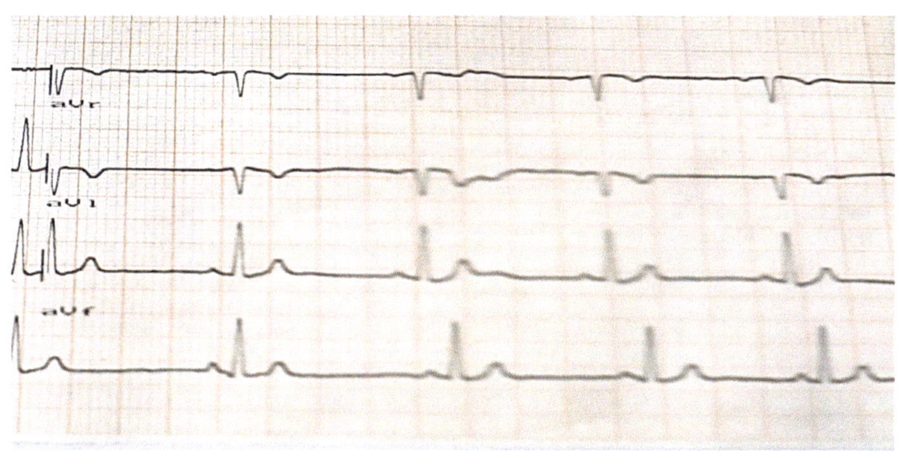

B

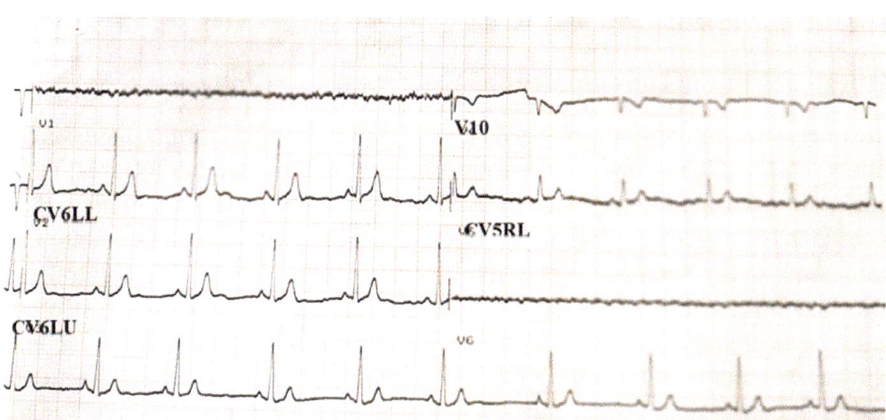
V10
CV6LL
CV5RL
CV6LU

C

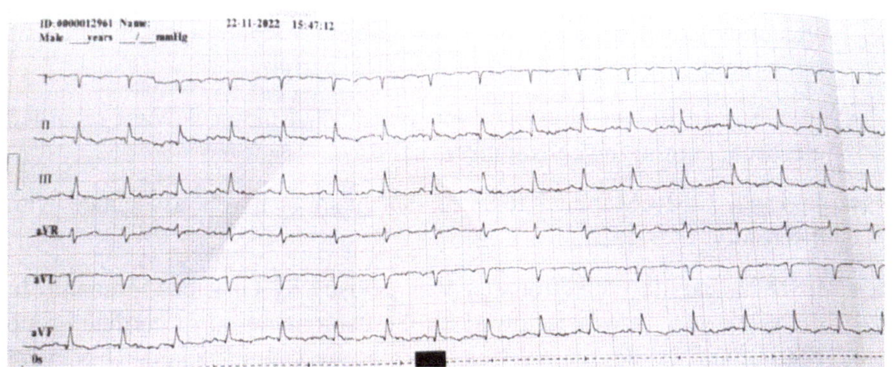
ID: 0000012961 Name:
22-11-2022 15:47:12
Male ___years ___/___mmHg
II
III
aVR
aVL
aVF

D

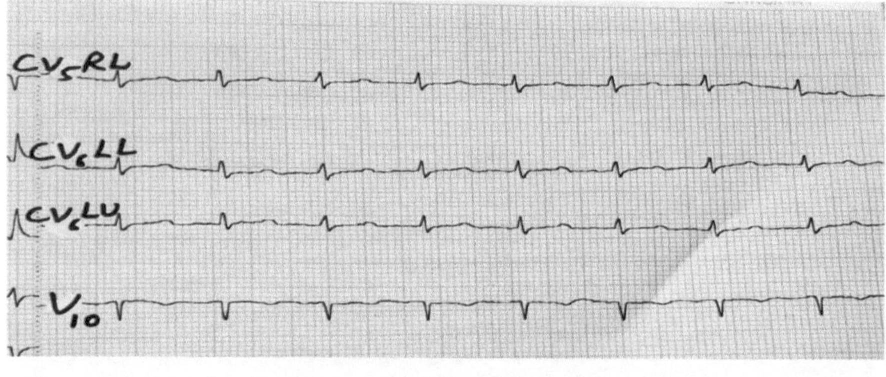

E

Fig. 4: A, B and C Electrocardiogram of a dog in different leads (Lead I,II,III, aVR, aVL, aVF, CV_6LL, CV_6LU, V_{10}, CV_5RL) . D and E. Electrocardiogram of a cat in different leads (lead I, II,III, aVR, aVL, aVF, CV_5RL,CV_6LL,CV_6LU and V_{10})

Milestones in the Development of Electrocardiography

Nowadays electrocardiography is an essential part of initial cardiac assessment among companion animals that are presented with dyspnea, marked weakness, seizures, syncope, shock, accident, trauma and any other emergency. The technique of electrocardiography is now much more developed and has witnessed many changes since its invention. It is always fascinating to understand the evolution of the technique to present day status and for future improvement. Application of technology along with history, physical and clinical examination has improved the evaluation process of both out-patients and in-patients, since last decade of 19th century. A brief history of important achievements in the development of electrocardiography is given below.

- The development of galvanometer in late 1700's was the first important step in the development of the modern electrocardiographic machine as it facilitated the measurement of electrical activity.
- In 1786, an Italian physician and physicist, Luingi Galvani recorded electrical current in skeletal muscle.
- In 1842, Carlo Matteuci realized that heart beat was associated with electricity.
- In 1873, capillary electrometer was devised by Gabriel Lippmann. In the same year, it was followed by the demonstration of cardiac group beating and 2nd degree AV block in frog by Luigi Luciani. This event was followed by the demonstration of AV block in human using apex

cardiogram by Alfred Lewis Galabin in the same year. Subsequently, with the invention of electrocardiogram, this group beating was known as "Wenckebach periodicity'.

- In 1876, Marey ,the Irish scientist, analyzed the electric pattern of frog's heart .
- The revolutionary invention was by Waller, who refined the capillary galvanometer and demonstrated its working on his dog-Jimmie. Because of slow instrument response time, tracings had to be converted mathematically. He developed dipole concept by recording various bipolar limb leads in cats. He was the person who demonstrated ECG for the first time using mercury capillary electrometer (refined capillary galvanometer) and toy train in 1887. He used five electrodes, one on each of the four extremities (both hands and both limbs) and one in mouth, with 10 leads derived from different combinations. This first electrocardiogram showed only two deflections which were termed as V1 and V2 to indicate ventricular activity. He considered electrocardiography as an experimental method useful to physiologists rather than physicians.
- In 1893, the term "electro-cardiogrammem "was introduced by Willem Einthoven. In 1895, he derived a correction formula to compensate inertia and friction when heart electrical activity was recorded using Lippmann capillary electrometer. He used the words A ,B,C,D to denote the words in uncorrected tracings. He later coined the words PQRS and T for the corrected derived deflections in 1906.
- Karel Frederik Wenckebach identified impairment of AV conduction in frog in 1899. It is now called as Wenckebach block or Mobitz Type I block.
- Einthoven, inspired from the work of Waller, refined the capillary electrometer and invented the string galvanometer in 1901 using quartz string coated in silver. He demonstrated five deflections. Initial old string galvanometer was the big machine and patients have to rinse their extremities in the cylindrical electrodes filled with electrolyte solution (Burch and DePasquale, 1964). He used three electrodes and dropped right leg and mouth electrodes. He placed positive leads on left arm and left leg to produce positive deflections on the electrocardiogram. These three leads were used to construct Einthoven triangle. This was the birth of clinical electrocardiogram.

- Einthoven published the first ECG in his article in year 1902. Later in 1905, he recorded normal and abnormal electrocardiograms using his string galvanometer and recording apparatus. He introduced U wave a few year later. 'U' wave was detected only in ECGs recorded with the string galvanometer. Electrocardiograms were also transmitted from patients in hospital to some distance away.
- With the passage of time, the weight of electrocardiographic machine reduced from 600 pounds in 1903 to 30 pounds in 1930 to only few kg in 2000 .There has been a trend over past decade towards a smaller and more compact mobile electrocardiographic monitoring equipment.
- In 1906 John Hay recorded simultaneous jugular venous and radial arterial pulses.
- In 1908, Thomas Lewis did experimental studies in dogs and clinical recordings in humans using the Einthoven's string galvanometer. He was honored as "Father of Clinical Cardiac Electrophysiology". He described atrial fibrillation in open chest horse and published his first book on "Electrocardiography" in 1913.
- In 1912, the concept of equilateral triangle formed by standard leads I, II and III (Einthoven triangle) was outlined by Einthoven.
- Lewis Lead (S5 –lead) electrode was developed by Sir Thomas Lewis in 1913 to detect atrial activity and its relationship to ventricular activity.
- Johannes Norr, German Veterinarian, worked on "Electrocardiogram in Horses" and submitted his doctoral thesis in 1913.
- In 1920, Louis Sigurd Friderica observed that the duration of QT interval was related to cube root of R-R interval. This is now termed as Friderica formula. On the other hand in the same year Henry Cuthbert Bazett observed that corrected QT interval was related to square root of R-R interval. His formula is known as Bazett Formula.
- Mobitz classified second degree AV block in 1924 in two separate groups as Mobitz type I and II.
- In 1924, Einthoven bagged the Nobel Prize in Physiology and Medicine for his work on the mechanism of the electrocardiogram and was recognized as " Father of Electrocardiography"
- First portable ECG machine was introduced in 1928. The machine was powered by a vehicle battery.

- In 1930, L. Wolff, J. Parkinson and P.D. White described the syndrome 'Bundle branch block with short P-R interval in healthy young people prone to paroxysmal tachycardia.
- Precordial lead was introduced by Charles C. Wolferth and Francis Clark Wood in 1931. He called it as Lead IV. The precordial electrode was placed on the chest over the apex of the heart. In the same year (1931) precordial lead IV was introduced by Frank Norman Wilson. Then CL, CR, CF, CB and V leads were introduced. There remained confusion on the placement of these leads until the V1 through V6 precordial or chest leads became a standard procedure all over the world.
- Augmented unipolar limb leads (aVR, aVL, aVF) were introduced by Goldberger in 1942.
- In year 1933, Wolferth and Wood suggested that the abnormal slurring of the initial part of QRS complex in Wolff-Parkinson –White syndrome and prolongation of QRS complex were not due to bundle branch block but to an acceleration of the passage of impulse from atrium to a part of ventricle.
- In 1937, Louis Nelson Katz and Hans Wachtel observed biphasic QRS complex (large R and S waves) in lead V2-5.
- In 1944 , a symbol (Δ)was proposed by Marcel Segers, J. Lequime and H.Denolin to represent the triangle shape at the base of up slopping QRS complex in pre excitation syndrome.
- In 1953, a distinct deflection at J point on the electrocardiogram was described by John J Osborn. It was termed as 'Current of injury' and commonly known as 'J' deflection or Osborn wave.
- Holter ECG (dynamic ECG) was developed in 1957 by Norman Holter. This was a portable device that facilitated continuous monitoring of electrical activities of cardiovascular system for more than 24 hours.
- First western portable defibrillator was invented by Frank Pantridge in 1965.
- In 1976, Erhardt Sjogren and Wahlberg described the use of CR_4 R or V4R lead in the diagnosis of right ventricular infarction.
- In 1977, epsilon wave was described by Guy Fontaine in patients with arrhythmogenic right ventricular dysplasia.
- Year 2013 has witnessed the progress and prosperity of wearable devices

and smart phone based ECG device that have become a new tool for self-diagnosis and remote diagnosis.

- Subsequently, during 2018 the application of Smart-phone based ECG has taken a revolutionary change in both human and veterinary medicine.
- With the advancement and research in the development of electrocardiograph unit, the future devices may provide a comprehensive diagnosis combining electrocardiogram with MRI, functional MRI, ultrasound, CT scanner, oxygen saturation, blood pressure, EEG, pulse oximetry, breathing and haemodynamic parameters.
- Big data mining for ECG holds strong promise and potential in future.
- Accuracy of diagnosis and application in evidence based medicine is another potent area of future research in electrocardiography.

Indications of Electrocardiographic Examination

Electrocardiographic examination is indicated for evaluation of cardiac functioning in health and diseases. It is of great assistance in following conditions.

- Routine examination of the dogs.
- Medical checkup of sports and sniffer dogs.
- Pre-surgical evaluation and monitoring of heart function during anesthesia and surgery.
- Differentiation of arrhythmias and conduction disturbances.
- Differential diagnosis of cardiac and respiratory diseases in dogs with signs of respiratory distress/ gasping/ panting/ dyspnea.
- Cardiac evaluation in cases of seizures/syncope.
- Evaluation of dogs suspected with cardiomyopathy.
- Cardiac monitoring and prognostication of dogs in non-cardiac emergencies such as severe heat stroke /sun stroke or with severe hypothermia.
- Evaluation of cardiac functioning in dogs with multi organ failure.
- Evaluation and monitoring of dogs in acute emergencies and in intensive care units.
- Evaluation of geriatric dogs.

- Cardiac evaluation of dogs with effusions (peritoneal, pericardial, pleural).
- Cardiac evaluation in dogs in cases of fall/ trauma/ accidents.
- Cardiac evaluation of dogs with electrolyte disorders.
- Monitoring the progress of treatment in cardiac and noncardiac emergencies.
- Creating database for differentiating nonspecific causes of weakness, fatigue, lethargy.

Advantages of Electrocardiography

- It is a simple non-invasive and easy to use diagnostic tool for monitoring the heart.
- Generally no sedative or any anesthesia is needed for electrocardiography.
- Electrocardiogram is immediately available for interpretation as soon as electrocardiographic recording is completed.
- Arrhythmic dogs can be evaluated quickly in a better way
- Electrocardiogram provides an additional data base to facilitate the diagnosis and treatment of disease of both cardiac and noncardiac origin.
- Evaluation of cardiac compromised animals in a better way.
- Electrocardiogram provides visual record of cardiac status of the animals.

Limitations of Electrocardiogram

Despite a very useful technique, it has its own limitations.

- Electrocardiogram cannot provide a definite diagnosis of congestive heart failure.
- Electrocardiogram cannot provide definite prognosis during anesthesia or surgical procedures.
- Myocardial wall thickness cannot be measured.
- Diagnosis of diseases of different cardiac valves , endocardium or pericardium is not possible.
- Diagnosis of obstructive blood flow diseases cannot be made.
- Body conformation and different breeds of the dogs can make the interpretation of electrocardiogram a little difficult.

- Normal electrocardiogram may not always rule out the possibility of cardiac disease. Therefore interpretation of electrocardiogram should be done in conjunction with the results of all other tests and examinations.

References

Burch, G.E. and DePasquale, N.P. (1964) . A history of electrocardiography. Chicago: Year Book Medical; 1964. (Google Scholar)

Further Readings

Jeon, B., Lee, J. and Choi, J. (2013). Design and implementation of a wearable ECG system. Int. J. Smart Home. 7: 61–70.(Google Scholar).

Varshney, J.P. (2020). Electrocardiography in Veterinary Medicine. Springer Nature, Singapore, Pte, Ltd.

Waller, A.D. (1889). On the electromotive changes connected with the beat of the mammalian heart, and of the human heart in particular. Phil. Trans. R .Soc. Lond. B.; *180*: 169–94. (Google Scholar).

2

Electrocardiographic Unit

An electrocardiographic unit has a compact electrocardiograph machine, power cord, patient cable, thermal recording ECG paper roll, and conducting gel.

Electrocardiographic Unit

The Electrocardiograph is a sensitive galvanometric device that is capable of recording difference in electric potential up to 1 mV (1/1000 of a volt). The machine has a voltage meter and amplifier combined with a strip recording device (Fig.5) to provide a permanent record. Various basic features viz. running (paper) speed of the machine , sensitivity, lead selector, off/on switch, filter etc are displayed on the screen (Fig. 5). Electrocardiographic machine can record electrocardiogram at the paper speed of 25 or 50 mm per second as per our selection. The sensitivity switch controls amplitude of the waves. The amplitude or sensitivity can be selected as 0.5,1. or 2. The sensitivity of 1 means that 1 mV input causes deflection of 1 cm or 10 mm on the ECG paper; the sensitivity of 2 means that 1 mV input causes deflection of 2 cm or 20 mm on the ECG paper; and the sensitivity of 0.5 means that 1 mV input causes deflection of 0.5 cm or 5 mm on the ECG paper . Lead selector switch/ touch spot is used to select the leads in single channel ECG machines.In automatic six channel machine or twelve channel ECG machines there is no need to select the leads manually. These features are minimal basic features that comes with every machine, however, they may vary with machine to machine and depend on the model. Hence, manufactureres' specifications or instructions given in the user manual should be followed before using any machine for better results. Eelectrocardiographic machines of different companies may have different set up but basics are same.

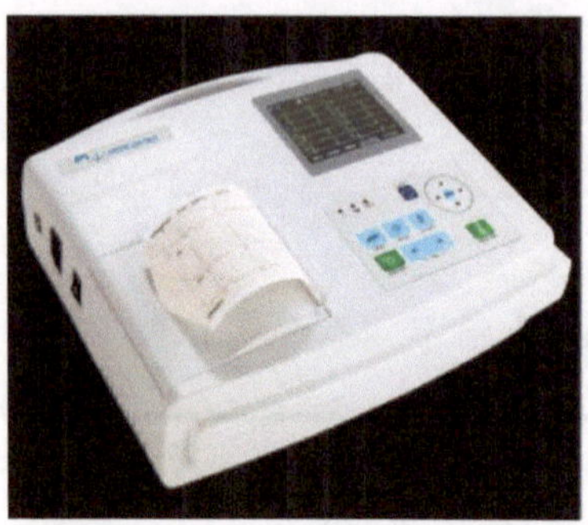

BPL Cardiart 6208 three channel ECG Machine

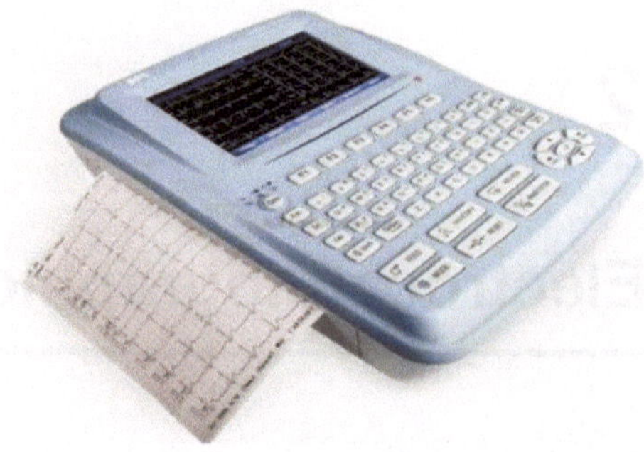

BPL 9108D twelve channel ECG machine

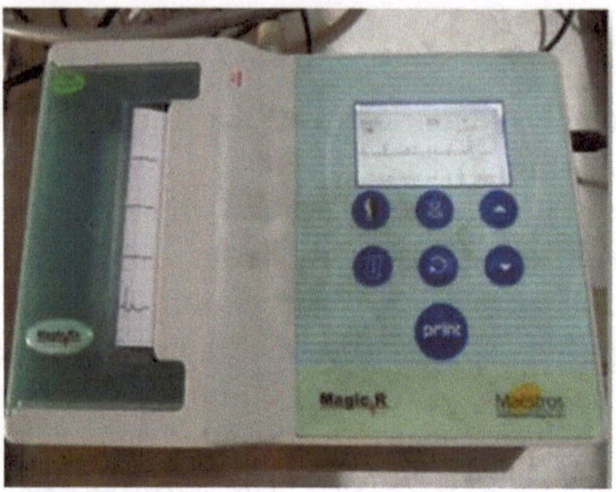

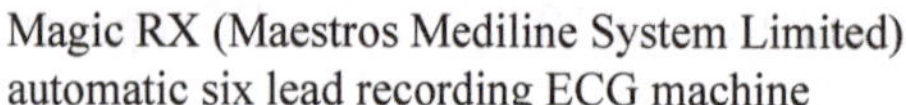

Magic RX (Maestros Mediline System Limited) automatic six lead recording ECG machine

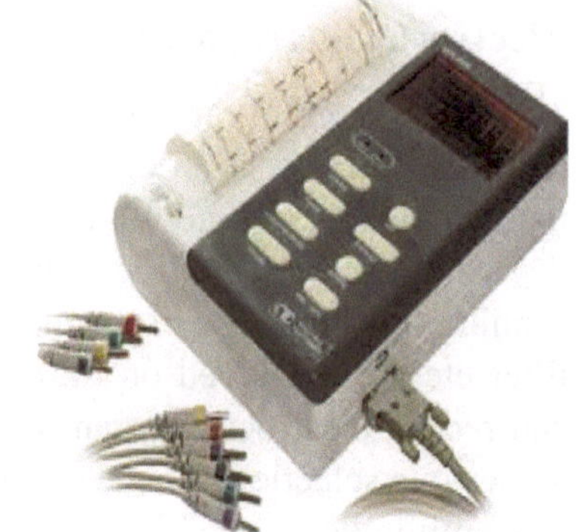

Maestros 12 channel ECG Machine

Fig. 5: Different types of the Elctrocardiographic machines

Availability of Electrocardiographic Machines in India

Though multiple brands of ECG machines are available in Indian market, all of them are designed for human use. However, the same are being used to record ECG in animals also, but measurements and interpretations are done by the Veterinarian.Few ECG machines dedicated for veterinary use along with interpretations are also available . These veterinary use ECG machines provide some interpretations also. Any machine can be used for recording ECG among veterinary patients that should invariably be analysed and interpreted by a veterinary specialist. The following are few of the models available in the Indian market.

1. BPL 6208 3 channel ECG Machine
2. BPL Cardiart 9108 12 channel ECG Machine

3. BPL Cardiart 108 T Digi ECG machine Single channel
4. BPL GENX 3 ECG 3 channel ECG machine
5. BPL 9108 D 12 channel ECG machine with 7 " display
6. BPL 8108 View 5 channel ECG Machine
7. BPL 6108 T Single channel ECG Machine
8. BPL Cardiart GENX1 single channel ECG Machine
9. Comen CM1200A 12 channel ECG Machine
10. Comen CM 300 3 channel ECG machine
11. Commen CM 1200 B 12 channel ECG Machine
12. Bionet Cardiocare 2000, 12 channel ECG Machine
13. Bionet Cardio 7 ECG machine 12 channel
14. RMS Vesta 301i 3 channel ECG Machine
15. RMS Vesta 101 Single channel Test ECG machine.
16. Philips TC 20 12 channelECG Machine
17. Philips Page writer TC 10 ECG Machine 12 channel
18. Contec 1200 12 channel ECG Machine touch screen.
19. Contec 100 G single channel ECG Machine
20. Contec 1200 G 12 channel ECG Machine
21. GE MAC 2000 12 channel ECG Machine
22. GE MAC 800 6 channel ECG Machine
23. Clarity True Beat 100 F 3 channel ECG Machine
24. Schiller 3 channel ECG Machine Cardiovit AT-1 G2
25. Magic RX (Maestros Mediline System Limited)automatic six lead ECG machine

Required Features in an Electrocardiographic Machine

A good electrocardiograph should have the following important features

- Machine should be light weight, compact with handle for portability.
- It should be compatible with the main power supply (220-240 V).

- It should have high performance rechargeable battery with built in charger. The battery backup should be sufficient to take 50 to 100 electrocardiograms without AC power.
- There should be digital filtering to remove interferences from electric line and muscle tremors.
- ECG machines are single, 3,6 or 12 channel display . Selection can be done as per choice/ requirement.
- ECG recording can be preferred with standard leads I,II,III ; augmented leads aVR, aVL, aVF, chest leads unipolar or V leads; or simultaneous acquisition from 12 leads.
- ECG unit should have facility for speed selection.
- Electrocardiograph should have facility of automatic adjustment of base line for optimal recording.
- A good electrocardiographic machine should have different filters (base line filter, EMG filter and AC filter).
- Modern electrocardiographs are also having built in facility for measuring ECG parameters and interpretating.
- There should be built in facility for high resolution thermal printing.

Standard Settings of an ECG Machine

- ECG machines have different types of display screen. Lead II should be visible, as this is the standard lead used for interpretation in dogs and cats. Good quality ECG machines allow the simultaneous display of 3 (I,II,III),6 (I,II,III, aVR, aVL, aVF) or 12 leads (all three standard bipolar leads, three unipolar leads and 6 chest leads) as per their inbuilt specifications.
- Standard sensitivity of ECG machine is 1 (1 mV = 1 cm or 10 mm). It can be changed to 0.5 or to 2 as per requirement. If the complexes are too big at sensitivity of 1, sensitivity should be changed to 0.5. In case complexes are too small at sensitivity of 1, then it should be changed to 2.
- Standard paper speed is 25 mm/second. This can be doubled (50 mm/second) to see complexes spaced out.
- Automatic setting of the machine is good for monitoring because it displays on screen only, and does not print. If a printed trace is required,

a manual option will need to be selected through the mode or menu button, and the 'run' or print button selected. Some machines have an analysis feature as well.

- If ECG machine has filter switch or button, it should be turn on, to dampen interference. It can also dampen all electrical activity. So care should be exercised.

ECG Cable and Electrodes

ECG cable is also known as patient cable or trunk cable. The cable has a monitor specific connection on one end that connects to ECG port on patient monitor. The other end the yoke connects to a set of lead wires to with a safety Din connection (Fig. 6).

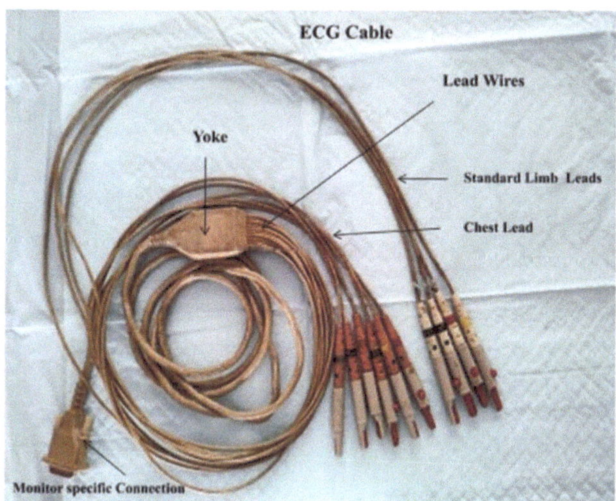

Fig. 6: Showing ECG cable, connector, lead wires, electrodes and clips.

One bundle of cable wires has four separate wires attached to four electrodes (limb electrodes) and other bundle has six wires attached to six chest electrodes (Fig.7 A and B) There are four separate limb electrodes labeled as, left arm (LA)-yellow coloured, right arm right (RA) – red coloured , left foot or limb (LL) –green colored and right foot or limb (RL)-black coloured. The other bundle of wire cable has six separate wires attached to six chest electrodes (Fig. 7 A and B) or one cable wire attached to only one exploring chest electrode (Fig. 7C) . Six separate chest electrodes are marked as V1,V2,V3,V4,V5 and V6. In dogs four chest electrodes (V1,V2,V3 and V4) are used as CV_5RL, CV_6LL, CV_6LU and V_{10} respectively. Only one exploring chest electrode is marked as C (Fig.7C). This chest electrode is manually placed at different chest locations to record ECG in different chest leads.

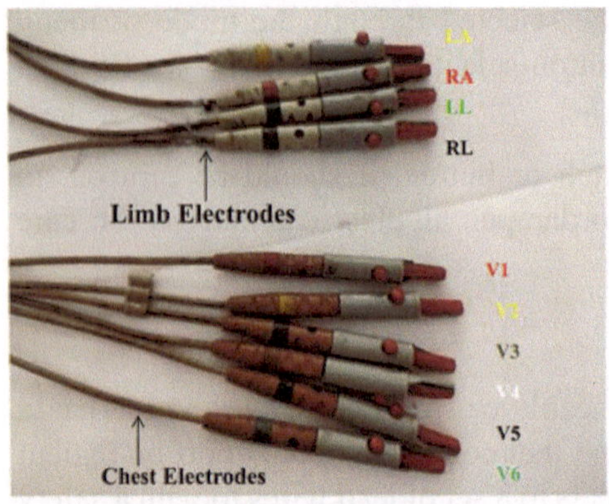

A

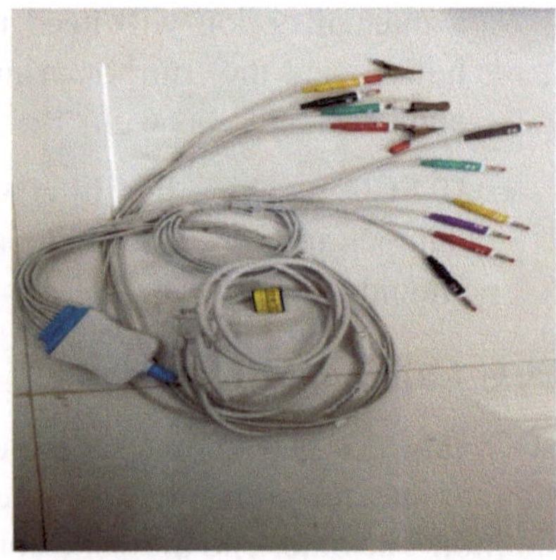

B

C

Fig. 7: Showing wire leads and different standard limb and chest electrodes

Electrode Attachment

There are various types of electrode attachment (Fig.8) such as flat contact alligator clips, needles, or cuffs that are attached to the electrodes on one end and to dog's skin on the other end.

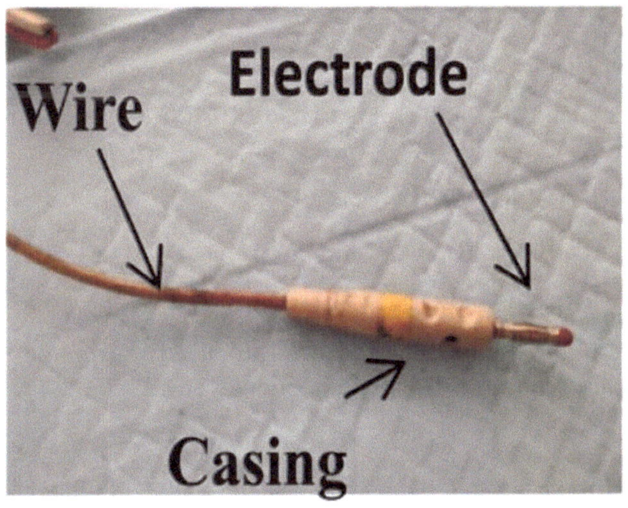

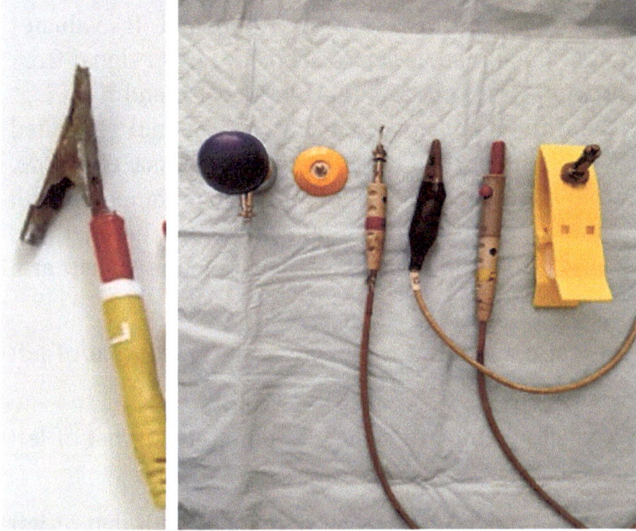

Fig. 8: Showing electrode , different types of electrode attachments as alligator clips , needle, cuff, for attaching to electrode on one side and skin of the dog on other side.

Lead System

A lead in ECG is created by analysing several electrodes and is defined as a graphical description of the electrical activity of the heart. It is computed by analysing the different electrical currents at different angle or pair of electrodes. Heart is evaluated in different leads. Each lead has definite direction and polarity. Leads record components of depolarization and repolarization aligned to them.

Leads

The different leads of an ECG are as follows:

1. Extremity Leads or Standard Limb Leads : Lead I,II,III, aVR,aVL and aVF
2. Chest Leads : CV_5RL, CV_6LL, CV_6LU, and V_{10}
3. Measuring Leads : I,II,III, CV_5RL, CV_6LL, CV_6LU, and V_{10}
4. Calculated Leads: aVR, aVL and aVF
5. Wilson's Central Terminus (WCT): the 'zero' lead produced by averaging signals from the limb electrodes. This is a directionless lead.

   WCT= 1/3 (RA+LA+RL)

Standard lead system or Bipolar lead system – It is also termed as Einthoven Lead system. This system consists of three leads (lead I, II and III). In this lead system , the potential difference of two limbs is compared. It evaluates activation of the heart in the frontal plane. Electrodes record ECG signal from four body locations (right arm –RA, Left arm –LA, left leg-LL and right leg-RL). The final output is the difference between electrical potential generated between two electrodes. Right limb or right leg is a ground reference electrode. Therefore the electric potential of right arm or right fore limb is compared with that of left arm or left fore limb; electrical potential of right arm or right fore limb with that of left leg or left hind limb; and electrical potential of left arm or left fore limb with that of left hind leg or limb.

Lead I compares the electrical potential of right fore limb (-)with that of left fore limb (+).

Lead II compares the electrical potential of right fore limb (-)with that of left hind limb (+).

Lead III compares the electrical potential of left fore limb (-) with that of left hind limb (+).

Einthoven triangle (Fig. 9) is an imaginary formation of three limb leads (lead I,II,III) in a triangle formed by right and left shoulders and pubis. It is an inverted equilateral triangle with the heart in the centre.

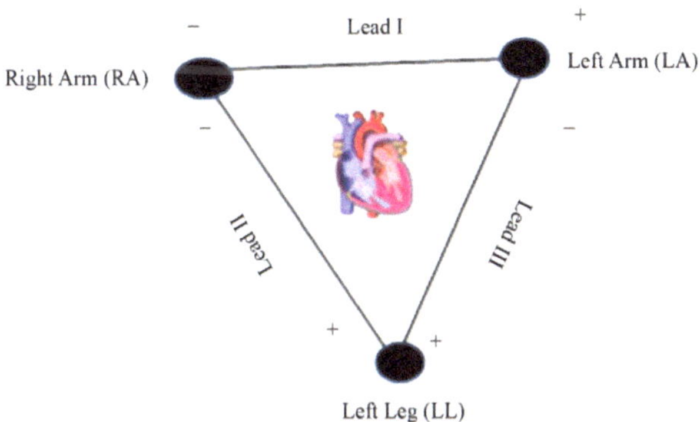

Fig. 9: Diagramatic representation of standard lead system and Einthoven trinagle.

Augmented unipolar limb lead system- The other lead system is augmented unipolar limb leads consisting of aVR, aVL and aVF leads (Fig. 10). The word 'a' stands for augmented , 'V' stands for vector and words R,L and F stand for right forelimb, left forelimb and left hind limb or foot respectively.They are derived from the same three electrodes as lead I,II and III but they use Goldberger's central terminal as their negative pole. The augmented leads are unipolar because there is a single positive electrode that is referenced against a combination of other two limb electrodes. The positive electrodes for these augmented leads are located on the right fore limb (aVR) , left left fore limb (aVL) and left hind limb (aVF).These leads provide an additional information about cardiac vector. In this system electrical potential at the reference limb is compared with the sum of electrical activity at the other two limbs.

aVR - Electrical potential of right forelimb (+) is compared to the sum of electrical potential of left forelimb and left hind limb (-).

aVL - Electrical potential of left forelimb (+) is compared to the sum of electrical potential of right fore limb and left hind limb (-).

aVF - Electrical potential of left hind limb (+) is compared to sum of electrical potential of right and left forelimbs (-).

Bailey's Hex-axial Lead system – This is most widely used lead system in canine and feline electrocardiography. It combines both bipolar standard and augmented unipolar lead systems (Fig.10).

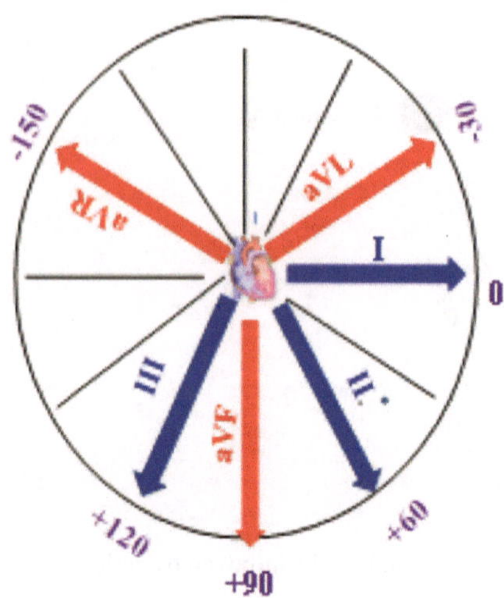

Fig. 10: Bailey's Hex-axial lead system comprised of three standard bipolar leads (I,II,III blue colour) and three augmented unipolar leads (aVR, aVL , aVF red colour) as shown in the figure. These leads record electrical activity along a single plane (frontal plane) relative to heart .

Special Leads

Unipolar precordial chest leads- In dogs four chest leads (CV_5RL, CV_6LL, CV_6LU, and V_{10}) are used. While in man, six chest leads (V1,V2,V3,V4,V5, and V6) are used. The chest leads view the heart from the transverse plane and provide important information for the diagnosis of heart enlargement (right or left), bundle branch blocks, ischaemic heart changes and arryhthmias.

Examination of lead II is very important in dogs and cats as it provides valuable information. Augmented unipolar leads are used to determine the position of the heart and confirming the changes observed in standard leads. The unipolar precordial chest leads are not well established in canines. V_{10} lead is most frequently used precordial chest lead to confirm changes in right heart.

Electrocardiographic paper

Electrocardiographic paper is simply a graph paper having horizontal and vertical lines making boxes (Fig.11). There are two types of boxes i.e. large and small. Small boxes are of 1 x 1 mm or 0.1 x 0.1 cm while large boxes are of 5 x 5 mm or 0.5 x 0.5 cm. Every fifth horizental and vertical line is darker as compared to other lines. Both horizontal and vertical lines are 1mm (0.1 cm) apart. The distance between two horizontal lines represents amplitude denoted as mV. When ECG machine is set at sensitivity of 1 (i.e.1.0 cm or 10 mm = 1 mV) the distance between two horizontal lines represents 0.1 mV.

The distance between two horizontal lines indicates 0.05 mV or 0.2 mV at the sensitivity of 2 or 0.5 respectively. The vertical lines are also 1 mm apart and represent the time interval or duration in seconds or mili seconds. The distance between two vertical lines represents time of 0.04 seconds or 0.02 seconds when ECG recording is done at the speed of 25 mm per second or 50 mm per second respectively. Voltage magnitude of electrocardiographic complexes is expressed in mV and duration in second or milisecond .

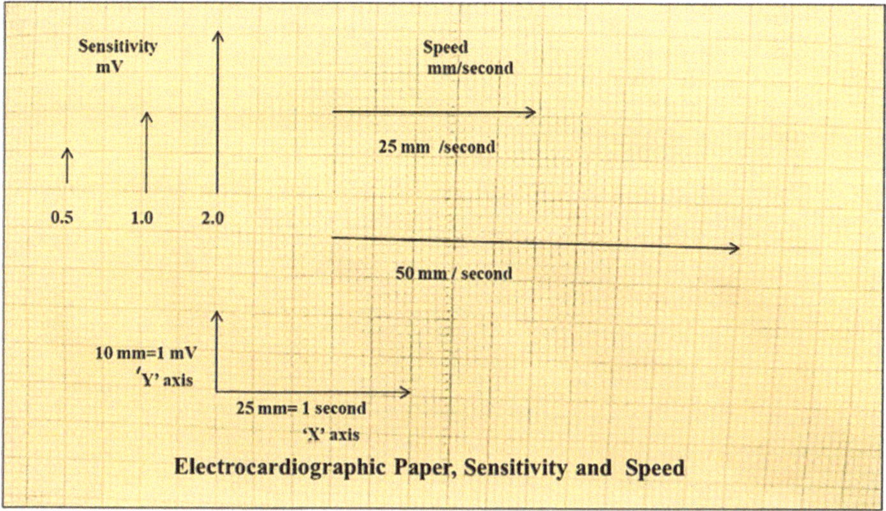

Fig. 11: Electrocardiographic paper and grid lines. Time is shown on the 'X' and voltage (amplitude) of the wave is shown on 'Y' axis of the graph paper. At the running speed of 25 mm or 50 mm per second ,the interval between two vertical lines is 0.04 seconds or 0.02 second respectively. At the sensitivity setting of 1 (1cm=1mV),2 (2 cm= 1 mV) or 0.5 (0.5 cm =1mV), the distance between two horizontal lines indicates 0.1 ,0.05 or 0.2 mV respectively.

Time and speed

Electrical activity of the heart is recorded by drawing traces on the moving ECG graph paper strip . All ECG machines can run at two speeds i.e. at 25mm/second (Fig.12) or 50 mm/second(Fig.13). Generally ECG machines are run at 25 mm/second. At this speed the interval between two vertical lines denotes 0.04 second (40 ms). When the paper output speed is doubled (50 mm/second), minor or subtle electrocardiographic findings hidden in the tracing become more evident and the interval between two vertical lines denotes 0.02 second (20 ms).

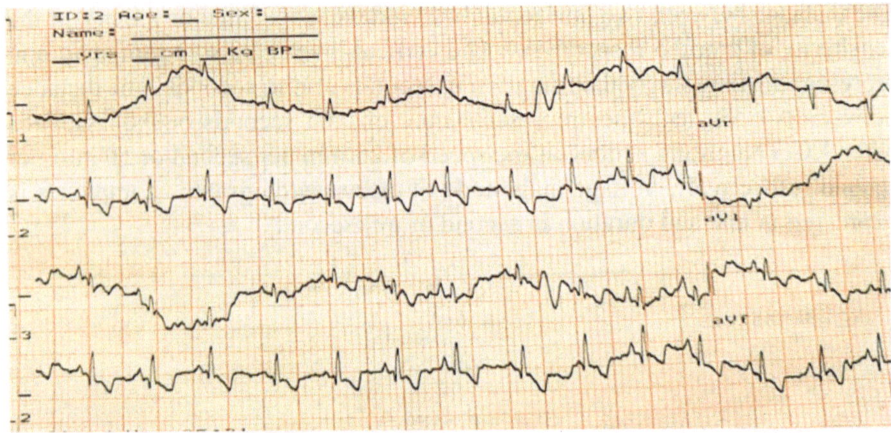

Fig. 12: Electrocardiogram of six month old non-descript dog taken at the speed of 25 mm/second.The distance between two vertical lines denotes 0.04 second

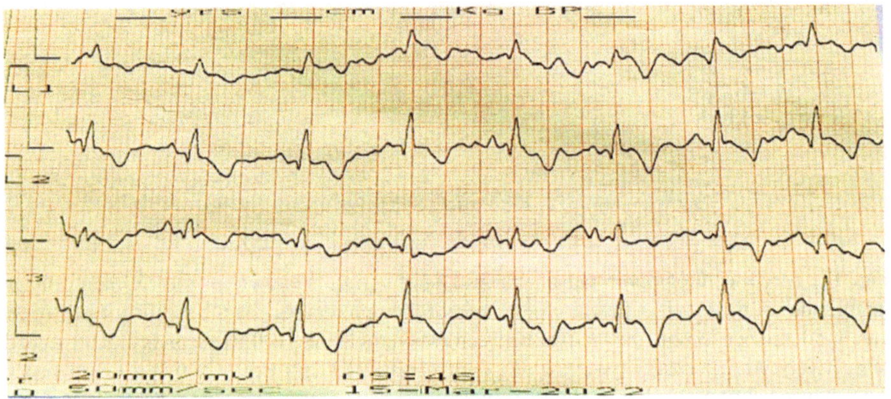

Fig. 13: Electrocardiogram of the same non-descript dog (as above) taken at the speed of 50 mm/second.The distance between two vertical lines denotes 0.02 second.

Sensitivity

In the ECG strip,voltage is plotted on the vertival axis (Y- axis) . The standard sensitivity calibration is 10 mm or 1 cm = 1 mV. When the complexes are too large , the sensitivity can be reduced to half i.e. 5.0 mm or 0.5 cm = 1 mV. If the complexes are too small the standard sensitivity can be doubled i.e. 20 mm or 2.0 cm = 1mV (Fig.14).

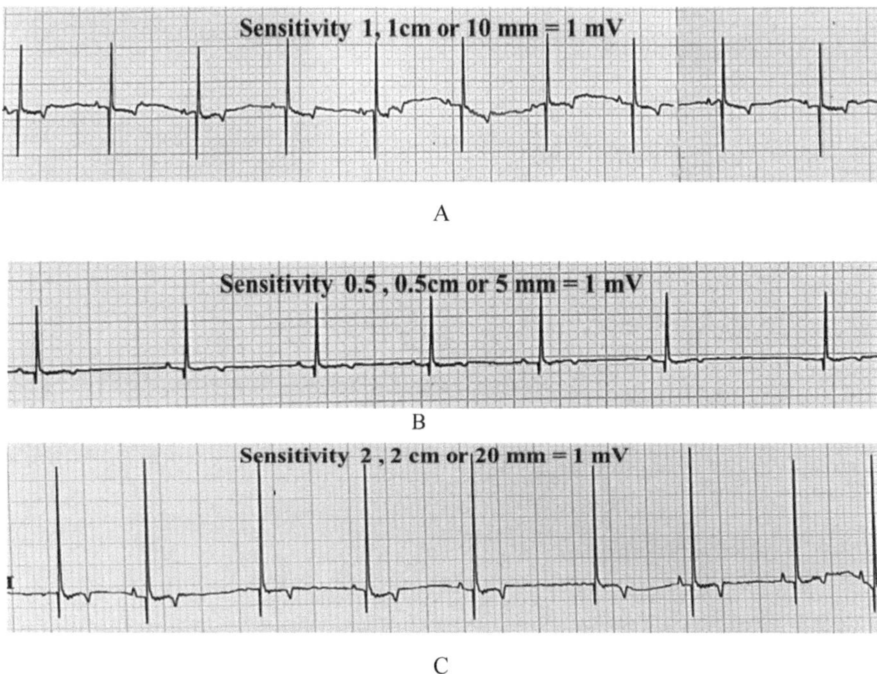

Fig.14: Electrocardiogram of an adult dog taken at different sensitivity. A at 1.0 (1.0 cm = 1 mV), B at 0.5 (0.5 cm = 1 mV) and C at 2.0 (2.0 cm = 1mV). The complexes are smallest at 0.5, largest at 2.0 sentitivity and intermediate at 1.0 sensitivity. Normally the electrocardiogram is recorded at sensitivity 1. If amplitude of the complexes is too large, sensitivity is reduced to 0.5. It is changed to 2.0 when amplitude of complexes is too small.

Further Readings

Varshney, J.P. (2020). Electrocardiography in Veterinary Medicine. Springer Nature, Singapore, Pte, Ltd.

3

Recording of An Electrocardiogram

The process of recording an electrocardiogram involves preparation of sites, application of conduction gel, positioning and restraining the patient, attaching the electrodes and then actual recording. Errors in placement of electrodes and artifacts during electrocardiography may generate erroneous electrocardiogram.

Sites for Placement of Electrodes in Dogs and Cats

There are definite sites (Fig. 15 and Fig.16) for placement of electrodes both in dogs and cats .Improper placement of electrode may lead to erroneous electrocardiogram.

A. Standard Limb Electrodes- Limb electrodes (Fig.15) are placed in dogs and cats as follows:

Right Fore Limb - Proximal to the olecranon on the posterior aspect.

Left Fore Limb - Proximal to the olecranon on the posterior aspect.

Right Hind Limb - Over patellar ligament on the anterior aspect.

Left Hind Limb - Over patellar ligament on the anterior aspect.

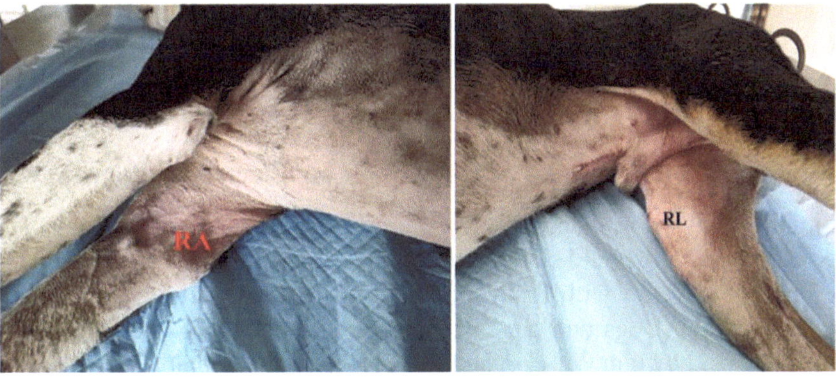

Fig. 15: Sites for placement of electrodes on fore limbs and hind limbs. RA=Right arm Electrode, RL= Right leg Electrode. LA and LF electrodes are placed on similar spots on the left arm and left leg as shown for right arm and right limb

B. Chest Electrodes- Chest electrodes (Fig.16) are placed as follows:

CV_5RL - 5th right intercostal space near edge of sternum.

CV_6 LL - 6th left intercostal space near edge of sternum.

CV_6LU - 6th left intercostal space at costo-chondral junction

V_{10} - Dorsal spinous process of 7th thoracic vertebra.

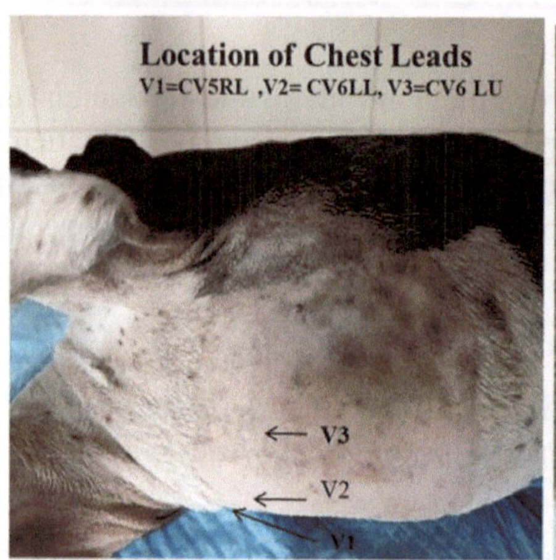

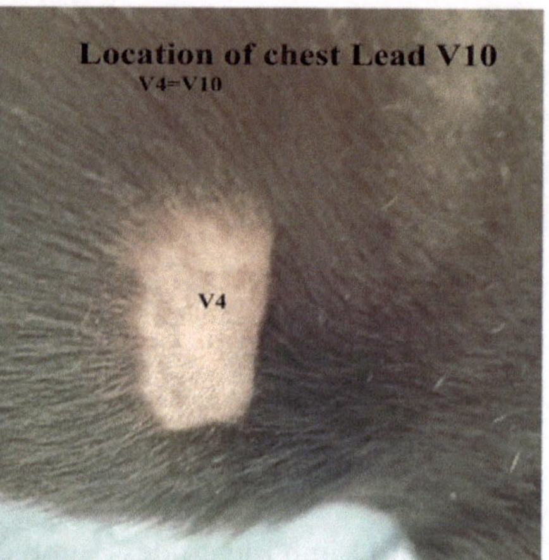

Fig. 16: Sites for placement of chest electrodes. V1= CV_5RL, V2= CV_6LL, V3= CV_6LU, V4 =V_{10}

Preparation of sites for Placement of Electrodes

The sites for placement of electrodes are prepared by cleaning and shaving the area for a good quality electrocardiogram. After cleaning, the sites and electrode alligator clips should be moistened with electrocardiographic gel, paste or alcohol. In odd circumstances when nothing is available water can be used to increase the contact between skin and electrodes. In emergency cases when there is no time for shaving, the skin and hairs may be wet with liberal application of electrocardiographic gel.

Positioning and Restraining of Dog or Cat for Electrocardiography

Positioning of the dog or cat is very important in electrocardiography. The electrocardiography should be done in a calm and comfortable room. Wooden table or table covered with foam mattress and non-conductive rubber sheet is most desirable. Dogs and cats are positioned on the table in right lateral recumbancy as shown in Fig.17 A and B. It is the most acceptable and standard position for taking electrocardiogram in dogs and cats. In some situations electrocardiography can also be done in left lateral (Fig.17 C) or in standing (Fig.17 D) positions. But altered body positions have effect on measurements of waves and also on mean electrical axis. The amplitude of Q and R waves is increased in lead I and II; amplitude of R and S waves is increased in aVR and aVL; amplitude of R and S waves is decreased in lead III; and MEA is shifted to left when ECG is taken in standing position (ST) as compared to right lateral (RL) recumbency (Rishniw *et al.*, 2002). When electrocardiogram is recorded in left lateral (LL) recumbency there is an increase in the amplitude of R wave in lead II,III and aVF; increase in amplitude of S wave in lead aVL; decrease in the amplitude of R wave in lead aVR; and no change in mean electrical axis (Rishniw et al.,2002). Generally no anesthesia or sedation is required for taking an electrocardiogram. Dog can be restrained by a person in right lateral recumbancy by keeping his right arm over the neck and left arm over the hind quarter of the dog in the manner that both legs (left and right) do not touch each other (Fig.17). The forelimbs should be kept perpendicular to the long axis of the body. Improper positioning of the fore limbs may yield erroneous results. For example: the form of 'QRS' complex in lead I appear like that of aVF (Fig.17 E) when left fore limb is pulled caudally; and it appears like that of aVR if the left fore limb is pulled cranially.

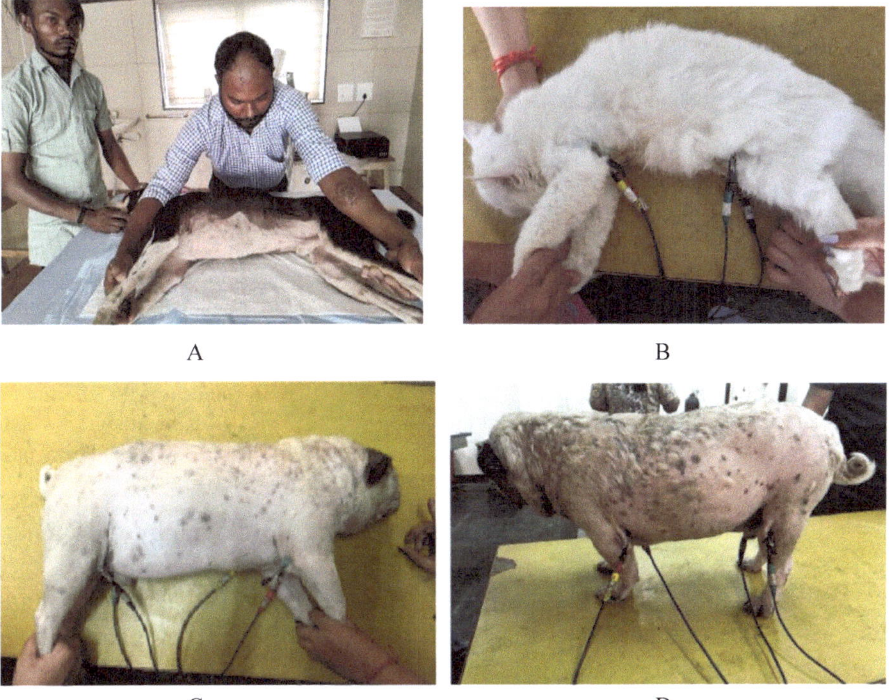

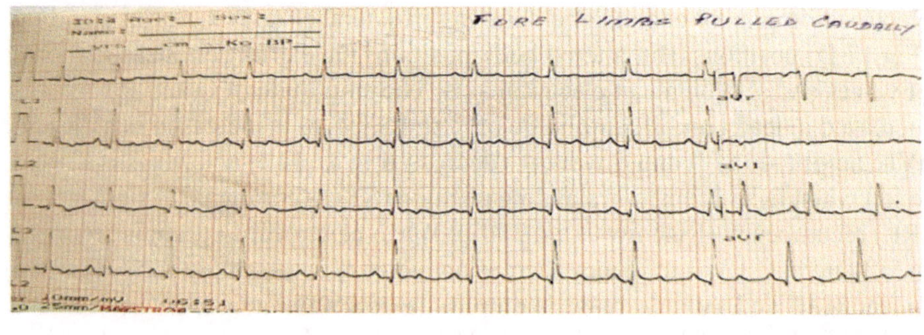

E

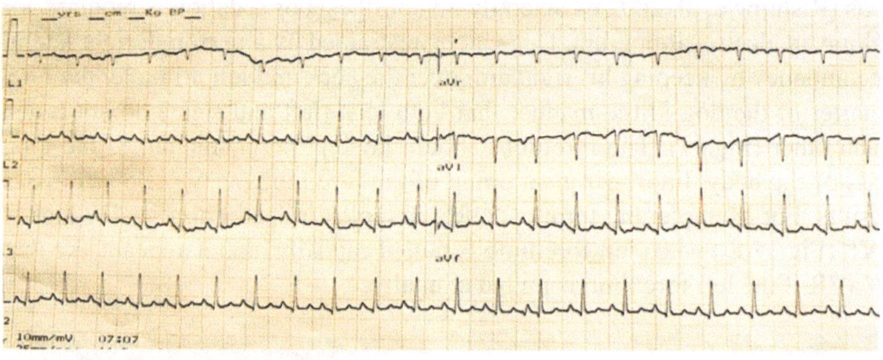

F

Fig. 17: A. Positioning and restraining of a dog in right lateral recumbency for electrocardiography. Note the positioning of both fore and hind limbs. It is the most accepted and widely used position for electrocardiography in dogs. B. Positioning and restraining of cat in right lateral recumbency for electrocardiography. Note the positioning of both fore and hind limbs. It is the most accepted and widely used position for electrocardiography in cats. C. Positioning of a dog in left lateral recumbency for electrocardiography. Electrocardiography can also be done in left lateral recumbency. Left lateral recumbency for electrocardiography affects measurements of the waves and mean electrical axis. D. Positioning of a dog in standing position for electrocardiography. The standing position for electrocardiography also affects measurements of the waves and mean electrical axis. E. Electrocardiogram (lead I, II, III, aVR, aVL, aVF; sensitivity 1, speed 25 mm/s) of a dog in right lateral recumbency but fore limbs pulled caudally. Note the complexes in lead I are almost like aVF . F. Electrocardiogram (lead I, II, III, aVR, aVL, aVF; sensitivity 1, speed 25 mm/s) of a dog in right lateral recumbency but fore limbs pulled cranially. Note the complexes in lead I are almost like aVR.

With the presence of owner at the table during electrocardiography, the animal feels comfortable. Therefore, owner should be allowed to remain with the dog/cat during the process of electrocardiography. Highly aggressive and nervous dogs are uncooperative and can be managed with diazepam (1 mg/Kg orally 1 hour before the procedure) or acetylpromazine (2 mg/Kg orally 1 hour before the procedure or 0.5 mg/Kg intramuscularly or intravenously 15 min before the procedure) to get a good quality electrocardiogram. Diazepam and acetylpromazine or acepromazine maleate are sedative/ tranquilizers usually make the dog comfortable without significantly affecting cardio-pulmonary functions. When any sedative is used, it is to be mentioned while interpreting the electrocardiogram. General anesthetics, tranquilizers in high doses or parasympatholytic drugs (atropine) are not recommended for taking an electrocardiogram as they can alter the physiologic state.

Attaching the Electrodes

Electrodes are attached with the help of flattened or modified alligator clips in dogs (Fig.18) and cats (Fig. 19) as detailed below:

RA Electrode - Attached proximal to the olecranon on the posterior aspect of the right forelimb.

LA Electrode- Attached proximal to the olecranon on the posterior aspect of the left forelimb.

RL Electrode - Attached over patellar ligament on the anterior aspect of the right hind limb.

LL Electrode - Attached over patellar ligament on the anterior aspect of the lcft hind limb.

The limb electrodes (RA,LA,RL, LL) make six leads as L I, II, III, aVR, aVL and aVF. These six leads are termed as frontal plane leads. Of these three (I,II,III) are actually rccorded and other three (aVR, aVL , aVF) are calculated one.

Apart from these limb leads , four V leads or unipolar precordial chest leads are also used in the dogs as detailed below :

CV_5RL (rV_2) Electrode - It is attached at 5th right intercostal space near the edge of sternum.

CV_6LL (V_2) Electrode - It is attached at 6th left intercostal space near the edge of sternum.

CV_6LU (V_4) Electrode - It is attached at 6th left intercostal space at costo-chondral junction.

V_{10} Electrode - It is attached over dorsal spinous process of 7th thoracic vertebra.

These V leads are horizontal plane leads. In electrocardiographic machines, chest electrodes are marked as V1,V2,V3,V4,V5 and V6.Out of these V1 to V4 can be used as CV_5RL,CV_6LL,CV_6LU and V_{10} respectively for dogs.

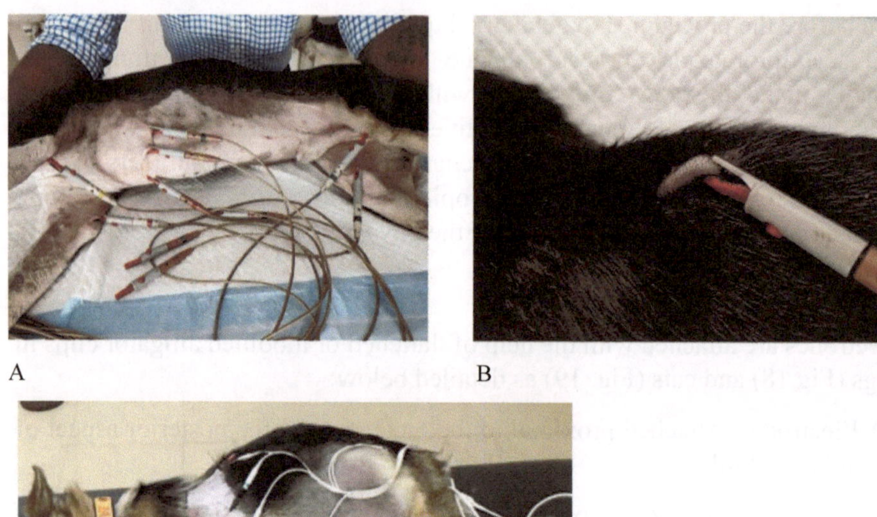

A B

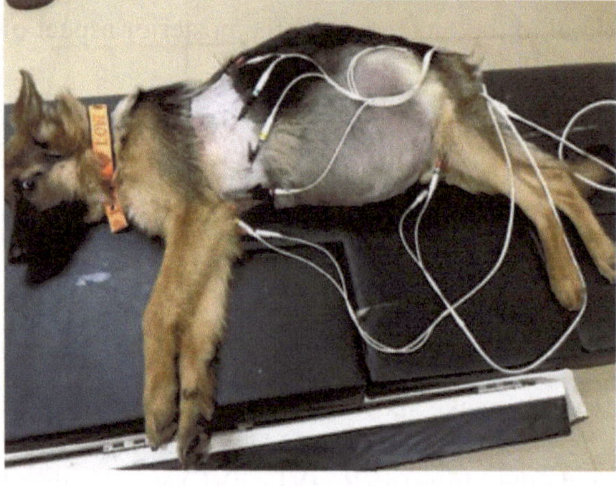

C

Fig. 18: Placement of electrodes on dog. Attach left arm (yellow) electrode to the skin proximal to olecranon on the caudal aspect of the left fore limb, right arm (red) electrode to the skin proximal to olecranon on the caudal aspect of the right fore limb, left limb (green) electrode to the skin over patellar ligament on the anterior aspect of the left hind limb, right limb (black) electrode to the skin over patellar ligament on the anterior aspect of the right hind limb; CV_5RL electrode at 5th right intercostals space near edge of sternum, CV_6LL electrode at 6th left intercostals space near edge of sternum, CV_6LU at 6th left intercostals space at costo-chondral junction (A and C) and V_{10} over dorsal spinous process of the 7th thoracic vertebra B and C).

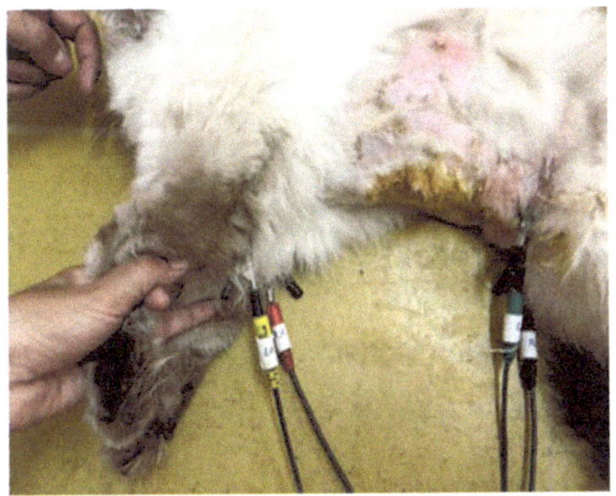

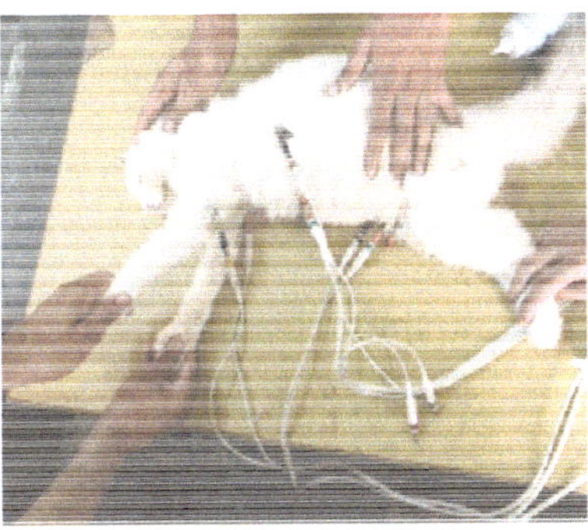

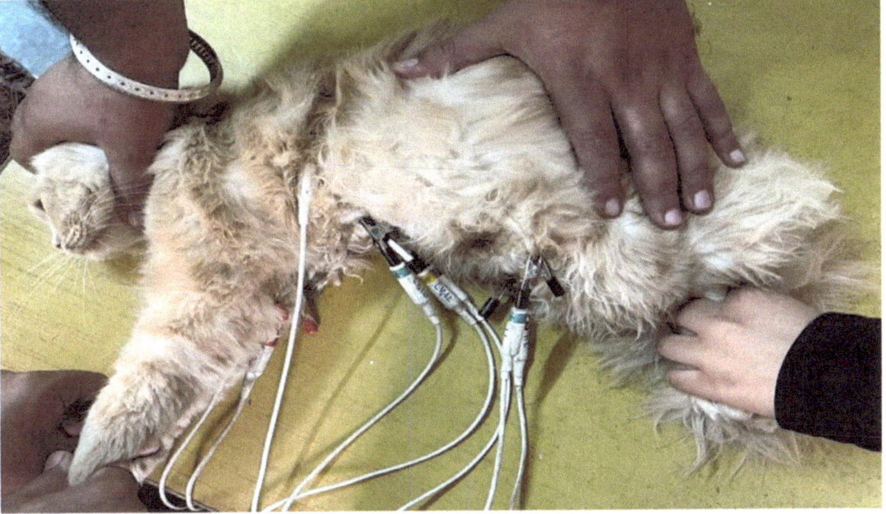

Fig. 19: Placement of electrodes on cat. Attach left arm (yellow) electrode to the skin proximal to olecranon on the caudal aspect of the left fore limb , right arm (red) electrode to the skin proximal to olecranon on the caudal aspect of the right fore limb, left limb (green) electrode to the skin over patellar ligament on the anterior aspect of the left hind limb, right limb (black) electrode to the skin over patellar ligament on the anterior aspect of the right hind limb ,CV_5RL electrode at 5th right intercostals space near edge of sternum, CV_6LL electrode at 6th left intercostals space near edge of sternum, CV_6LU at 6th left intercostals space at costo-chondral junction and V_{10} over dorsal spinous process of the 7th thoracic vertebra as similar to that of dogs

Features of Limb and Chest Leads

- Standard limb leads are frontal plane leads and examine the electrical activity of the heart in the frontal plane of the body.
- Chest leads are horizontal plane leads and determine the electrical activity of the heart in sagittal and horizontal planes of the body.

- V lead records the direction and voltage of electrical activity from the heart to the electrode position.

Recording of an Electrocardiogram

1. Generally instructions given by the manufacturer are to be followed.
2. Connect the power cord if machine is to be used on main electric supply.
3. Connect the earth clip to some metal plate/sheath/object.
4. Load the electrocardiographic paper.
5. Connect the patient cable to the patient cable socket of the ECG machine.
6. Connect the lead wires of the patient cable to the electrodes.
7. Clean the electrode area on the body surface with 75% alcohol.
8. Apply electrocardiographic gel on electrodes and electrode area.
9. Attach the electrodes to the patient.
10. Press the on/off to turn on the device.
11. Enter details of the dog.
12. Set the standard sensitivity at position 1. Sensitivity can be changed to 0.5 or 2.0 as per need.
13. Set the standard paper speed at 25 mm per second. It can be changed to 50 mm/second if needed.
14. Press print / start as per machine.
15. Display and printing of electrocardiogram will begin and will stop as soon as all the leads are recorded.
16. Turn power off.
17. Remove the lead electrodes from the dog or cat.
18. Clean the gel with the help of a towel or tissue paper.
19. Electrocardiographic machines from different companies have different settings. Therefore machines should be operated as per instructions in the manual.

Errors in Placement of Electrodes

Relationship between limb leads and electrodes placed at correct places making the Einthoven triangle is shown in Fig. 20 A. The normal electrocardiogram when the leads are correctly placed is shown in Fig.20 B. Misplacement of limb lead electrodes is a common cause of ECG abnormality and may simulate pathology. When three limb leads (LA,RA ,LL) are misplaced or exchanged without disturbing the neutral electrode (RL or right hind limb), Einthoven triangle (Fig. 20) is flipped or rotated, leading to inversion of the switching leads. Reversal of one of the limb electrode with the neutral electrode (RL or right hind limb electrode) disrupts Einthoven triangle and disrupt the zero signal received from Wilson's central terminal, altering the appearance of both limb leads.

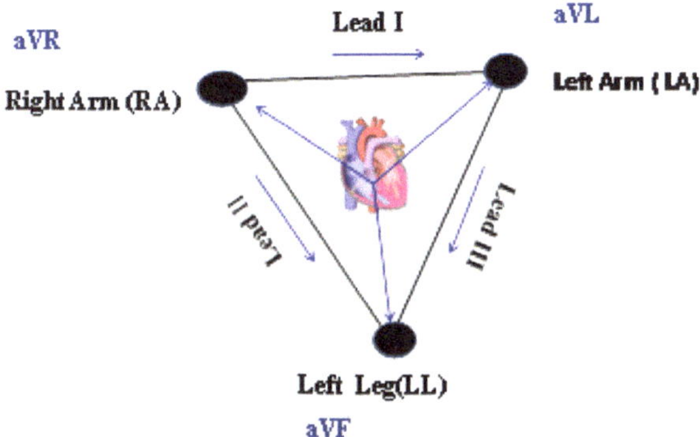

A

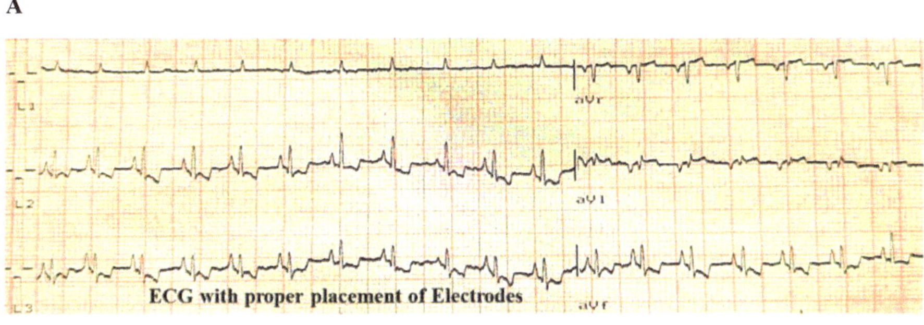

B

Fig. 20: Relationship between limb leads and electrodes and formation of Einthoven triangle (A) and a normal electrocardiogram with proper placement of elctrodes (B).

1. Reversal of LA and RA – When fore limb electrodes (RA and LA) are reversed (Fig.21 A), the following changes are seen in the electrocardiogram (Fig.21 C) as Einthoven triangle flips 180^0 horizontally around an axis formed by the lead aVF (Fig.21 B).

- There is an inversion of Lead I. All three waves in lead I (P, QRS and T) become inverted.
- Leads II and III switch their place.
- Leads aVL and aVR also switch their place.
- Lead aVR, normally negative, becomes positive.
- There is no change in the position of Lead aVF.
- Marked right axis deviation may be seen.

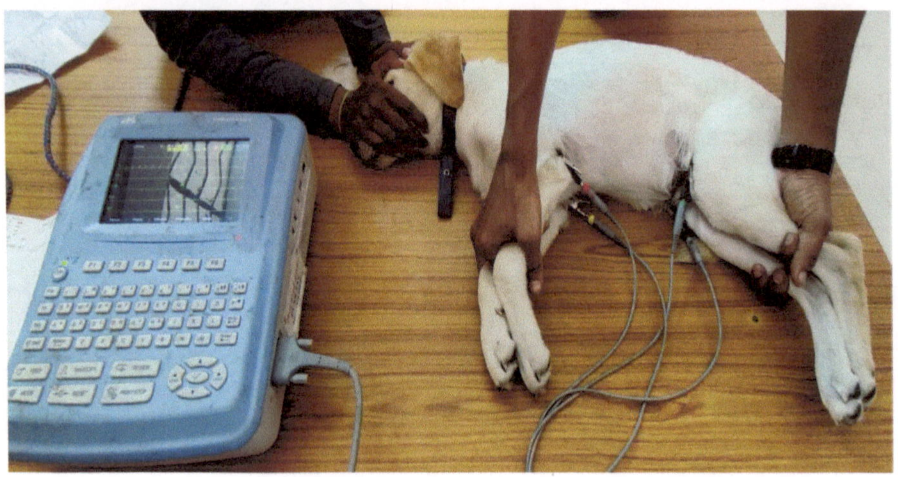

A

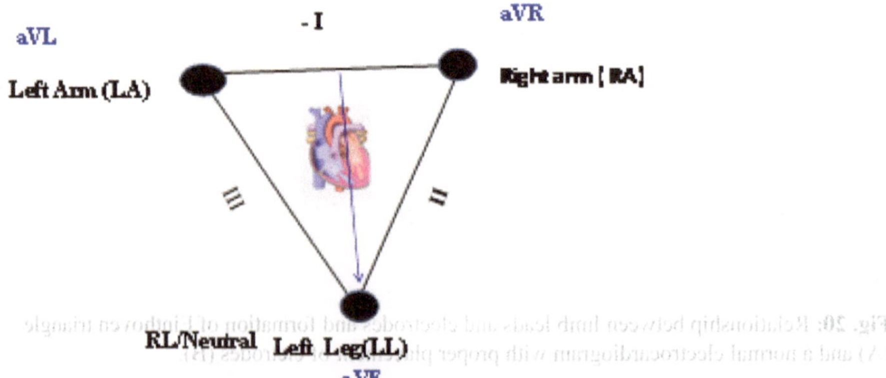

B

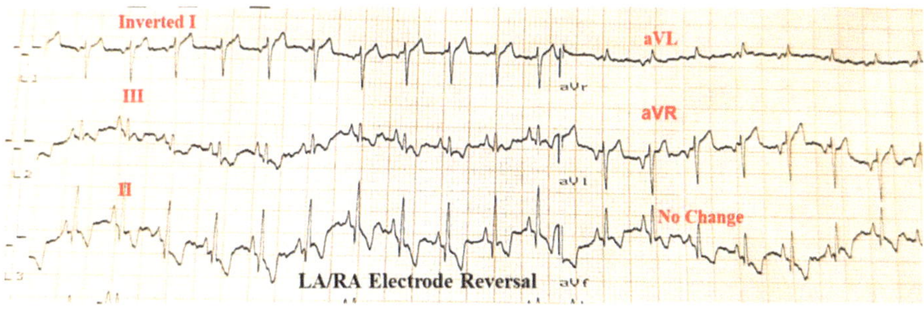

C

Fig. 21: Reversal of LA and RA electrodes. Relationship between limb leads and electrodes and electrocardiogram produced when electrodes of LA/RA are reversed.

2. Reversal of LA and LL – When left fore limb electrode (LA) is reversed with left hind limb electrode (Fig.22 A) following changes are seen in the electrocardiogram (Fig. 22 C) as Einthoven triangle rotates 180 ^{0} vertically around an axis formed by the lead aVR (Fig. 22 B).

- There is inversion of Lead III. All three waves in lead III (P, QRS and T) become inverted.
- Leads I and II switch their place.
- Leads aVL and aVF also switch their place.
- There is no change in the position of Lead aVR.
- 'P' wave is larger in lead I than lead II.

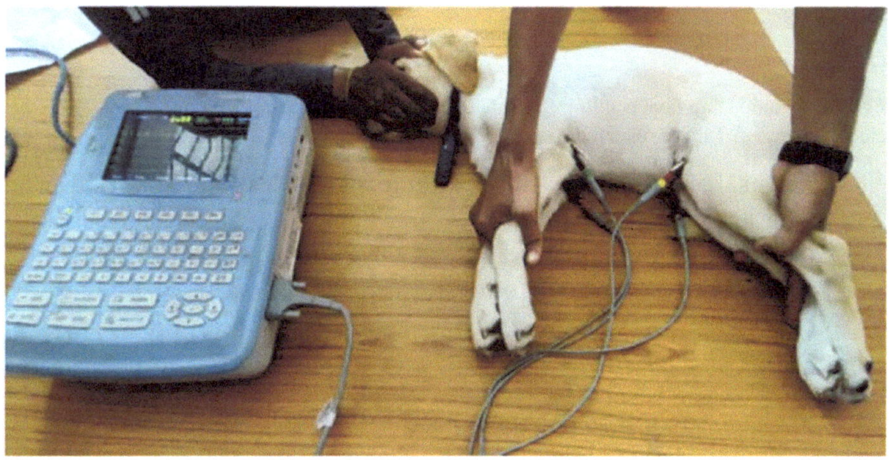

A

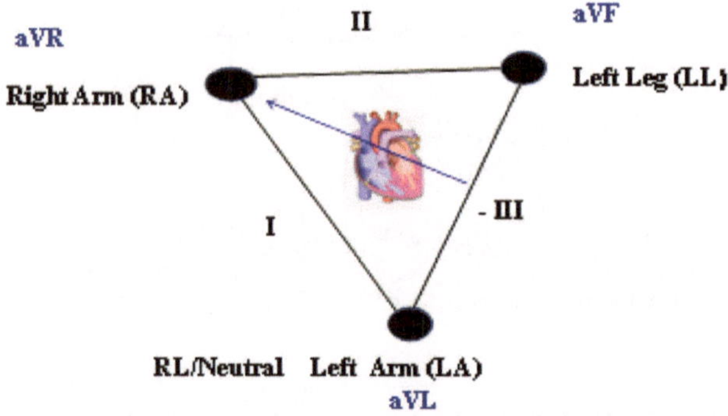

B

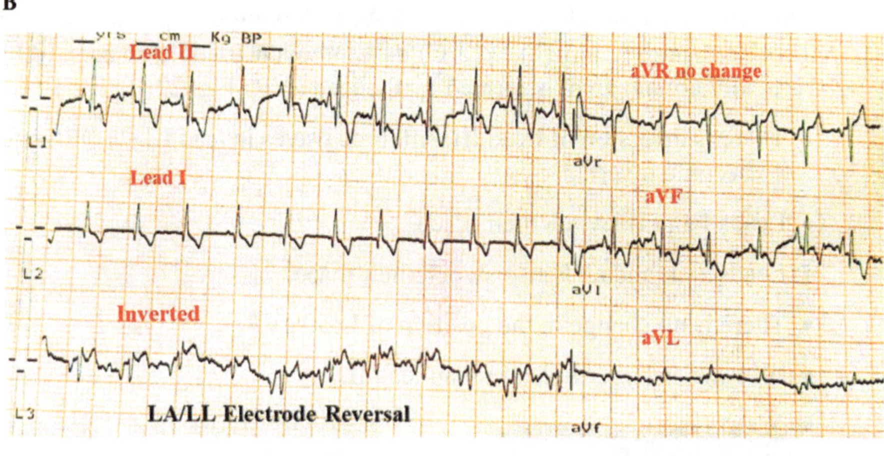

C

Fig. 22: Relationship between limb leads and electrodes and electrocardiogram produced when electrodes of LA/LL are reversed.

3. Reversal of RA and LL – When right fore limb electrode (RA) is reversed with left hind limb electrode (Fig.23 A), following changes are seen in the electrocardiogram (Fig.23 C) as Einthoven triangle rotates 180 vertically around an axis formed by the lead aVL (Fig.23B).
   - There is inversion of Lead II. All three waves in lead II (P, QRS and T) become inverted.
   - Leads I and III switch their place and also become inverted.
   - Leads aVR and aVF also switch their place.
   - There is no change in the position of Lead aVL

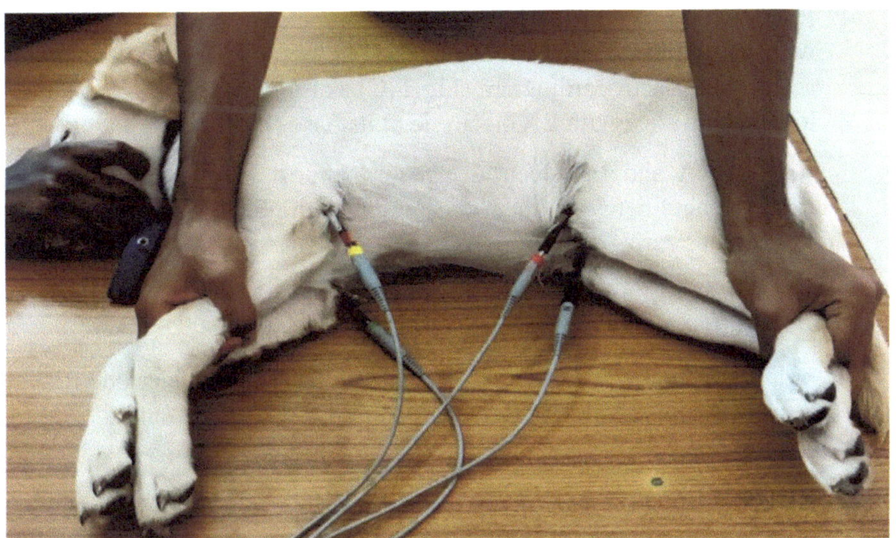

A

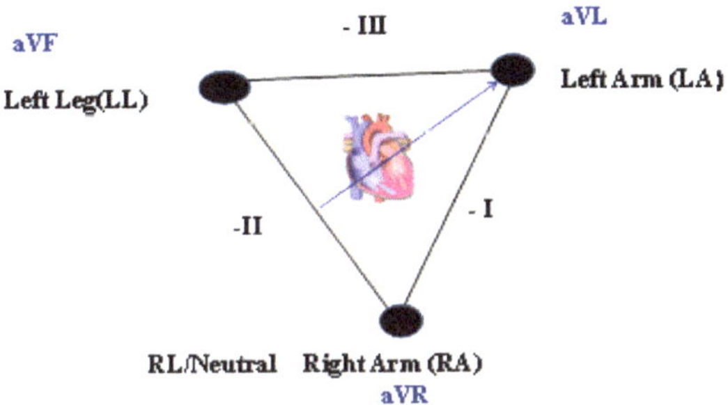

B

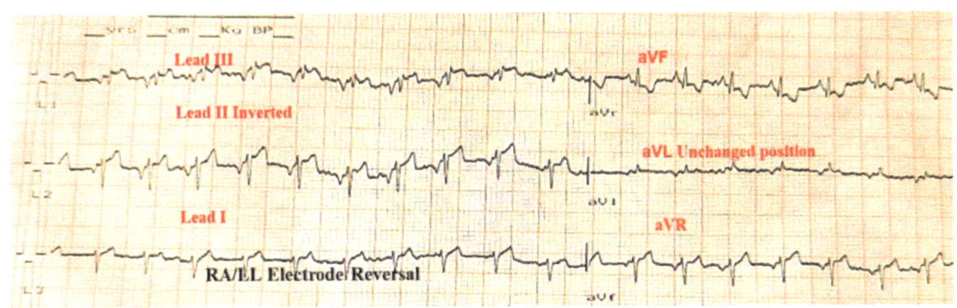

C

Fig. 23: Relationship between limb leads and electrodes and electrocardiogram produced when electrodes of RA/LL are reversed

4. Reversal of RA and RL – When right fore limb electrode (RA) is reversed with right hind limb neutral electrode (Fig.24 A), following changes are seen in the electrocardiogram (Fig.24C) as Einthoven triangle collapses to very thin slice with LA electrode at its base (Fig.24B).
   - Both RA and LL electrodes record almost identical voltages and difference between them becomes negligible. Therefore lead II becomes zero.
   - Lead aVL runs between thin slice facing approximately opposite to lead III.
   - Displacement on right hind limb electrode (neutral electrode RL), to right fore limb (RA) electrode position, makes aVR and aVL leads identical.
   - Lead I becomes an inverted lead III (-III).
   - Lead II records zero potential.
   - The position of lead III remains unchanged.

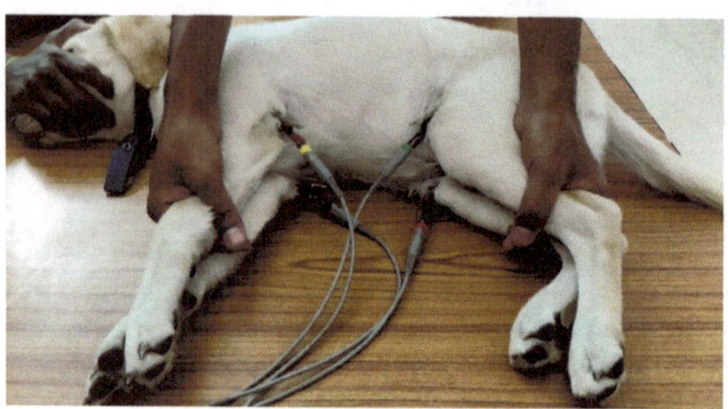

A

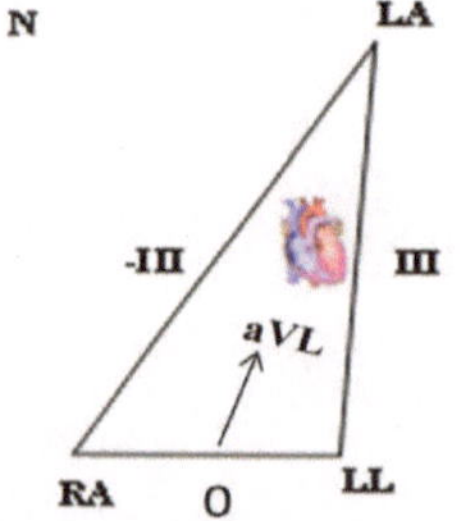

Relationship Between Limb Leads and Electrodes
RA/RL Reversal

B

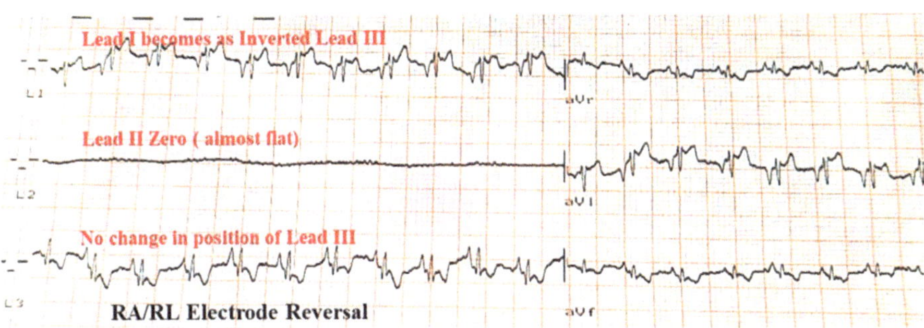

C

Fig. 24: Relationship between limb leads and electrodes and electrocardiogram produced when electrodes of RA/RL are reversed

5. Reversal of LA and RL – When left fore limb electrode (LA) is reversed with right hind limb (RL) neutral electrode (Fig. 25 A), following changes are seen in the electrocardiogram (Fig.25C) as Einthoven triangle collapses to very thin slice with RA electrode at its base (Fig.25B).

   - Both LA and LL electrodes record almost identical voltages and difference between them becomes negligible. Therefore lead III becomes zero.
   - Lead aVR runs between thin slice facing approximately opposite to lead II.
   - Displacement on right hind limb electrode (neutral electrode RL), to left fore limb (LA) electrode position, makes aVL and aVF leads identical.
   - Lead I becomes identical to lead II
   - No change in lead II.
   - Lead III records flat line with zero potential.
   - Lead aVR approximate to an inverted lead II.
   - Leads aVL and aVF becomes identical.

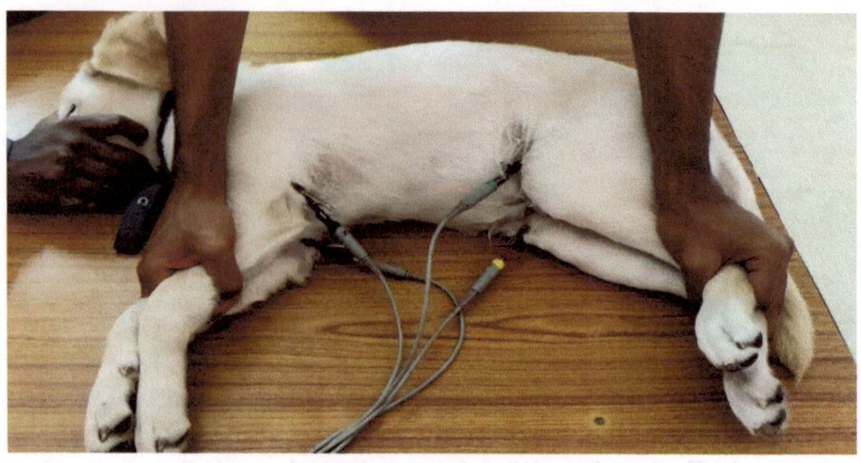

A

RA RL (Neutral)

II II aVR

LA 0 LL

Relationship Between Limb Leads and Electrodes
LA/RL Reversal

B

Identical to II
Approximate to inverted II
I
aVr
No change in position of Lead II
Identical to aVF
II
aVl
Lead III zero (almost flat
Identical to aVL
III LA/RL Electrode Reversal
aVf

C

Fig. 25: Relationship between limb leads and electrodes and electrocardiogram produced when electrodes of LA/RL are reversed

Common Artifacts observed during Electrocardiography

Abnormalities crept in during the process of taking an electrocardiogram, are termed as artifacts. These abnormalities are not related to cardiac diseases. In fact these defects are due to technical or mechanical errors or from malfunctioning of the electrocardiograph during the process of recording an electrocardiogram .The artifacts in electrocardiogram strip creates unnecessary confusion. The artifacts generally observed in an electrocardiogram strip are of four type's viz. electrical interference, muscle tremors, wandering base line or poorly defined base line. These artifacts need to be managed for a good electrocardiogram.

***Electrical interference*:** The electrical interference artifact is also called as 60 cycle interference or disturbance. This type of artifact appears as a regular sequence of 60 sharp up and down waves per second (Fig.26). The base line assumes the shape of regular saw tooth (Fig.26).The main cause of this type of artifact is due to improper grounding of the patient, electrocardiograph or electrical source. The interpretation of an electrocardiogram becomes difficult in the presence of electrical interference artifacts.

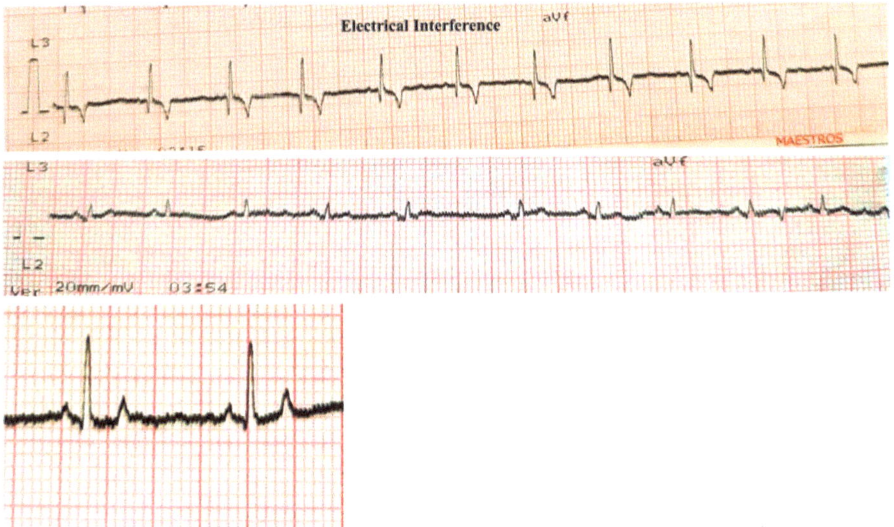

Fig. 26: Electrical Interference or 60 cycle disturbance in electrocardiogram. The base line has assumed the shape of regular saw tooth appearance. Nothing can be said about 'P' wave and 'P-R' interval when electrical interferences are present.

The electrical interference artifact can be corrected by proper grounding of power cord, secure attachment of all electrodes, liberal application of electrocardiographic gel on the skin, secure attachment of electrodes to the cable, switching off the fluorescents lights in the room, holding legs of the dog apart, not allowing electrode clips to touch each other, ensuring no touch of leads by any attendant during electrocardiography, proper cushioning of metal table with foam mattress and rubber sheet, avoiding electric watches in the vicinity of dog undergoing electrocardiography, ensuring no touch of electric cords with metal table, preventing hair or skin contact with the electrodes on the adjacent limb, or removing metal collar or halter from the body, if any.

Muscle Tremors: Muscle tremors/fasciculation or trembling of the body of the dog, panting, shivering or purring during electrocardiography can produce artifacts in the electrocardiogram (Fig.27). The muscle tremor artifacts are irregular, rapid saw-tooth vibrations of the base line and make the reading of electrocardiogram a difficult task.

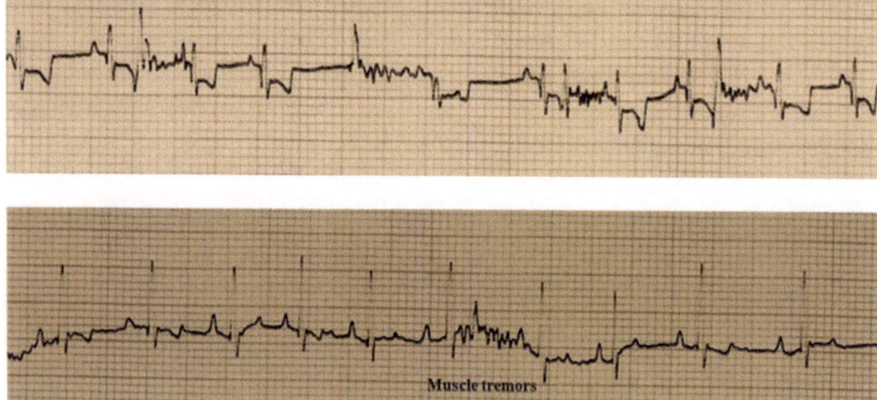

Fig. 27: Electrocardiograms showing muscle tremors.

Muscle tremor artifacts can be corrected by ensuring comfortable positioning of the dog, keeping the owner with the dog during electrocardiography, using mild tranquilizers in uncooperative dogs (tranquilizers may influence heart rate, hence interpretation of electrocardiogram should be done cautiously), placing hand over the chest, or reducing the sensitivity to ½.

Wandering base line: Base line may become wandering if there is change in the resistance between the electrode and skin of the dog. (Fig.28) .Respiratory movements, coughing or panting cause wandering baseline.

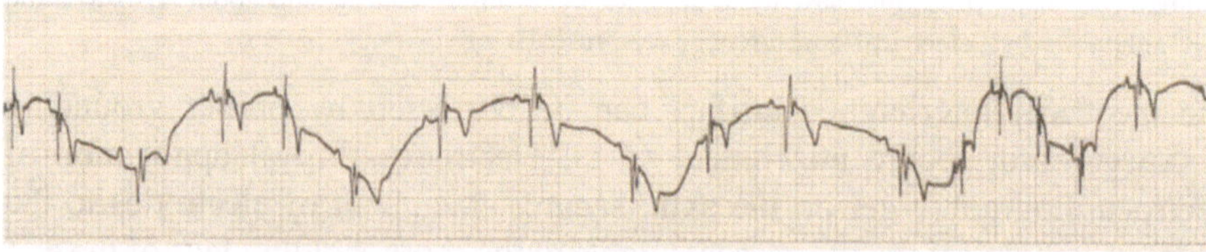

Fig. 28: Electrocardiogram showing wandering base line.

Wandering base line can be corrected by making the dog comfortable. ECG of the dogs with heart failure can be taken in the position in which the dog is comparatively comfortable as lateral recumbency is not comfortable. Other measures such as closing the mouth of the dog for 3-4 seconds during electrocardiography, by placing the electrode cable on the table with the dog, keeping a towel between front legs or applying pressure with palm on the thorax.

Poorly defined baseline: Poorly defined base line is another artifact that is generally seen with large waves such as 'R' wave (Fig.29).

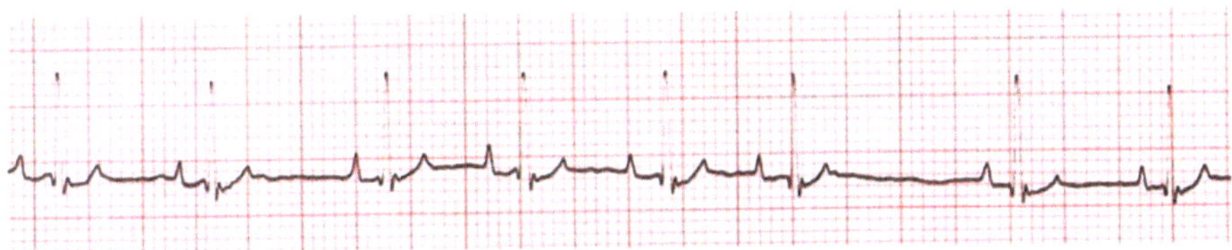

Fig. 29: Electrocardiogram of a dog taken at sensitivity of 1.0 and paper speed of 25 mm/ second. Note the poorly defined 'QRS' complex. The 'R' wave is poorly defined as compared to other waves.

Poorly defined base line can be corrected by reducing the sensitivity of the machine, if wave is large. In manual machines stylus may be cleaned or stylus heat may be increased.

Other Artifacts: Some other artifacts may also crept in (Fig. 30)

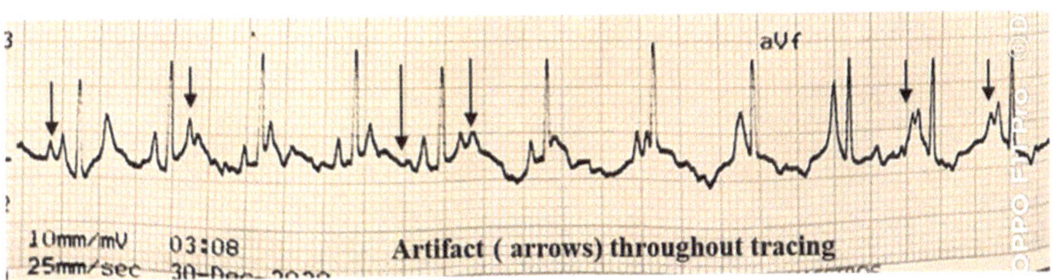

Fig. 30: Electrocardiogram of a dog taken at sensitivity of 1.0 and paper speed of 25 mm/ second. Note the artifacts throughout the strip.

Placement of Electrodes in Ruminants

Electrocardiogram in ruminants (Cow, Buffalo, Goat, and Sheep) is generally recorded in standing position. These animals are kept standing on a rubber mat .The sites for attaching electrodes are left jugular furrow two third down in the neck, over the apex of the heart just behind the left elbow and wither. The sites for applying alligator clips are prepared by shaving and cleaning with alcohol. Gel is applied liberally on the areas of attachment of electrodes. Base- apex lead system is generally practiced in ruminants for large appreciable complexes. In this lead system, the right arm electrode (Red) is attached to neck in the left jugular furrow two third down in the neck, left arm electrode (Yellow) is placed over the apex of the heart just behind left elbow and right hind limb electrode (earth electrode) is attached at wither (Fig.31). Electrocardiogram is recorded in a calm and quite surroundings using electrocardiographic machine at a paper speed of 25 mm per second and amplitude of 1 mV = 10 mm or 1 cm. The recording is done in lead 1.

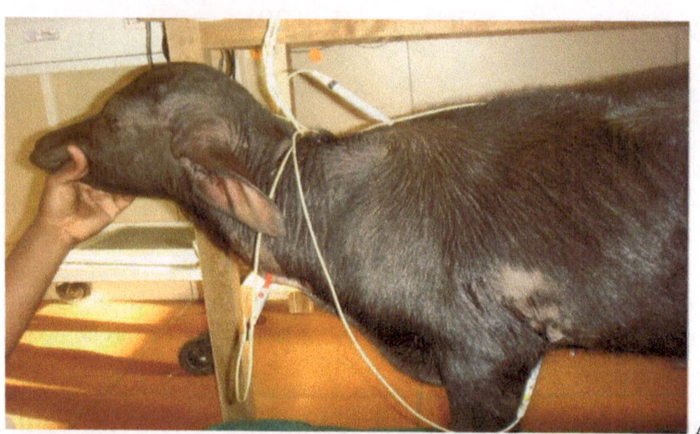

A

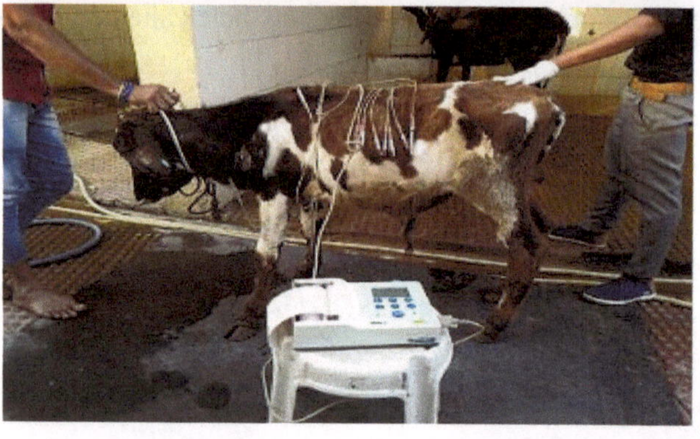

B

Fig. 31: Showing sites and placement of electrodes in a buffalo calf **(A)** and cow calf **(B)**. The sites are prepared by clipping and shaving. Gel is applied liberally on the sites and electrode clips. The left arm electrode (yellow) is placed over the apex of the heart just behind left elbow; right arm electrode (red) is attached to neck in the left jugular furrow two third down in the neck; and right hind limb electrode (earth electrode) is attached at wither.

Placement of Electrodes in Equines

Base-Apex lead system is more appropriate in equines as in case of ruminants. The procedure is almost similar to that followed in the ruminants. The horses or donkeys are kept in standing position on a rubber mat. The sites for attaching electrodes are right jugular furrow two third down in the neck, over the apex of the heart just behind the left elbow and wither or in the right side in front of scapula. The sites are prepared by shaving and cleaning with alcohol. Gel is applied liberally on the areas of attachment of electrodes. In base-apex lead system , the right arm electrode (Red) is attached to neck in the right jugular furrow two third down in the neck, left arm electrode (Yellow) is placed over the apex of the heart just behind left elbow and right hind limb electrode (earth electrode) is attached at wither or in the right side in front of scapula (Fig.32). Electrocardiogram is recorded in a calm and quite surroundings using electrocardiographic machine at a paper speed of 25 mm per second and amplitude of 1 mV =10 mm or 1 cm . The recording is done in lead 1 and is analyzed for amplitude and duration of waves, duration of intervals and heart rate.

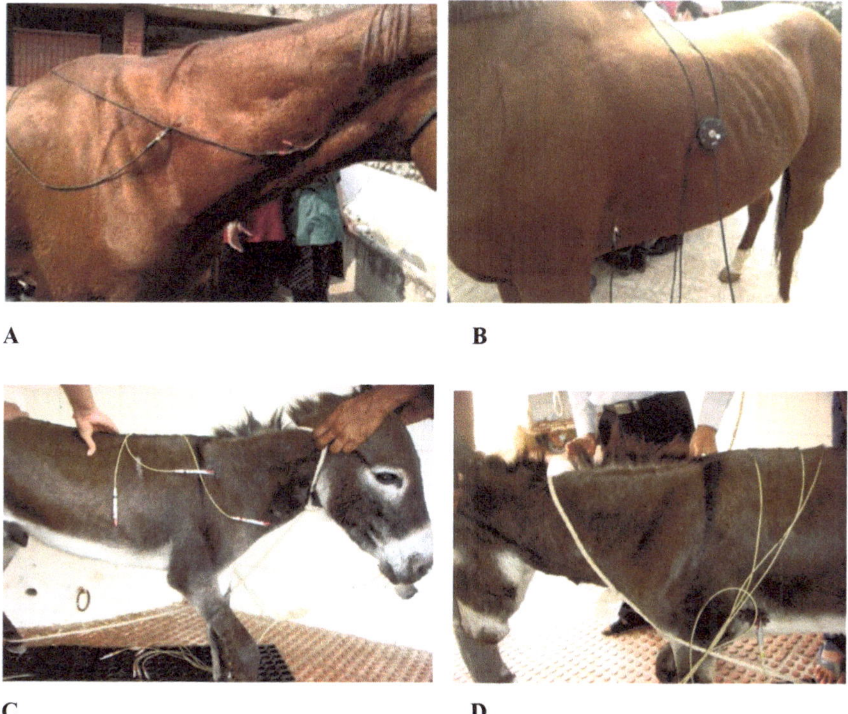

Fig. 32: Showing sites and placement of electrodes in horse (A and B) and donkey (C and D) . The sites are prepared by clipping and shaving. Gel is applied liberally on the sites and electrode clips. The left arm electrode (yellow) is placed over the apex of the heart just behind left elbow (B and D) ; right arm electrode (red) is attached to neck in the right jugular furrow two third down in the neck; and right hind limb electrode (black -earth electrode) is attached at wither or in the right side in front of scapula (A and C).

Reference

Rishniw, M., Pociello, F., Erb, H.N. and Fruganti, G. (2002). Effect of body positions on 6 lead ECG of dog. J.Vet.Int. Med. 16:69-73.

Further Reading

Varshney, J.P. (2020). Electrocardiography in Veterinary Medicine. Springer Nature, Singapore, Pte, Ltd.

4

Morphology of An Electrocardiogram

Electrocardiogram (ECG)

Electrocardiogram is a graphic record of electrical events of the heart recorded by the electrocardiograph. It represents the sum up surface voltage and direction of electrical activity produced during cardiac muscle depolarization and repolarization plotted against time (Fig. 33). The time is represented on the X- axis (horizontal line) and amplitude of voltage is represented on the Y-axis (vertical line) of the graph. The potential difference occurring over the surface of the body (at different lead placement locations) is associated with depolarization and repolarization of heart muscle (myocardium). The amplitude of the potential difference is measured as milli volt (mV) and their duration is measured in second or milliseconds. Electrocardiogram provides information about heart rate and its rhythm; chamber enlargement in dogs and humans; defects in generation and conduction of the current ; electrolyte changes (hypocalcaemia, hypokalemia, hypercalcaemia or hyperkalaemia); and some drug toxicities. Amplitude and duration of different electrocardiographic waves and intervals varies in different breeds of the dogs.

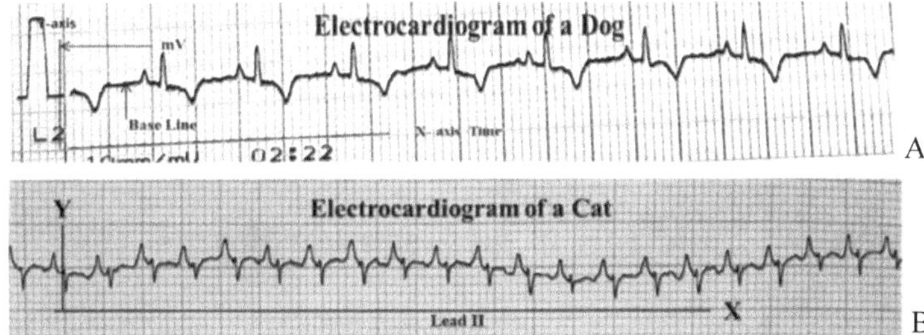

Fig. 33: Electrocardiogram of dog **(A)** and cat **(B)**. It is a graphic representation of the sum up surface voltage plotted against the time. Direction of the electrical activity produced during depolarization and repolarization of cardiac muscle cells is also indicated. X axis of the graph (horizontal line) represents time and Y axis of the graph (vertical) represents surface voltage and direction of current. Deflections above the base line indicates that the current flows toward the positive electrode and deflections below the base line indicates that the current flows away from the positive electrode.

Morphology of Electrocardiogram

Morphologically an electrocardiogram consists of waves (P, QRS, and T), intervals (P-R, Q-T, R-R) and segments (P-R, S-T, T-P) as shown in the Fig.34.

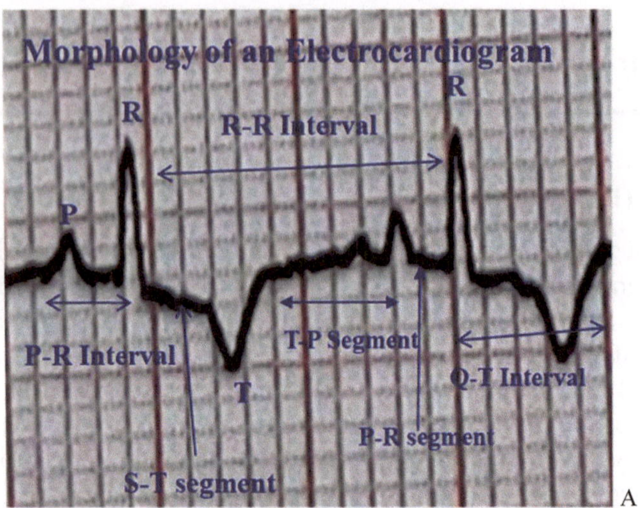

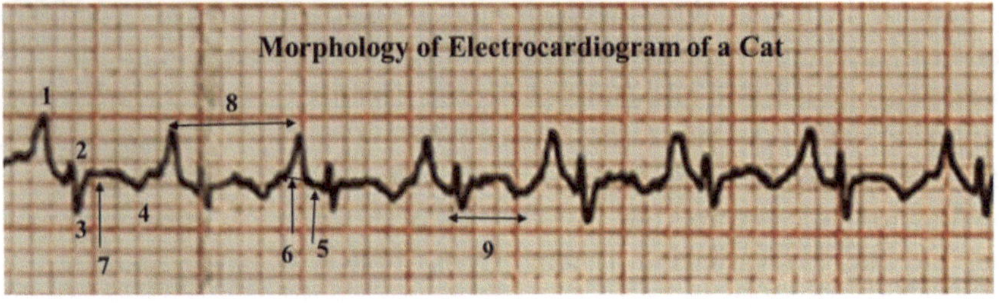

Fig. 34: Electrocardiograms showing morphology of an electrocardiogram of a Dog **(A)** and a Cat **(B)**. In figure B the numbers 1,2,3, 4 ,5,6,7,8, and 9 denote 'P' wave, 'r' wave, 'S' wave,'T' wave, 'P-R' segment, 'P-R' interval, 'S-T segment, R-R interval, and 'Q-T' interval respectively. Morphology of electrocardiographic complexes of dogs and cats is largely similar except size of complexes in cats is small and heart rate in cats is fast.

Recognizing Waves and Intervals in an Electrocardiogram (Fig. 33 and 34)

- The first small upward (positive) deflection in an electrocardiogram is designated as 'P' Wave
- A short base line after first positive deflection is termed as 'P- R' segment.
- Duration from the beginning of 'P' wave to the beginning of 'Q' or 'R" wave is termed as 'P-R' interval.

- The first small downward (negative) deflection is designated as 'Q' wave.
- A large positive (upward) deflection after 'Q' or 2nd positive deflection is termed as 'R' wave.
- The second small negative (downward) deflection is termed as 'S' wave.
- The baseline after 'S' wave or second base line in electrocardiogram is designated as 'S-T segment.
- The positive or negative deflection following 'S-T' segment is termed as 'T' wave.
- Duration from the beginning of 'Q' to the end of 'S' wave is designated as 'QRS' duration.
- Duration from the beginning of 'Q' to the end of 'T' is termed as 'Q-T' interval.
- Duration between two 'R' waves is termed as R-R interval.
- Duration between 'T' and next 'P' is termed as T-P segment.

Measuring Waves and Intervals in the Electrocardiogram

The measurements of waves and intervals are taken as follows as shown in the following figures.

P wave: 'P' wave is measured vertically (from top to bottom) for current amplitude and horizontally (from beginning to the end) for its duration (Fig.35).

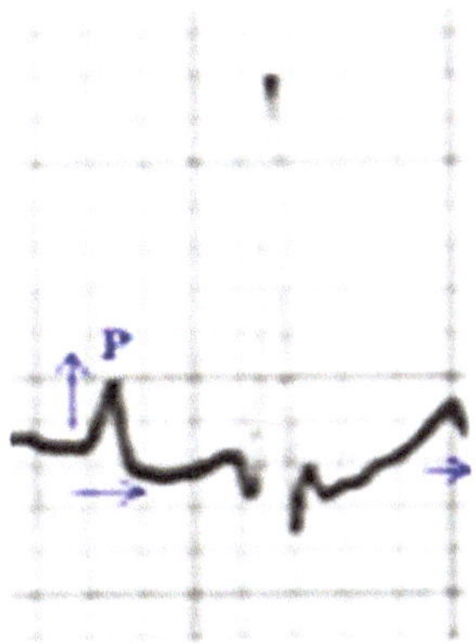

Fig. 35: Showing measurement of 'P' wave

P-R segment: It is measured from end of 'P' wave to beginning of 'QRS'. (Fig.36)

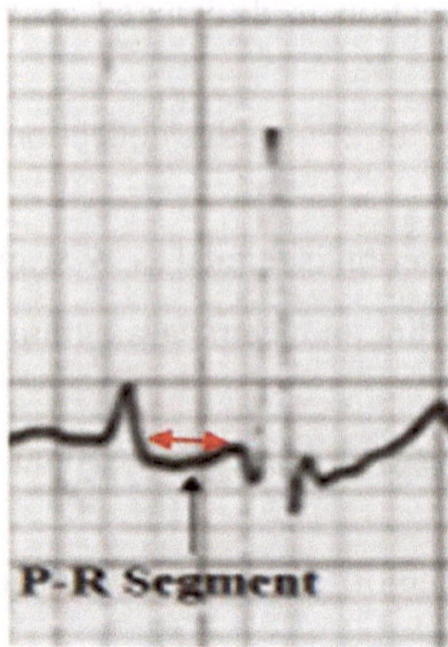

Fig. 36: Showing measurement of 'P-R' segment

P-R interval : It is measured from beginning of P wave to beginning of QRS complex (Fig.37).

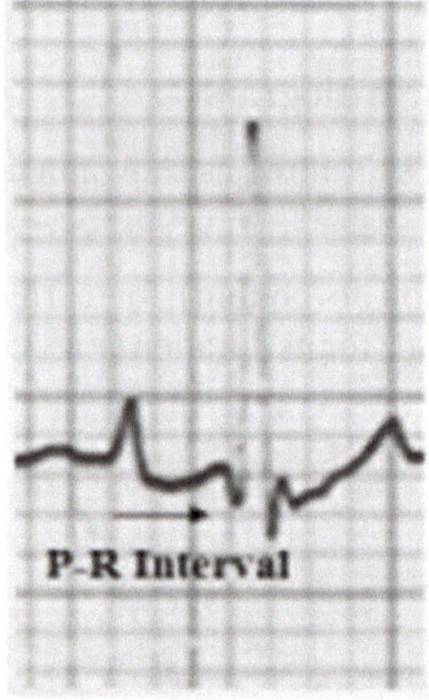

Fig. 37: Showing measurement of P-R interval.

Q wave : First small negative deflection is 'Q' wave. It is measured from the base line downward to the end of the deflection (Fig.38).

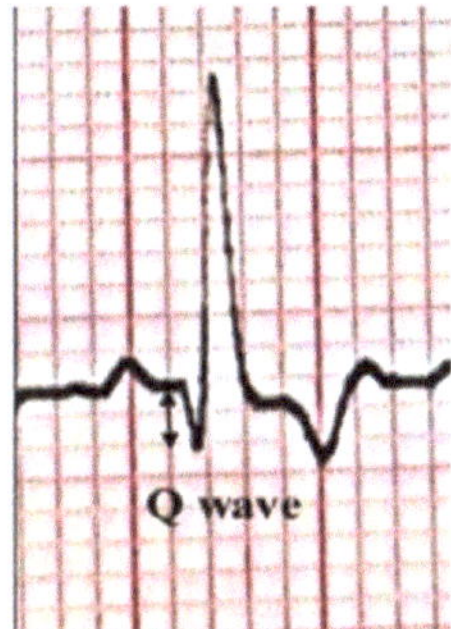

Fig. 38: Showing measurement of 'Q' wave

R Wave : It is measured from top to bottom of the wave for its current amplitude (Fig.39).

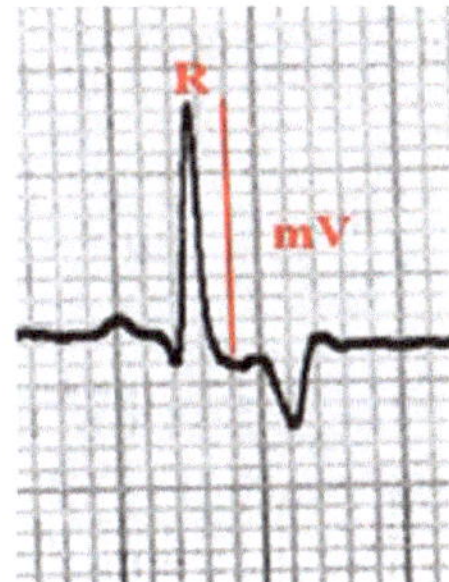

Fig. 39: Showing measurement of 'R' wave.

S wave : It is a negative deflection after 'R' wave. It is measured from the base line downward to the end of the deflection (Fig.40).

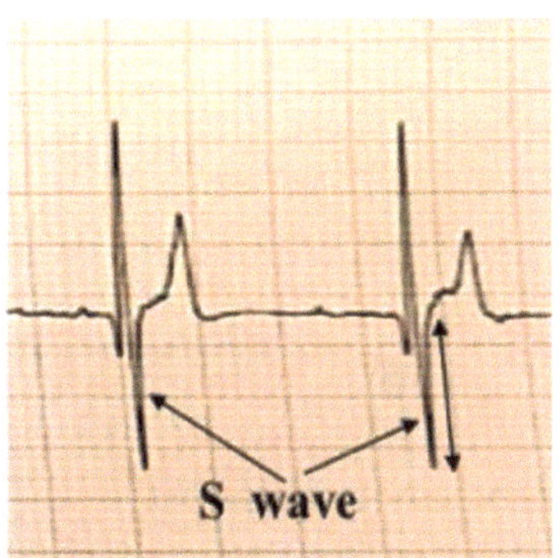

Fig. 40: Showing measurement of 'S' wave.

QRS complex : It is measured from the beginning to the end of QRS complex horizontally for its duration (Fig.41).

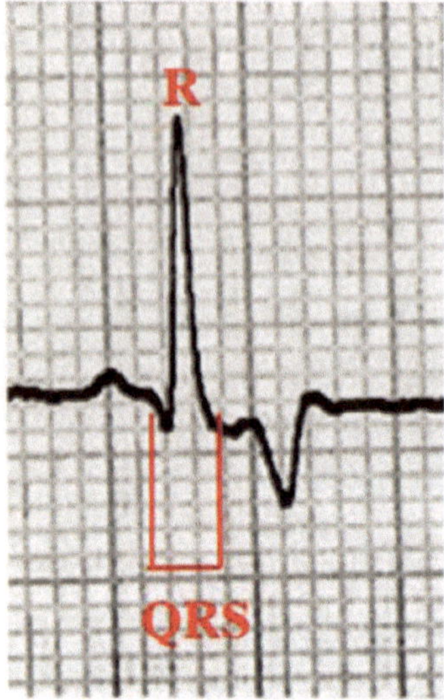

Fig. 41: Showing measurement of 'QRS' complex

S-T segment : It is measured between end of 'S' wave to beginning of 'T' wave. It runs along with the baseline before going into the 'T' wave (Fig.42).

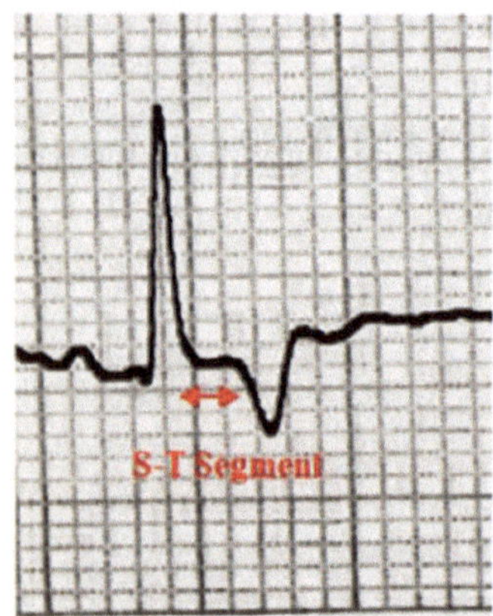

Fig. 42: Showing measurement of S-T segment.

T wave : Duration of 'T' wave is measured horizontally from the end of S-T segment to the end of T wave and from top to bottom for its current amplitude (Fig.43).

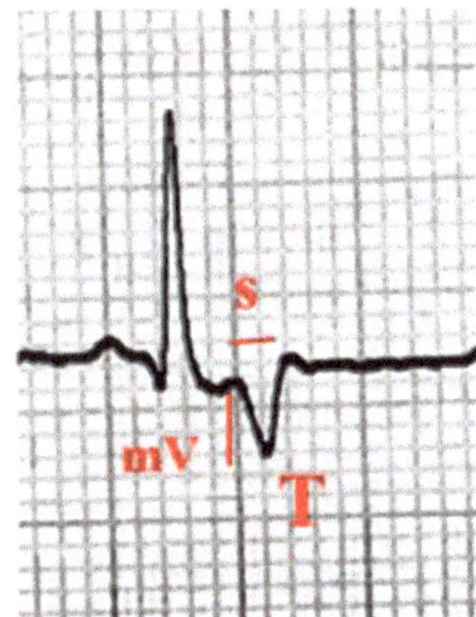

Fig. 43: Showing measurement of 'T' wave

Q-T interval : It is measured horizontally from beginning of 'Q' wave to end of 'T' wave (Fig.44).

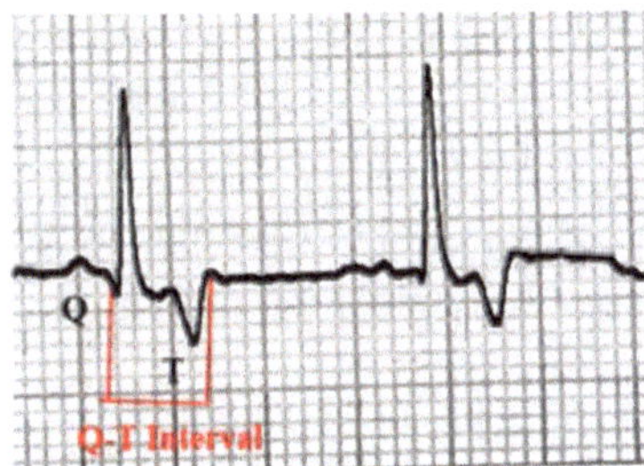

Fig. 44: Showing measurement of Q-T interval

R-R interval : It is measured horizontally between two R waves (Fig.45).

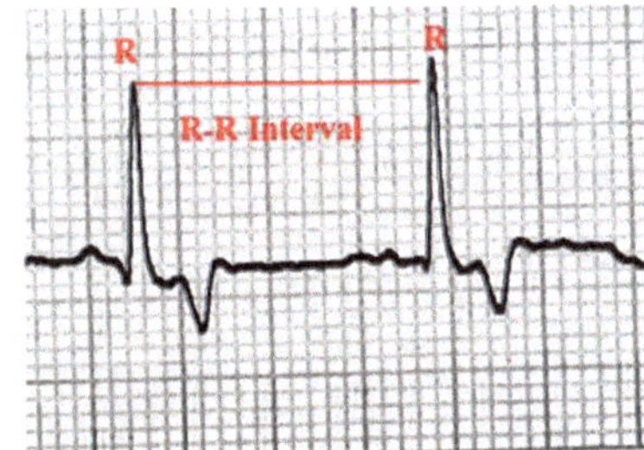

Fig. 45: Showing measurement of R-R interval.

T-P Segment : It is measured horizontally from the end of 'T' wave to the beginning of next 'P' wave (Fig.46).

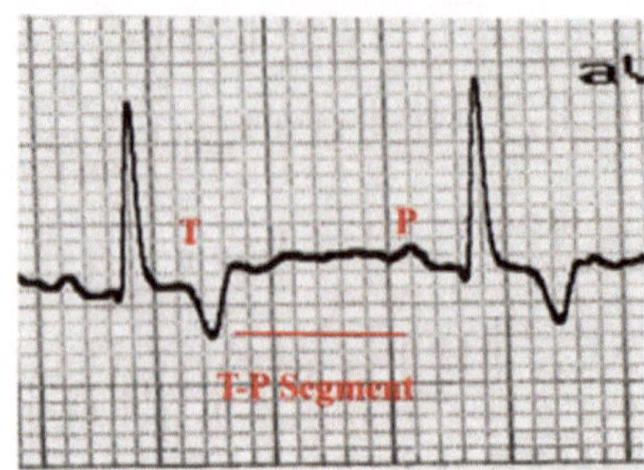

Fig. 46: Showing measurement of T-P segment

Morphology of the Electrocardiographic Waves in Different Leads

In routine practice, Bailey's Hex-axial lead system is used in dogs and cats. In which electrocardiogram is recorded in three standard bipolar limb leads (I, II, III) and three unipolar augmented leads (aVR, aVL and aVF). For more detail investigations four other chest leads (CV_5RL, CV_6LL,CV_6LU and V_{10}) are also employed. The morphology and, polarity of the waves in different leads of dogs and cats is given below.

- In lead I, 'P' and 'R' wave are positive and 'Q' and 'S' are negative. Deflection of waves is very small. 'T' wave can be positive or negative or very small (Fig.47).

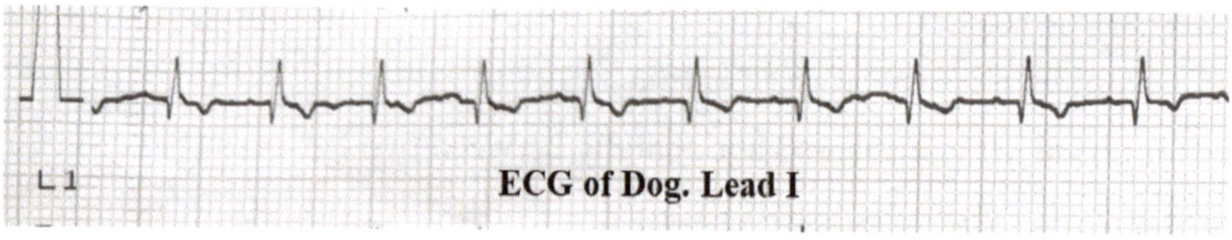

A

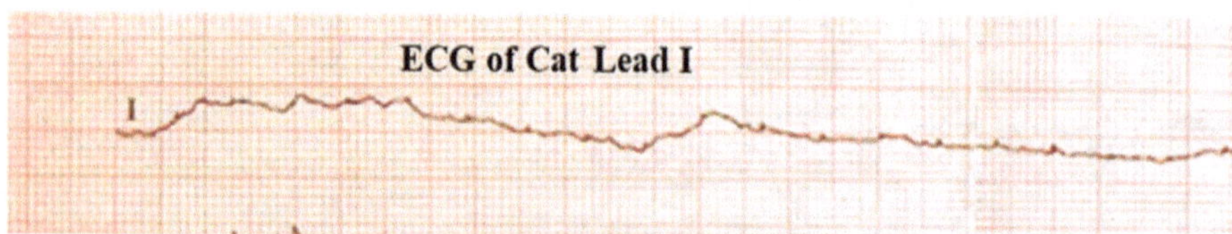

Fig. 47: Electrocardiographic complexes of dog **(A)** and cat **(B)** in Lead I.

- In lead II, deflections are largest. 'P','R' are positive. Q' and 'S' are negative. 'T' wave can be positive or negative (Fig.48).

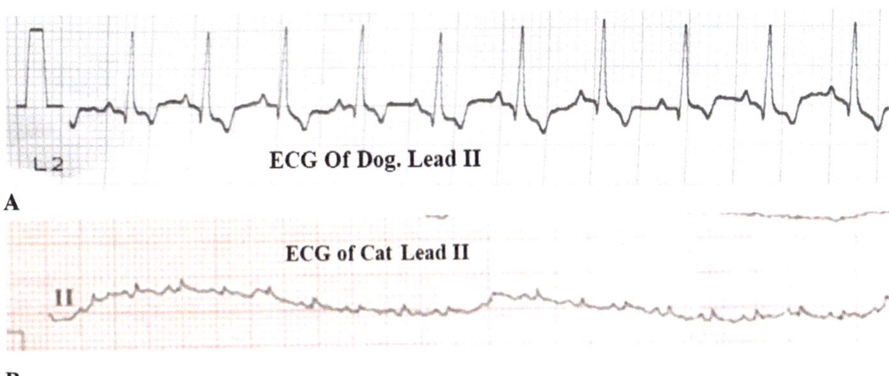

Fig. 48: Electrocardiographic complexes of dog (A) and cat (B) in Lead II.

- In lead III, waves are same as in lead II. Deflection are small than the lead II (Fig.49).

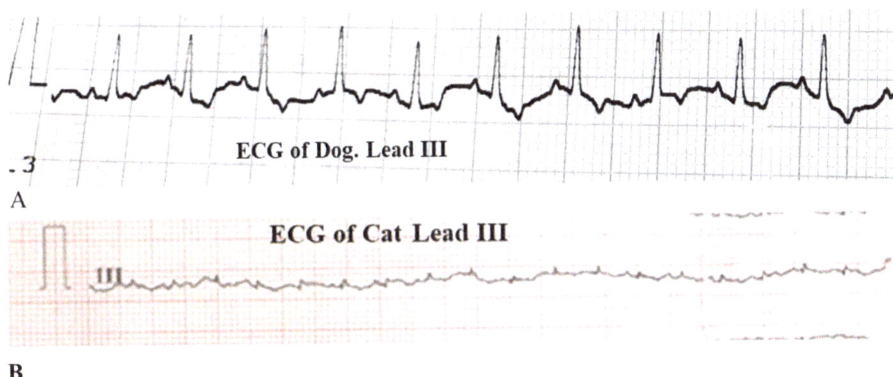

Fig. 49: Electrocardiographic complexes of dog **(A)** and cat **(B)** in Lead III.

- In lead aVR, the polarity of the waves is reversed (Fig.50) as compared to lead II. The positive waves in lead II are negative in lead aVR and waves negative in lead II are positive in lead aVR. The size of the wave is small as compared to lead II.

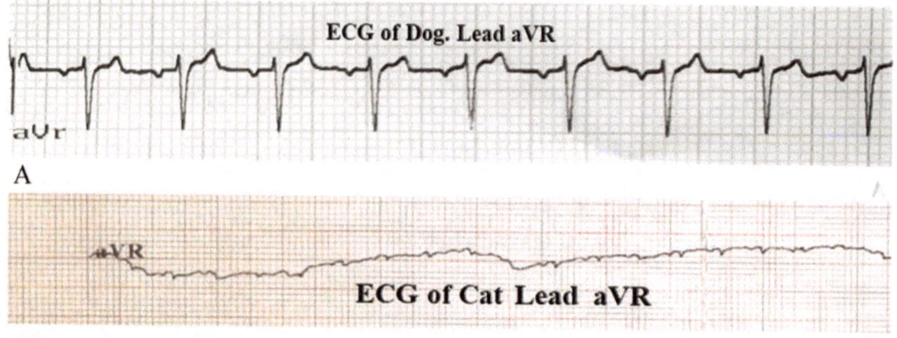

B

Fig. 50. Electrocardiographic complexes of dogs and cats in Lead aVR.

- In lead aVL, all waves (Fig.51) are similar to lead aVR in polarity but their size is small as compared to lead aVR.

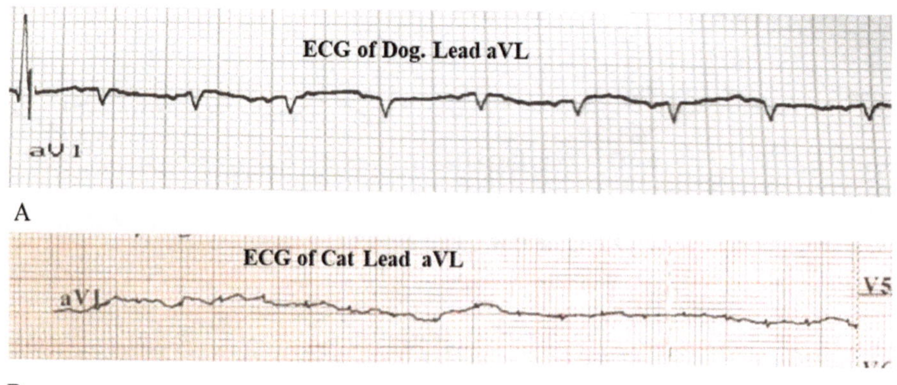

B

Fig. 51: Electrocardiographic complexes of dogs and cats in Lead aVL.

- In lead aVF, all waves follow the pattern of lead II. The size of the complexes may be a little small or almost equal to lead II (Fig.52).

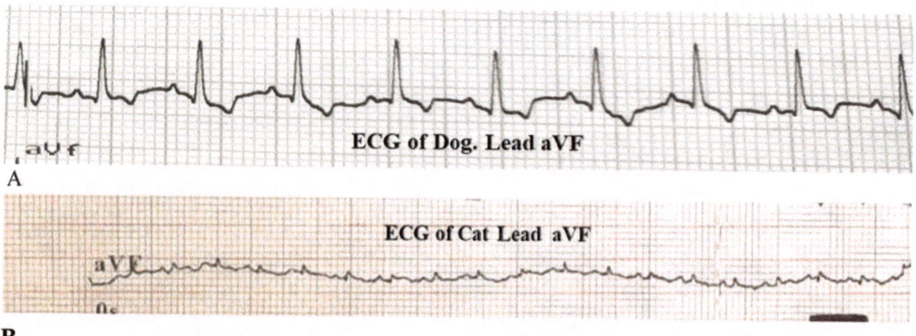

B

Fig. 52. Electrocardiographic complexes of dogs and cats in Lead aVF

Morphology of Waves

'P' wave - In lead II 'P' wave is small pointed (Fig. 53 A) or rounded (Fig. 53 B). It may be notched or biphasic also. The 'P' wave is usually positive in lead I, II, III, and aVF. If the 'P' wave is negative in lead II, it is abnormal. However, 'P' wave is normally negative in leads aVR and aVL (Fig.53 C).

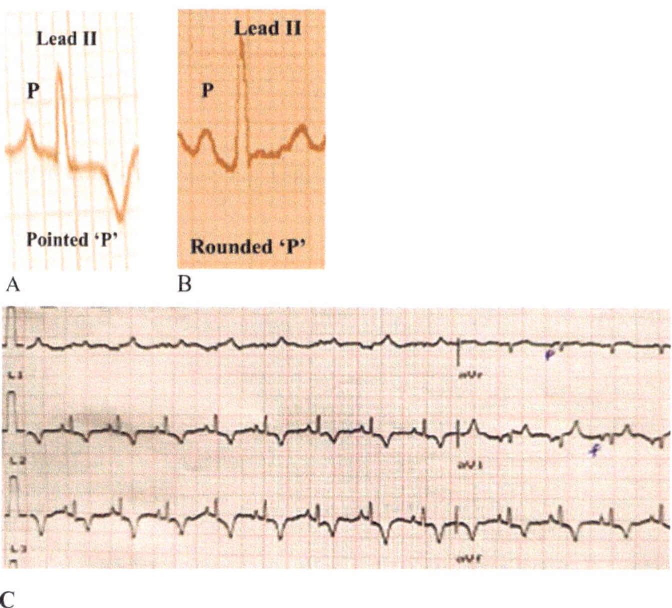

Fig. 53: Electrocardiograms are showing configuration of 'P' wave. It is small pointed (A) or rounded (B) wave. It is positive in lead II, III, and aVF and negative in lead aVR and aVL (C). It may not be very conspicuous in lead I.

'Q' wave – It is a first negative deflection (below the base line) reflecting depolarization of right ventricle (Fig.54).

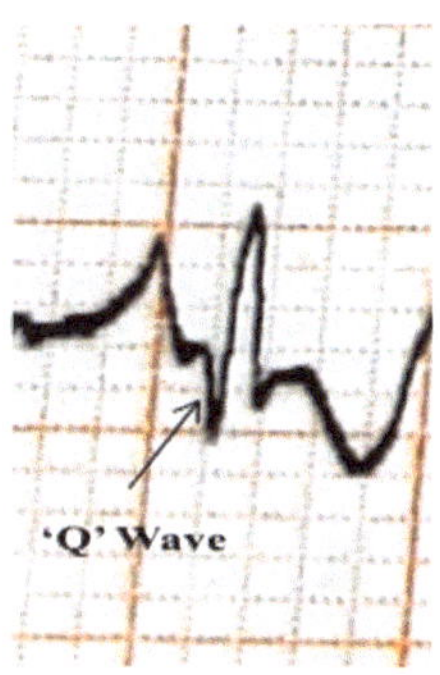

Fig. 54: Electrocardiogram is showing 'Q' wave (marked with arrow). It reflects depolarization of right ventricle. It is a part of 'QRS' complex.

'R' wave - It is a large positive deflection (Fig.55) after 'P' wave. When 'Q' wave is present, it is the upward deflection in continuation of the 'Q' wave. It is positive in lead I, II, III, and aVF and negative in lead aVR and aVL.

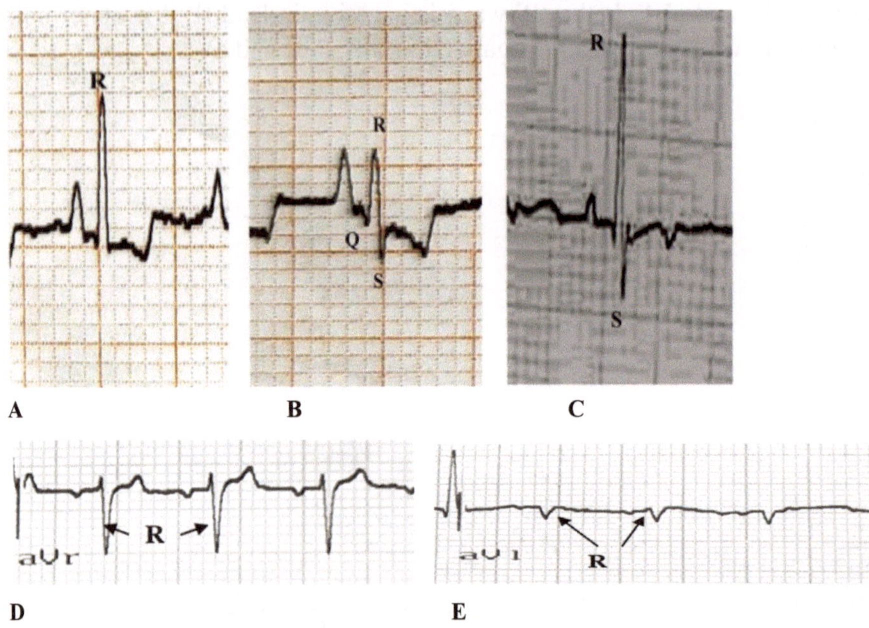

Fig. 55: Electrocardiograms are showing 'R' wave in Lead II (A, B, C) . 'R' wave is first positive deflection after 'P' wave. R wave is negative in lead aVR (D) and aVL (E) and is positive in rest of the leads.

'S' wave – 'S' wave (Fig.56) is the deflection below the base line (negative) following 'R' wave. It represents right ventricle depolarization. It is negative in lead II, III, aVF.

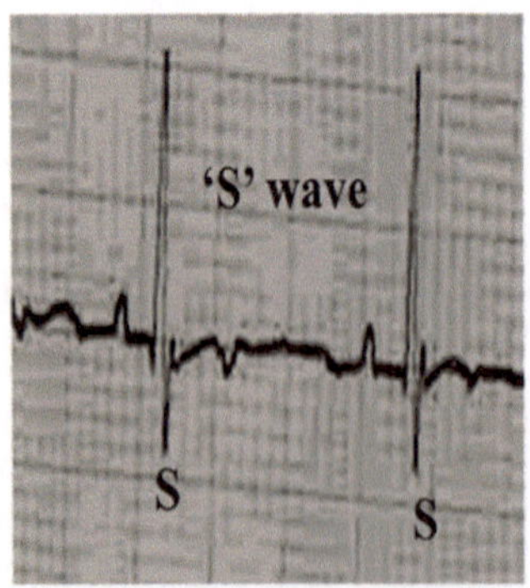

Fig. 56: Electrocardiogram is showing 'S' wave (marked as S) in lead II. It is negative deflection (below base line) that follows 'R 'wave.

'QRS' complex- 'R' wave is much more prominent. There are various forms of 'QRS' complex in limb leads (Fig.57) as shown below:

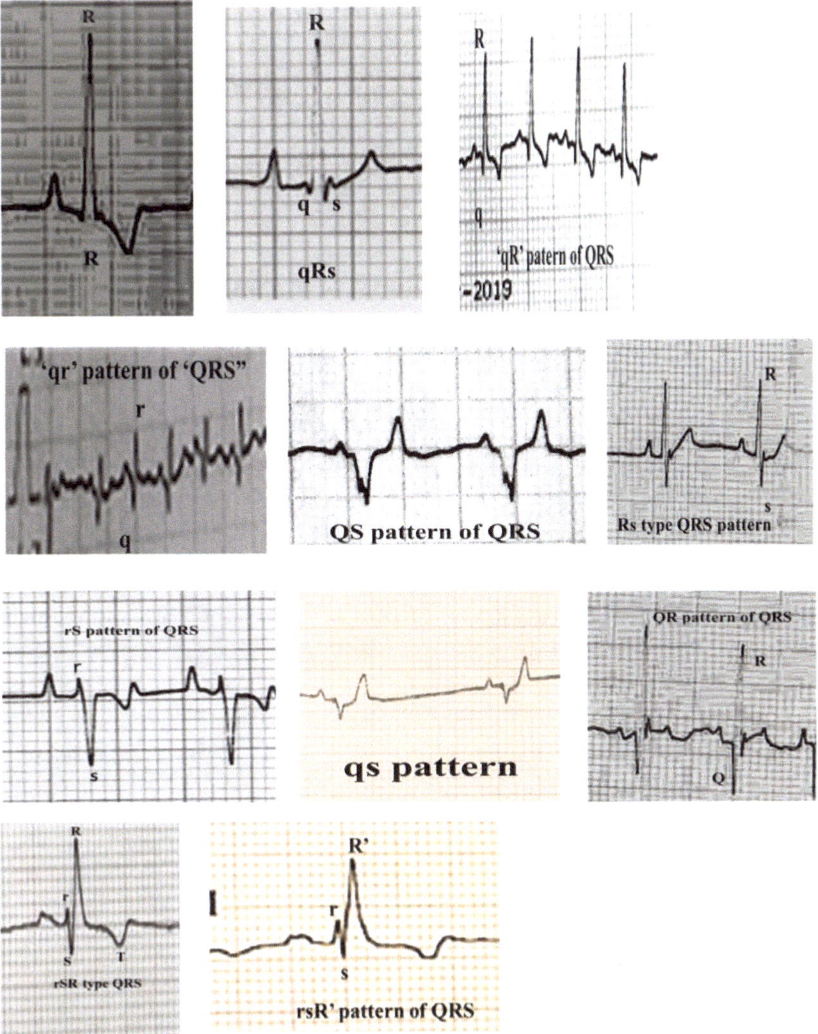

Fig. 57: Electrocardiograms are showing different types of 'QRS' pattern

'T' wave – It is the first major positive or negative deflection after 'QRS' complex (Fig.58).

'T' wave represents repolarization of ventricles. There are many configurations of the 'T' wave. It is seen as positive, negative, notched, biphasic, or almost flat. It is negative in lead V10 in all breeds of dogs except Chihuahua. It is positive in CV_5RL.

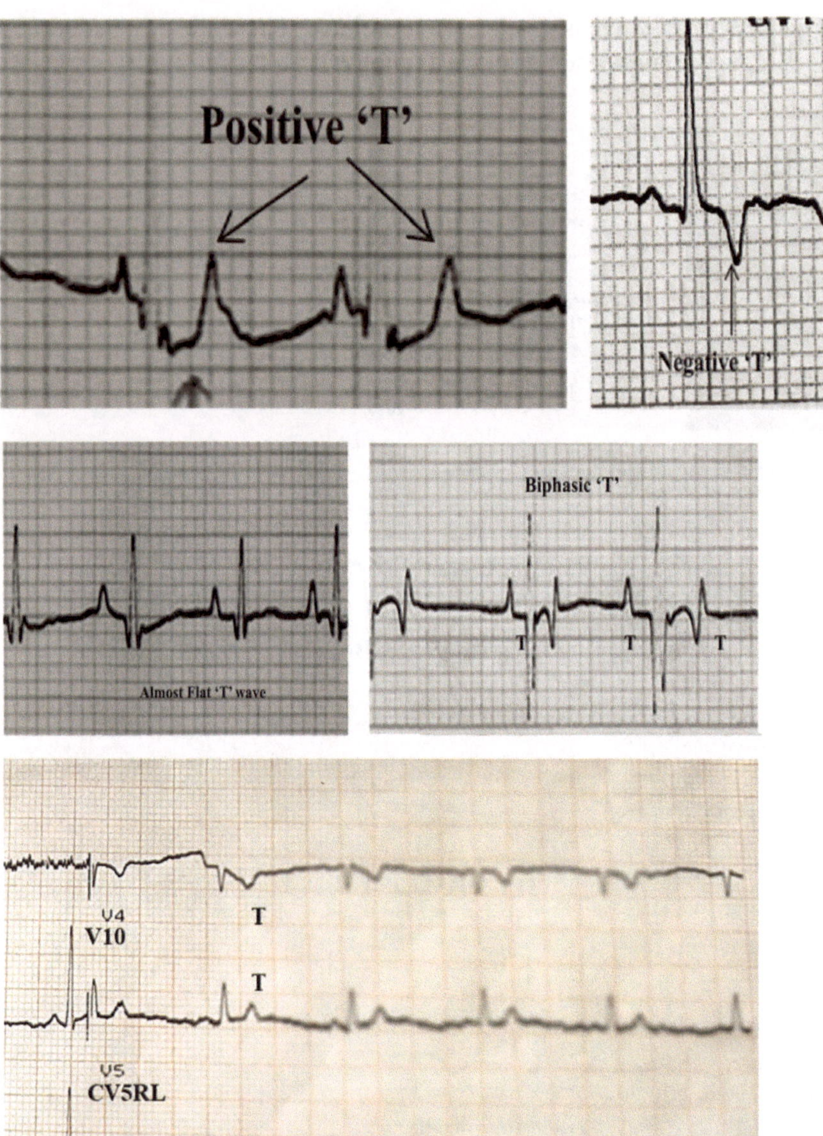

Fig. 58. Electrocardiograms are showing different types of 'T' wave. It is the first major deflection after 'QRS'. It may be positive, negative, flat or biphasic. It is negative in lead V_{10} in all breeds of dogs except Chihuahua. It is positive in lead CV_5RL.

Morpholgy of Segments

P-R segment- It is a straight base line after the 'P' wave (Fig.59). It is measured from the end of 'P' wave to the beginning of 'QRS' complex. P-R segment is different from P-R interval. The important factor in analyzing segments is their change from isoelectric line (elevation or depression) and their duration also. The P-R segment represents the electrical conduction through the atria and delay of the electrical impulse in the AV node. It is a straight line and the current wave is too weak to be recorded on volt meter. Abnormalities of P-R segment are very limited. In humans, depression in PR segment has been reported to be a signal for pericarditis or atrial infarction.

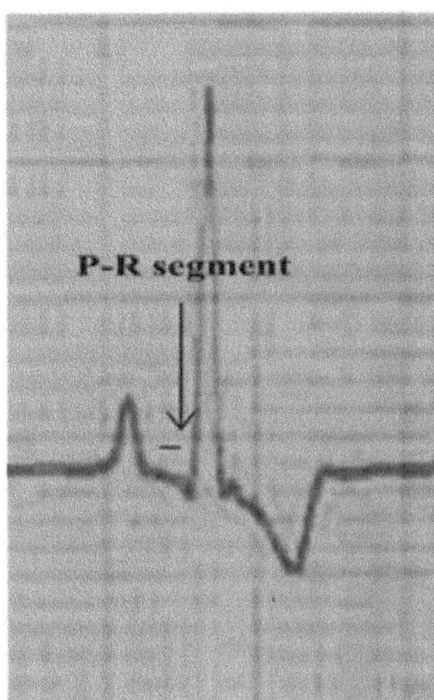

Fig. 59: Electrocardiogram is showing P-R segment. It is a straight line that follows 'P' wave

S-T segment – It begins at the end of QRS wave and ends at the beginning of 'T' wave. It is isoelectric line that follows 'QRS' complex (Fig.60). It is measured from the end of 'QRS' complex to the beginning of 'T' wave.

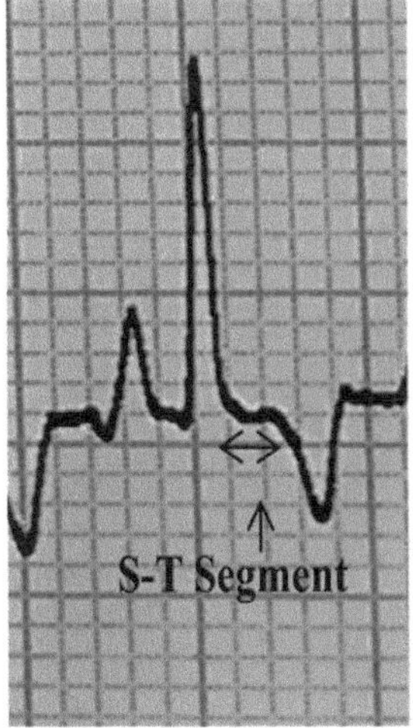

Fig. 60: Electrocardiogram is showing S-T segment. It is a straight line following 'QRS' complex.

T-P segment- It starts at the end of T wave and ends at the beginning of next 'P' wave and therefore measured from the end of the 'T' wave to the beginning of the 'P' wave (Fig. 61). It is an isoelectric line.

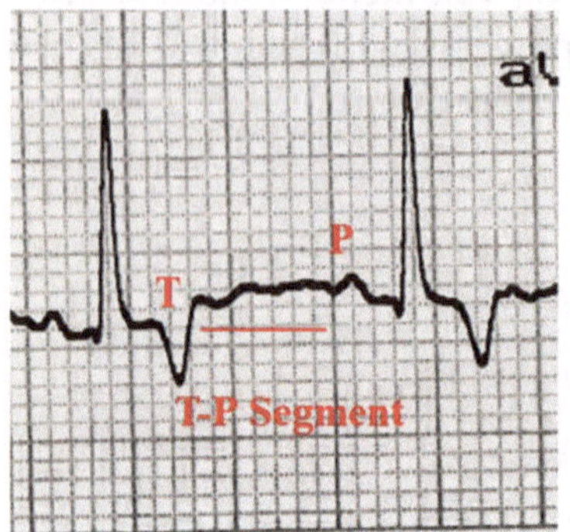

Fig. 61: Electrocardiogram is showing T-P segment. It is a straight line starting from the end of 'T' wave to the beginning of 'P' wave.

Morphology of Intervals

An interval in the electrocardiogram is a duration of the time. It includes one segment and one or two waves.

P-R interval or P-Q interval – It begins at the start of the 'P' wave and ends at the beginning of 'Q' or R wave (Fig.62). It is the time from the beginning of 'P' wave (atrial depolarization) to the beginning of 'QRS' complex. It indicates the conduction of the current impulse from atrium to Purkinje fibers. Usually P-R interval is almost same from complex to complex. Variation in P-R interval in different complexes indicate conduction disturbance.

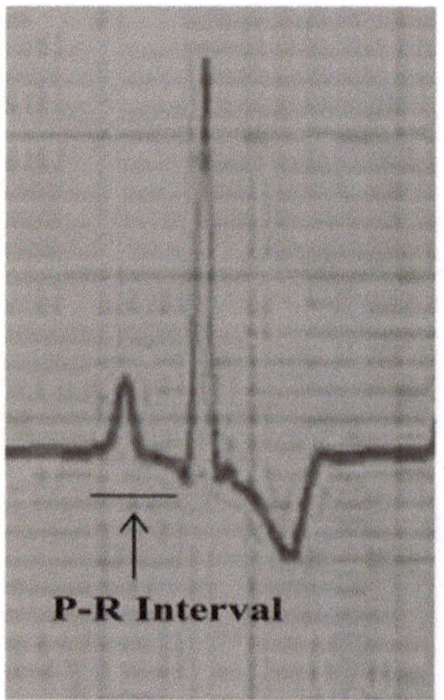

Fig. 62: Electrocardiogram is showing P-R interval. It is a duration that includes the duration of 'P' wave and the duration of P-R segment.

Q-T interval – It begins at the start of QRS and ends at the end of 'T' wave (Fig.63) combining 'QRS' duration, S-T segment and 'T' wave duration. It includes beginning of the ventricular depolarization through the plateau phase to the ventricular repolarization. The duration of Q-T interval depends on the heart rate. It is shortened when heart rate is fast and is lengthened when heart rate is slow.

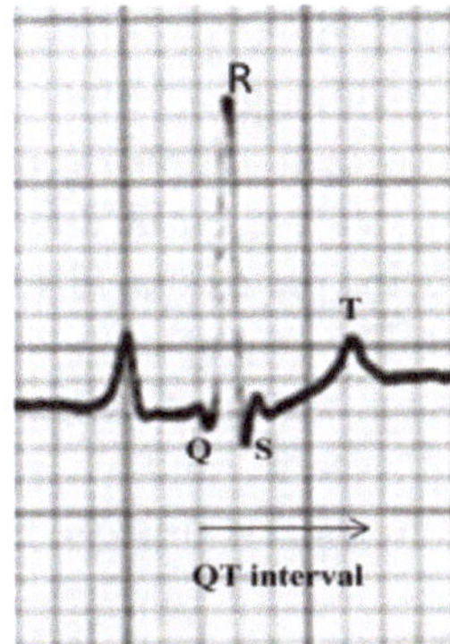

Fig. 63: Electrocardiogram is showing Q-T interval. It includes duration of 'QRS', S-T segment and duration of 'T' wave and represents the total period of ventricular depolarization and repolarization.

R-R Interval – It is the time elapsed between two successive R waves (Fig. 64) . Heart rate can be calculated by measuring R-R interval. If R-R interval is not uniform, it indicates arrhythmia.

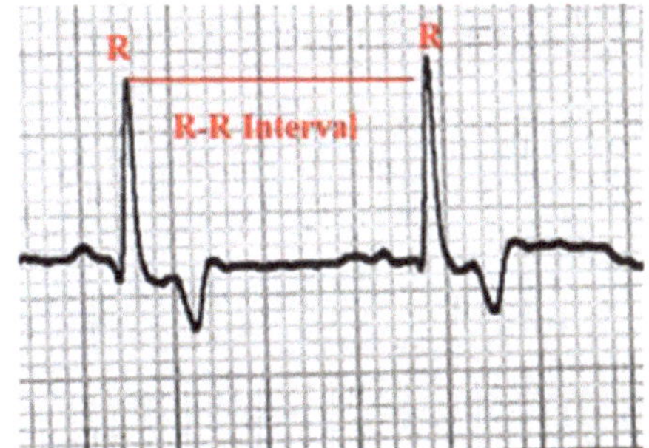

Fig. 64: Electrocardiogram is showing R-R interval. It is time elapsed between two R waves.

Heart Rate Variability (HR variability)

It is known that instantaneous heart rate fluctuates from beat to beat. The fluctuation in normal heart rate is called heart rate variability. Heart rate variability is a measure of variation in time between each beat. It is a physiological phenomenon .With aging and/or disease conditions, a constant heart rate is not maintained and beat to beat variability in heart rate occurs. The variability is under the influence of autonomic nervous system (ANS). Though the fluctuations in beat to beat are undetectable except with the help of specialized devices, can indicate current or future health problems. Fluctuations in parasympathetic nervous system plays major role in heart rate variability (Binkley *et al.*, 1991). Variations in blood pressure, thermoregulation, respiration, RAS (rennin-angiotensin system) and circadian rhythm influence the R-R interval that is a measure of heart rate variation (Stein *et al.*, 1994). Heart rate variability is a normal occurrence and is not arrhythmia. It is also being considered as a useful indicator of emotional states even in dogs (Katayama *et al.*, 2016). Heart rate variability is also being investigated in relation to cognitive psychophysiology. Heart rate variability can be of high frequency (correlated with parasympathetic nervous system activity) or low frequency (correlated with sympathetic nervous system activity and vagal activity). Decreased parasympathetic or increased sympathetic nervous system activity results in reduced heart rate variability.

In fact, heart rate variability is a statistical analysis of small variations in time intervals between heart beats. Vasovagal tonus index (VVTI) is a natural logarithm of the variance in R-R interval and therefore is a reliable indicator of heart rate variability. It is a time domain indicator of heart rate variability and can be calculated according to formula (Haggstrom *et al.*, 1996; Doxey and Boswood , 2004) given below ;

$$VVTI = L_n(SD_{R\text{-}R})^2$$

Where L_n = Mean of 10 consecutive R-R interval

$(SD_{R\text{-}R})^2$ = Variance of R-R interval

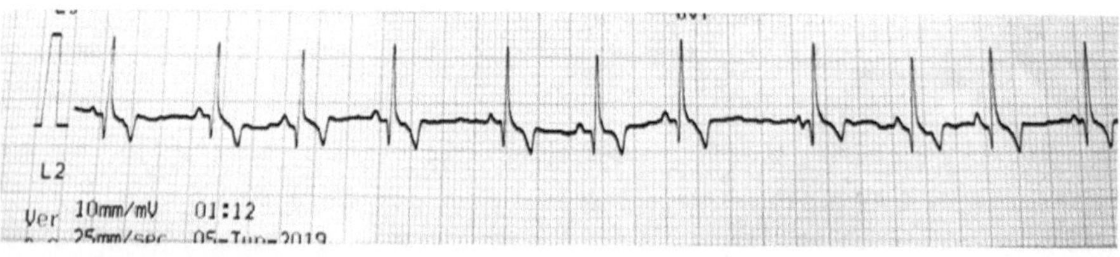

Fig. 65: Electrocardiogram of a dog (Lead II, sensitivity 1, speed 25 mm/s) is showing heart rate of 100 bpm and R-R interval is varying from 0.52 to 0.82 second (0.72,0.52,0.56,0.72,0.56,0.52,0.82,0.60,0.48,0.62 seconds)with a mean of 0.612 second. In this case VVTI is 0.067 second or 67 millisecond. VVTI is a reliable indicator of heart rate variability. It means there is beat to beat difference of 67 millisecond.

Q-T Interval Variability

Q-T interval variability is a physiological phenomenon and refers to beat to beat fluctuations in Q-T interval of electrocardiogram. There is inverse relationship between heart rate and Q-T interval and it is dependent on preceding R-R interval (Simonson *et al.*, 1962). Q-T interval needs to be interpreted in relation to heart rate. Lengthening of Q-T interval indicates abnormality in ventricular repolarization predisposing to arrhythmias. Q-T interval may also provide non-invasive assessment of sympathetic nervous system activity (Baumert *et al.,* 2016) and higher Q-T interval variability is associated with sudden death.

A number of correction formulae, derived from analyzing human data, are currently used, some for analyzing anaesthetized animals or animal models for toxicology assessments. Little information, however, is available on how to correct the QT interval for clinical practice, considering different HR ranges (due to different breeds) in conscious healthy dogs. It may be calculated using Bazett's formula (Bazett, 1920) given below. The Bazett's formula corrects the measured Q-T interval to a value (Q-Tc) attributable to heart rate of 60 bpm. This mathematically driven formula provides the value of the Q-Tc in the same unit of Q-T, generally milliseconds (Molnar *et al.*, 1995).

Q-T c = Q-T / √R-R

Where Q-T c = Q-T interval corrected

Q-T = Mean of 10 Q-T intervals

√R-R= Squarc root of R-R interval (mean of 10 intervals)

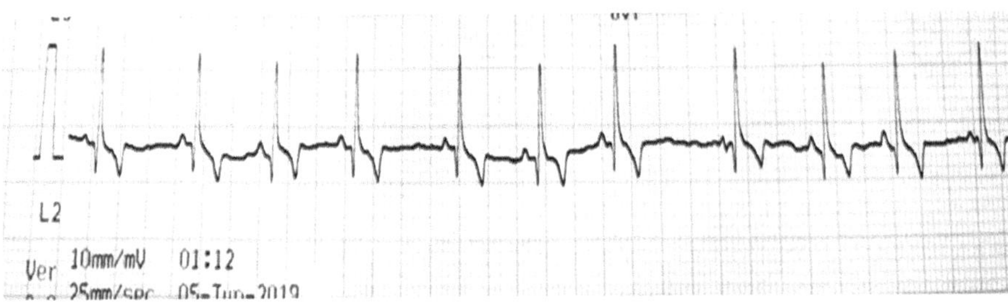

Fig. 66: Electrocardiogram of a dog at sensitivity 1 and speed 25 mm/s. Heart rate 100 bpm. Mean R-R interval is 0.612 second (mean of 10 consecutive R-R interval). Mean of 10 consecutive Q-T interval is 0.234 second or 234 millisecond (Q-T interval 0.24,0.22,0.20,0.24, 0.24,0.24,0.22,0.24, 0.26,0.24 second) . Q-T –c in this case is 0.299 second or 299 millisecond.

Current Generation and its Transmission in the Heart

From electrical point of view canine heart is considered as having two units as atria (right and left) and ventricles (right and left). The depolarization (contraction) of one unit (both atrium) is followed by the depolarization (contraction) of the other unit (ventricles). Sino-atrial node (SA node) is the seat of current generation in the heart for each cardiac cycle because primary pacemaker is located in the SA node. It is also known as the power house of the heart. The Sino-atrial' node (SA node) is a banana shaped compact muscular strap of pace maker cells located at the junction of the cranial (superior) vena cava and right atrium centered around SAN artery (James *et al*.,1966) . The sinatorial node, the interatrial bundle, the atrioventricular node (AV node), the common bundle of His, the right and left bundle branches and the Purkinje fibers are the units of cardiac conduction system. (Fig. 67). Depolarization process is initiated at SA node. From SA node depolarization wave is spread across the atria and through internodal fibers to the AV node. The AV node is situated on the right side of the lower part of the interatrial septum. Depolarization of right atrium begins first followed by depolarization of left atrium. There is about 0.01 second difference in the depolarization of right and left atrium (Friedberg, 1966) as right atrium is near to the SA node. In atrium, depolarization wave spreads from muscle to muscle though inter atrial conduction fibers. The depolarization wave is checked by non-muscular tissue at the junction of the atrium and the ventricles except at atrio-ventricular node (AV node). Current passes within the AV node from cell to cell. The P-R segment (straight line following P wave) in electrocardiogram represents this delay in passing of current from atrium to ventricles. The current or wave of depolarization passes in sequence from AV node to the bundle of His to bundle branches (right and left) to Purkinje fibers to ventricular myocardium. Current passes from bundle of His down the right ventricle side of the muscular septum to the anterior papillary muscle through right bundle branch. The left bundle branch passes the current wave from the bundle of His down the left ventricular side of the septum just below the cups of aortic valve. The left bundle branch further divides into anterior and posterior fascicles passing the current to the bases of corresponding papillary muscles. The fascicles divide further into Purkinje fibers .Which are distributed to ventricular myocardium. The wave of depolarization passes more rapidly through Purkinje fibers. Entire ventricular muscle mass contracts synchronously. After completion of depolarization, repolarization of ventricles begins and it is represented by 'T' wave in the electrocardiogram. The other subsidiary pacemakers are located in the atrium, AV node, Bundle of His, bundle branches, Purkinje system and ventricles (Fig.68) and have potential to take over the role of primary pacemaker when it fails. Activation of subsidiary pacemakers results in the formation of ectopic beat.

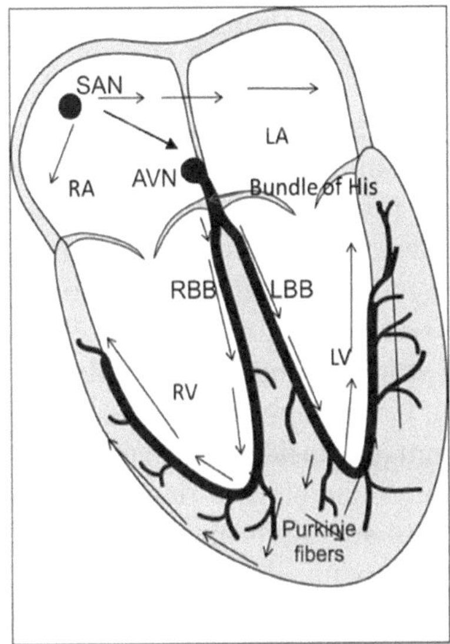

Fig. 67: Diagrammatic representation of the seat of current generation and its flow in the heart. The seat of current generation is SAN (Sino-atrial node) node. From here current spreads across atria and through internodal fibers to the AVN (Atrio-ventricular node) to Bundle of His to right and left bundle branches to Purkinje fibers to ventricular myocardium.

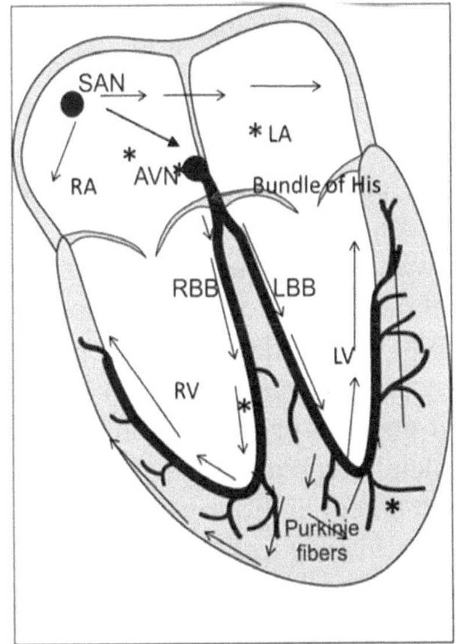

Fig. 68: Showing the hierarchy of different pacemakers in the heart. The primary pacemaker is in the SA node. Other subsidiary pacemakers (marked as *) are located in atria, AV node, Bundle of HIS, Purkinje system and ventricles . The velocity of impulse transmission from different pacemakers is different. Activation of subsidiary pacemaker results in formation of ectopic beat. Areas of potential ectopic foci in myocardium are represented by black asterisks.

Electrogram of cardiac cell during Resting, Depolarization and Repolarization

During resting phase the exterior surface of cardiomyocyte is positively charged and interior of the cell is negatively charged (Fig.69. 1.). The most important ions that contribute to the membrane potential are Na^+, K^+, Ca^{++} and Cl^- The variation in electrical charge of the interior and exterior of the cardiac cell is due to gradient of ions across the cell membrane. Potassium ion (K^+) concentration is much higher inside the cell as compared to outside the cell. In contrast the concentration of Na^+, Ca^{++} and Cl^- is higher outside the cardiac cell. Cardiomyocytes are capable of differentiating between potassium and sodium ions. By keeping sodium ions out and potassium ions inside the cell membrane (sodium potassium pump), cardiac cells are able to maintain resting membrane potential of ~90 mV. With the stimulation of cardiac cell, its membrane resting potential reduces suddenly causing alteration in permeability of cardiac cell membrane (Fig.69.2). This alteration in cardiac cell membrane permeability facilitates the entry of Na + into the cell and exit of K + ions from the cell. The movement of Na+ from outside to inside and of K + from inside to outside the cell membrane results in the alteration of electrical charge. The surface of cardiac cell starts becoming negative and interior of cell membrane starts becoming positive leading to the event of depolarization. When entire exterior of the cell membrane becomes negative and interior becomes positive, the process of depolarization is completed (Fig. 69. 3). This event is recorded as an upward deflection (if depolarization flows towards positive electrode) or downward deflection (if depolarization wave flows away from positive electrode) in the electrocardiogram. With the completion of depolarization process, there is no potential difference between various portions of the cell surface and deflection returns to baseline. Now the next event of repolarization begins with the exit of Na^+ from the interior of the cell and entry of K^+ from the exterior into the cell and the exterior surface of the cardiac cell starts getting positive charge and interior starts getting negative charge (Fig.69 .4) leading to the deflection as per current flow toward positive or away from positive electrode. When cardiac muscle cell is completely repolarized, it assumes the state of resting and cell is polarized having no potential difference (Fig.69.5). The exterior cell surface assumes positive and interior cell surface assumes negative charge. In this stage the electrogram remains at base line without any deflection.

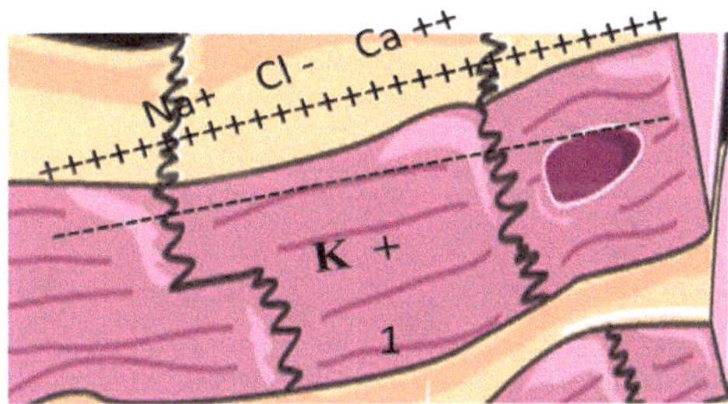

1. Electrogram of resting cardiomyocyte. The exterior surface of resting cardiac cell is positively charged and its interior surface is negatively charged. The cell is electrically polarized with no electrical activity and electrogram remains at base line without showing any deflection. The concentration of K+ is more inside the cardiomyocyte and of Na^+, $Ca^{++}$and Cl^- is more outside the cardiomyocyte.

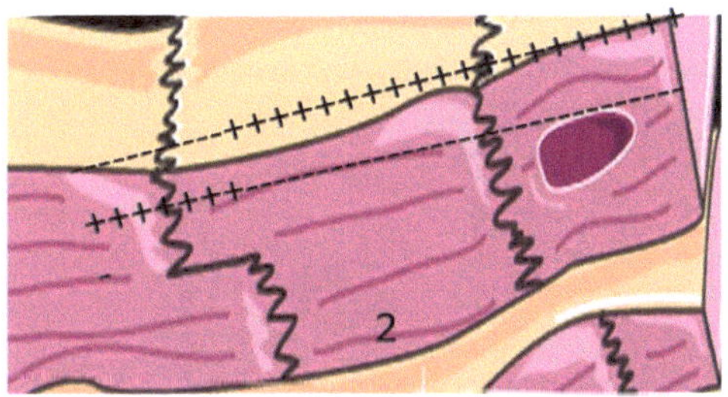

2. Electrogram of cardiomyocyte with stimulus .With stimulation of cardiac cell, the process of depolarization begins from left to right. The permeability of cardiac cell changes permitting the entry of Na+ into the cell and exit of K+ ions from the cell with altering the surface charge. The charge of the depolarized surface area (exterior surface of cardiac cell) with K + becomes negative and charge of the same area inside of the cells with Na + becomes positive resulting in to an upward deflection (if the depolarization wave flows towards positive electrode).

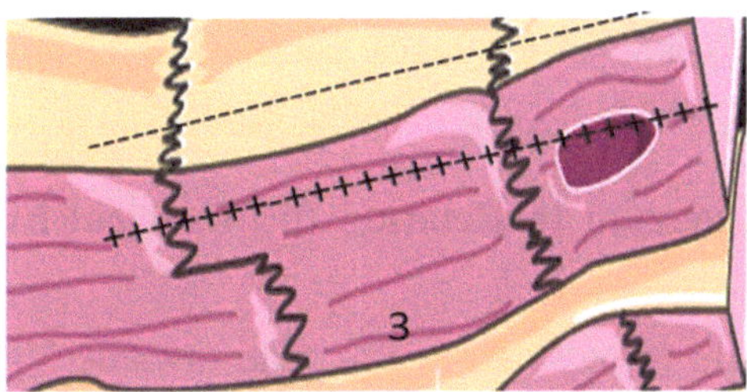

3. Electrogram of completely depolarized cardiac muscle cell. With complete depolarization of cardiac muscle cell, exterior of cell surface becomes negatively charged (because of exit of K^+) and interior of the cell surface becomes positively charged (because of entry of Na+ inside the cell) with no potential difference in various portions of cardiac muscle cell . This stage is similar to resting stage and electrogram recording comes to base line.

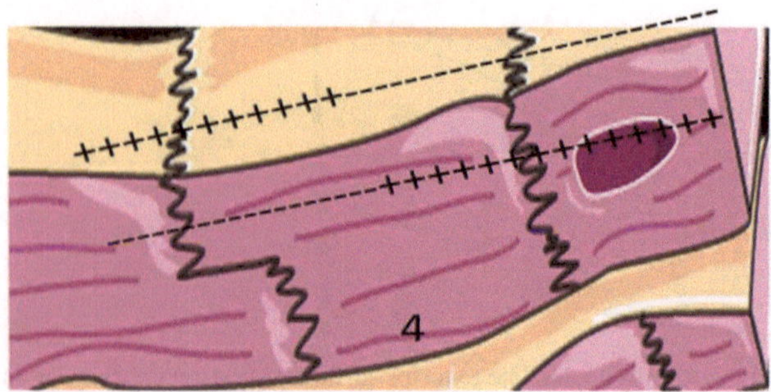

4. Electrogram of cardiac muscle cell with the beginning of repolarization. After completion of depolarization of cardiac muscle cell , repolarization begins at the same point (from where depolarization has started i.e. from left to right) with the entry of K+ into the cell and exit of Na+ from the cell .The exterior cell surface starts resuming positive charge and interior cell surface starts resuming negative charge leading to difference in electric potential at different portions of cardiac cell and current flows. If it flows away from positive electrode downward deflection occurs and if current flows towards positive electrode upward deflection occurs.

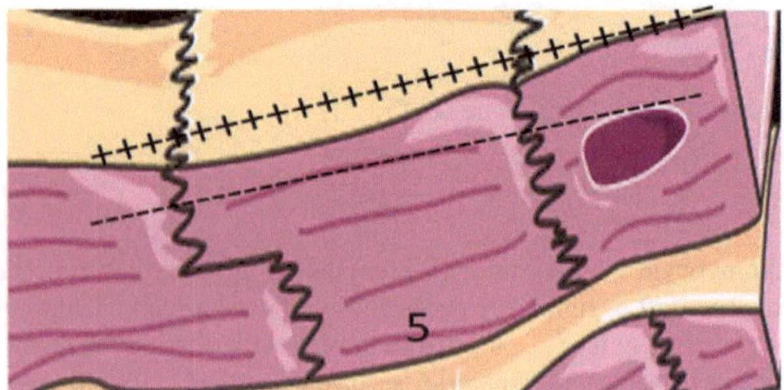

5. Electrogram of completely repolarized cardiac muscle cell. When cardiac muscle cell is completely repolarized, it assumed the state of resting and cell is polarized having no potential difference. The exterior cell surface assumes positive and interior cell surface assumes negative charge. In this stage electrogram remains at base line without any deflection.

Fig. 69: Electrical activity in the single cardiac muscle cell is illustrated in five steps (1to 5).

Generation of Electrocardiogram in Relation to Electrical Events in the Heart

Transmission of depolarization impulse from SA node towards left atrium and AV node through right atrium leads to the formation of 'P' wave in electrocardiogram (Fig.70). Its formation ('P' wave) denotes the total sum of all electrical forces produced during depolarization of both atria. The ascending arm of the 'P' wave (first half of the 'P' Wave) represents the depolarization of the right atrium and the descending arm of the 'P' wave (second half of the 'P'wave) represents the depolarization of the left atrium. The straight line following ‘P’ wave (P-R segment) denotes the delay in passing of the current at AV node. Total time of depolarization of both atria and delay in passing of the current in AV node is represented as P-R interval in the electrocardiogram. Depolarization impulse passes into ventricle only through bundle of His. ‘Q’, ‘R’ and ‘S’ deflections in electrocardiogram are produced by three phases of electrical activity representing septal activation, ventricular free wall myocardial activation and depolarization of basal septal and ventricular basilar portions of the heart respectively. After ventricular depolarization, the phase of repolarization begins. Between the ventricular depolarization (QRS complex) and repolarization, there is an electrically neutral area termed as S-T segment represented by the isoelectric line in the electrocardiogram. It is a time lag between depolarization and repolarization. Repolarization of ventricles is represented by ‘T’ wave. Each normal cardiac cycle is represented in the electrocardiographic tracing by three successive complexes- the P-wave, the QRS- complex and the T-wave corresponding to atrial depolarization, ventricular depolarization and ventricular repolarization respectively.

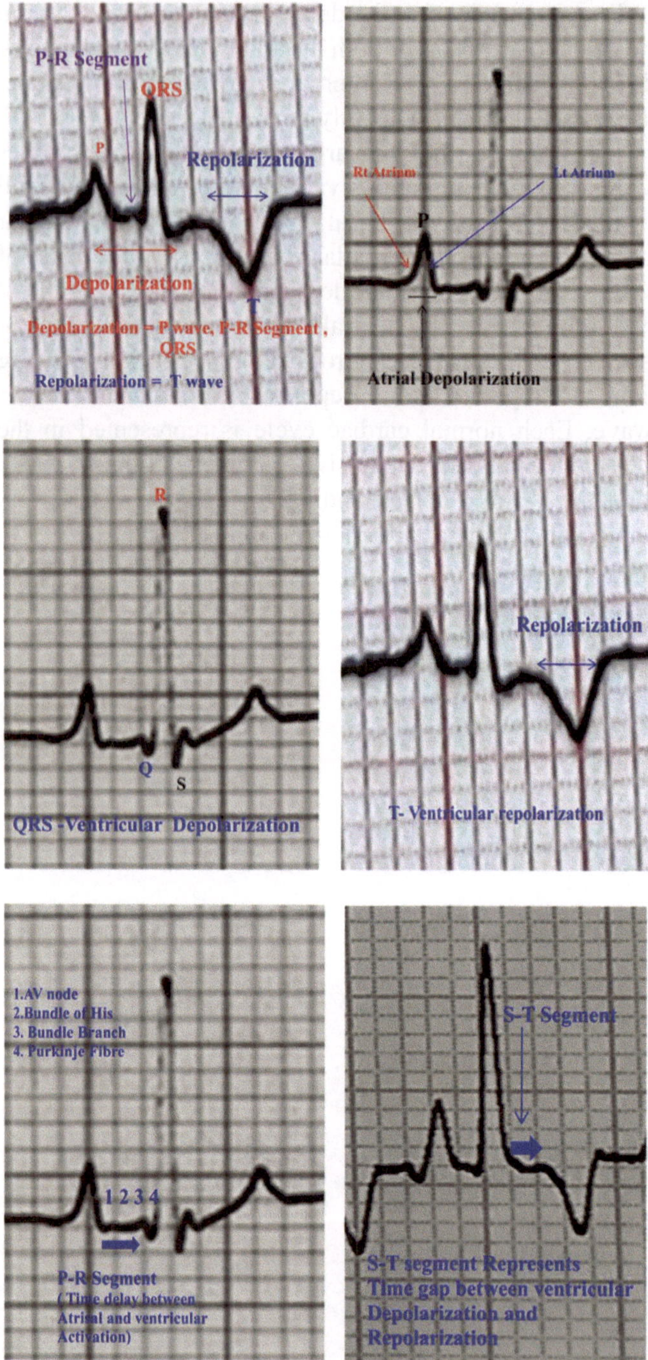

Fig. 70: Electrocardiograms are showing generation of electrocardiogram in relation to depolarization and repolarization of cardiac muscle fiber.

References

Baumert, M., Porta, A; Vos, M. A., Malik, M., Couderc, J., Laguna, P., Piccirillo, G., Smith,G.L., Tereshchenko, L.G. and Volders, P.G.A. (2016). QT interval variability in body surface ECG: measurement, physiological basis, and clinical value: position statement and consensus guidance endorsed by the European Heart Rhythm Association jointly with the ESC Working group on Cardiac Cellular. Electrophysiology. Europace 18:925-944. Doi:10.1093/europace/euv405.PMC 4905605, PMID 26823389.

Binkley, P.F., Nunziata, E., Hass, G.J., Nelson, S.D. and Cody, R.J. (1991). Parasympathetic withdrawal is an integral component of autonomic imbalance in congestive heart failure: demonstration in human subjects and verification in a paced canine model of ventricular failure. J. Am. Coll. Cardiol .18: 464–472.

Doxey, S. and Boswood, A.(2004) .Difference between breeds of dog in a measure of heart rate variability. Vet Rec 154:713–717

Friedberg, C.K. (1966) .Diseases of Heart, 3rd edn. W.B. Saunders Company, Philadelphia

Haggstrom, J., Hamlin, R.L., Hansson, K. and Kvart, C. (1996) .Heart rate variability in relation to severity of mitral regurgitation in Cavalier King Charles Spaniels. J. Small Anim. Pract. 37:69–75

James, T.N., Sherf, L., Fine, G. and Morales, A.R. (1966) .Comparative ultrastructure of the sinus node in man and dog. *Circulation* 34:1391–63. [PubMed] [Google Scholar]

Katayama,M.,Kubo,T.,Mogi,K.,Ikeda,K.,Nagasawa, M., and Kikusui, T. (2016). Heart rate variability predicts the emotional state in dogs. Behav. Processes. 128:108-112. doi: 10.1016/j.beproc.2016.04.015. Epub 2016 Apr 26.

Molnar, J., Weiss, J. S., and Rosenthal, J. E.(1995). The missing second: What is the correct unit for the Bazctt corrected QT interval ? Am. J. Cardiol. 75:537-538. https://doi.org/10.1016/S0002-9149 (99)80603-1 Simonson, E., Minn, M. and Cady, L.D. Jr. (1962) .The normal Q-T interval. Am. Heart J. 63:747–753.

Stein, P.K., Bosner, M.S., Kleiger, R.E. and Conger, B.M. (1994). Heart rate variability: a measure of cardiac autonomic tone. Am. Heart J. 127:1376–1381.

Further Reading

Varshney, J.P. (2020). Electrocardiography in Veterinary Medicine. Springer Nature, Singapore, Pte, Ltd.

5

Reading of An Electrocardiogram

After successful recording of the electrocardiogram, the next step is its reading, analysis, interpretation and report writing. It is the most important part of electrocardiography. Patients details (name, species of animal, breed, age ,sex, owners' name and address with E-mail and mobile number) and date of tracing are to be mentioned in the electrocardiograph prior to actual recording of the electrocardiogram or can be jotted down on the ECG strip after completion of recording as per available facility in the electrocardiographic machine. Clinical complaints and observations should be kept in mind while interpreting the electrocardiogram. Modern automatic electrocardiographic machines have facility to mark the leads on the strip. If the machine is manual or single channel leads are to be marked on the electrocardiographic strip as I,II,III, aVR, aVL , aVF ,CV_5RL, CV_6LL, CV_6LU and V_{10}. Speed (25 mm per second or 50 mm per second) and sensitivity (0.5, 1 or 2) are to be specified for calculating heart rate and measurements of different wave forms in case of manual machines. Modern automatic machines mark these details as per their setting automatically. Recording of an electrocardiogram is not a difficult or complicated task. One can acquire the skill of electrocardiographic recording easily. Casual reading of an electrocardiogram may mislead the diagnosis. Proper reading and interpretation of an electrocardiogram requires fundamental knowledge of cardiac anatomy, physiology and cardiology. An electrocardiogram should not be interpreted in isolation of other details but due weightage should be given to the history and clinical manifestations of the patient as well as other investigations. Anatomical heart defects or change in physiological states may not always be predictable by an electrocardiographic examination. It is an attending clinician who can interpret electrocardiogram better in the light of all other investigations. Wide variations in the normal electrocardiographic indices of different breeds of the dogs and overlapping ECG patterns between various conditions should also be kept in mind while interpreting an electrocardiogram.

Reading an Electrocardiogram

Reading and analysis of an electrocardiogram provide valuable information about cardiac rate, cardiac rhythm, amplitude and duration of waves, duration of intervals and mean electrical axis of the heart on frontal plane.

1. *Heart rate*

Heart rate is usually calculated from the observations of the lead II (Fig.71) of ECG strip as complex are large and well defined in this lead. The number of complexes (QRS) are counted in 3 seconds (15 large squares i.e.75 small squares when ECG machine is running at the standard speed of 25 mm per second or 30 large squares i.e. 150 small squares when ECG machine is running at the speed of 50 mm/second). The number of the complex is multiplied by 20 to get heart rate per minute. It is the simplest and easiest way of finding heart rate.

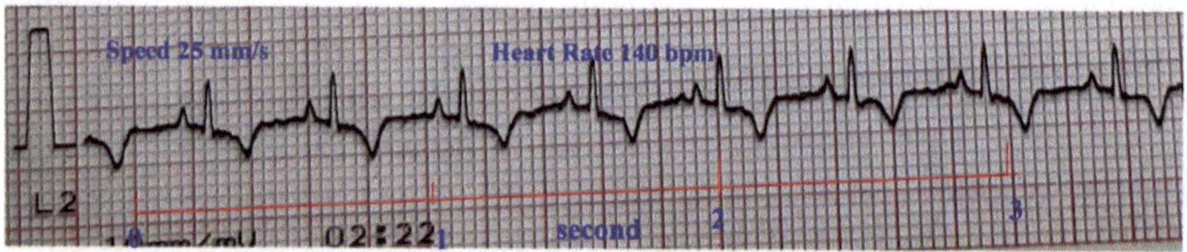

Fig. 71: Electrocardiogram of a dog taken at 25 mm/s speed. Five large or 25 small squares denote 1 second as marked in the above electrocardiogram. There are 7 complexes in 3 second. Its multiplication by 20 gives a heart rate of 140 beats per minute.

2. *Cardiac rhythm*

In an electrocardiogram of a healthy dog each complex consists of a ‘P’ wave, P-R segment, ‘QRS’, S-T segment and ‘T’ Wave (Fig. 72). Cardiac rhythm is said to be normal or sinus rhythm if every ‘QRS complex has a ‘P’ wave and normal uniform P-R or R-R intervals (Fig. 73). Frank arrhythmias have gross irregularities that can be detected at first sight (Fig.74) and measuring of ‘P-R’ and ‘R-R’ intervals may reveal small fine irregularities.

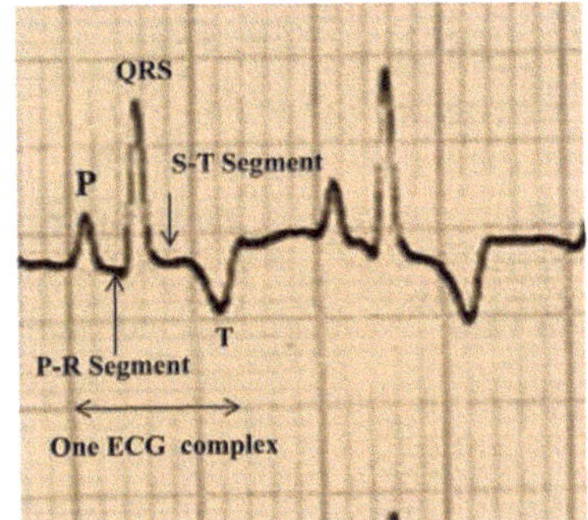

Fig. 72: Electrocardiogram of a dog is showing one ECG complex consisting of 'P', P-R segment, 'QRS', S-T segment and T wave.

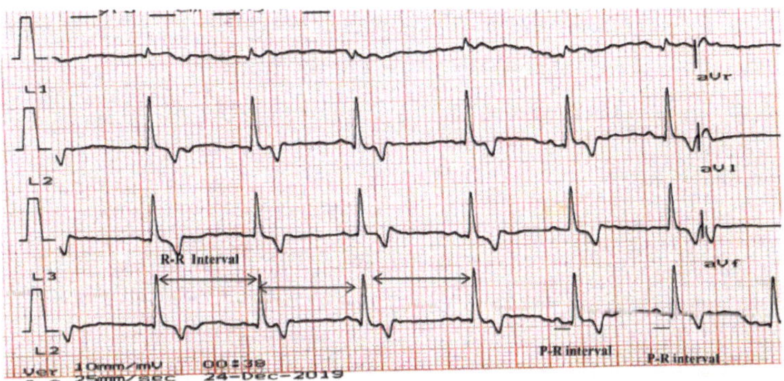

Fig.73: Electrocardiogram of a dog taken at the speed of 25 mm/s and sensitivity of 1 is showing almost uniform P-R interval (0.10 to 0.12 s) and R-R interval (0.6 to 0.64 s) in all complexes indicating sinus or normal rhythm.

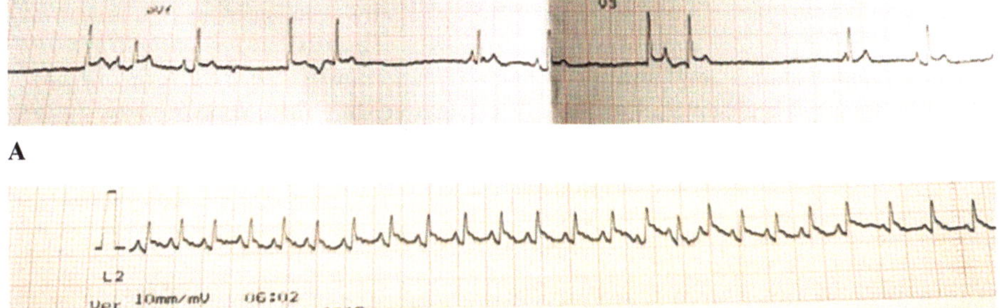

A

B

Fig. 74: Electrocardiograms (Lead II, sensitivity 1, speed 25 mm/s) of dogs are showing gross abnormalities such as long pauses **(A)** and mixing of T and P waves **(B)**.

3. *Reading Waves, Intervals and Segments*

Reading of all waves, intervals and segments is generally done in Lead II. Amplitude of waves is measured as height and their duration as width. In case of abnormalities, other standard leads (I, III), augmented leads (aVR, aVL, aVF) and chest leads (CV_5RL, CV_6 LL, and CV_6LU and V_{10}) are also examined. Reading of lead I and III is helpful in finding out mean electrical axis (MEA) on frontal plane.

Waves

The height (amplitude) of the waves ('P', 'Q', 'R' 'S', T), positive or negative, is measured from the base line to the top of the wave (in case of positive waves as 'P','R' 'T') or from base line to the bottom of the wave (in case of negative waves as 'Q' 'S' 'T') and their width or duration ('P','QRS, T) is measured from beginning to the end of the wave as shown in the Fig. 75.

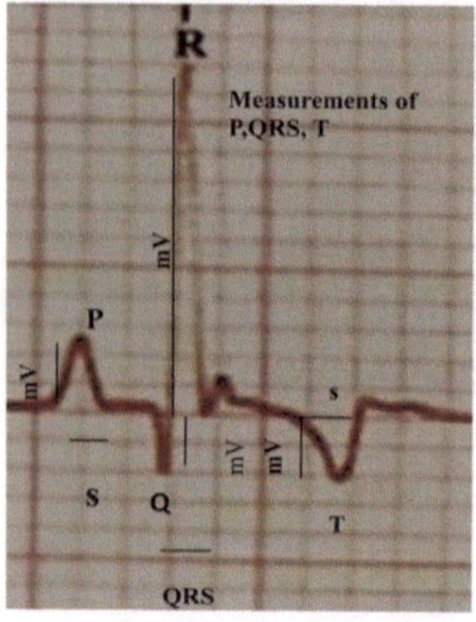

Fig. 75: Electrocardiogram of a dog, taken at the speed of 25 mm/s and sensitivity of 1, is showing measurements of 'P', 'Q' ,'R' and T waves. The 'P' wave is of 0.25 mV (2.5 mm height) and 0.04 s duration. (1mm width). The 'Q' wave is 0.2 m V (2 mm below base line). It is first negative wave. The 'R' wave is positive and of 1.2 mV (12 mm height). There is no 'S' wave in this electrocardiogram. The 'QRS' duration is of 0.04 s (1 mm width). The 'T 'wave is negative and is of 0.2 mV (2 mm below base line) and of 0.05 s duration (slightly > than 1 mm width).

Segments

Examination of duration of segments (P-R segment, S-T segment, T-P segment) and intervals (P-R interval, R-R interval and Q-T interval) is shown in the following figures. It provides valuable information for detecting arrhythmias and conduction defects.

P-R segment is examined from the end of 'P' wave to the beginning of 'QRS' complex (Fig. 76).The important factor in analyzing segments is their change from isoelectric line (elevation or depression) and their duration also. The P-R segment represents the electrical conduction through the atria and delay of the electrical impulse in the AV node. It is a straight line and the current wave is too weak to be recorded on volt meter. Abnormalities of P-R segment are very limited. In humans depression in PR segment has been reported to be a signal for pericarditis or atrial infarction.

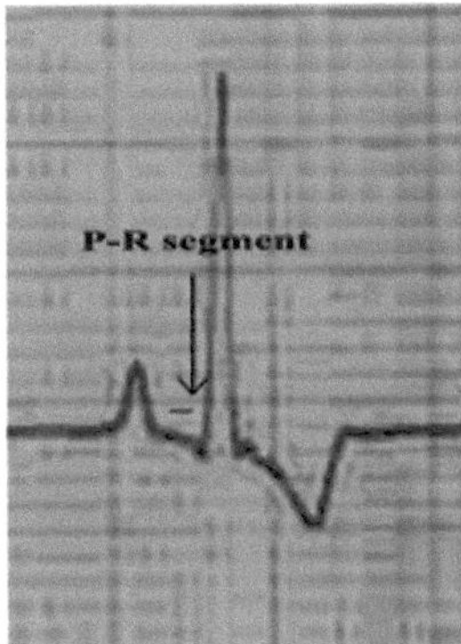

Fig. 76: Electrocardiogram of a dog is showing P-R segment of 0.08 s.

S-T segment is examined from the end of QRS complex to the beginning of 'T' wave (Fig.77). It is also an isoelectric line. Its duration, elevation or depression (deviation from isoelectric line) is noted.

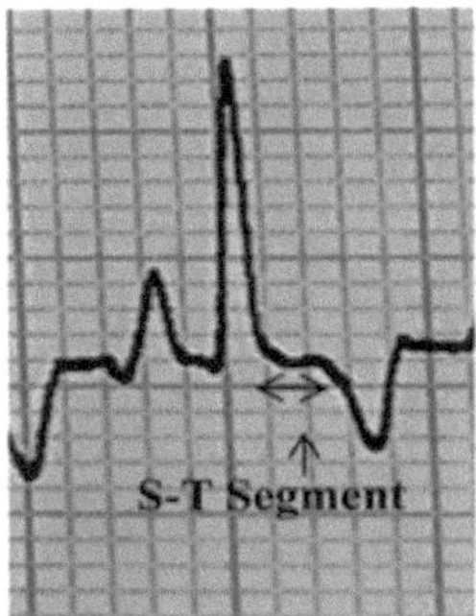

Fig. 77: Electrocardiogram of a dog is showing S-T segment of 0.06 s. In normal electrocardiograms it is an isoelectric line.

T-P segment is examined from the end of the 'T' wave to the beginning of the 'P' wave (Fig.78). It is also an isoelectric line. Its duration is also noted.

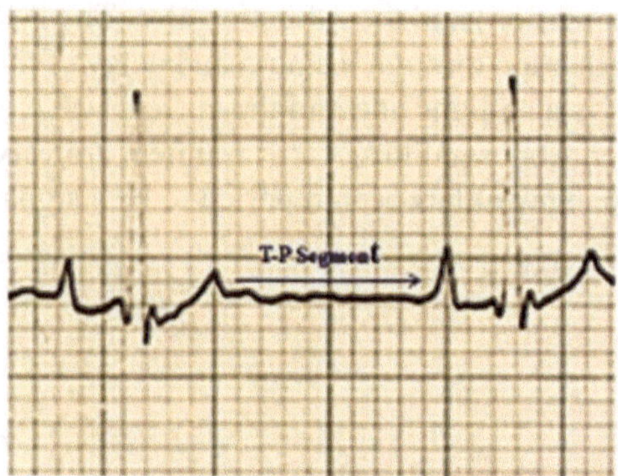

Fig. 78: Electrocardiogram of a dog is showing T-P segment of 0.32 s. In normal electrocardiogram it is an isoelectric line.

Intervals

An interval in the electrocardiogram is a duration of the time. It includes one segment and one or two waves.

P-R interval or P-Q interval is the duration of time from the beginning of the 'P' wave to the beginning of 'Q' or R wave (Fig.79). Its prolongation is indicative of delayed conduction of electrical impulse (wave of depolarization).

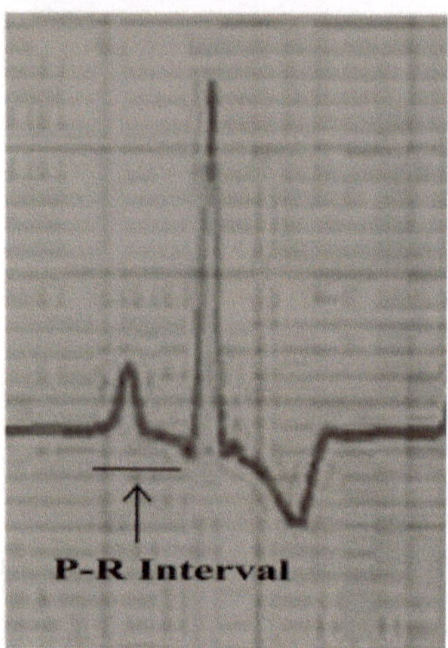

Fig. 79: Electrocardiogram of a dog is showing P-R interval of 0.12 s. It includes duration of 'P' wave and P-R segment.

Q-T interval starts from the beginning of the 'QRS' to the end of 'T' wave (Fig.80). It includes 'QRS' duration, S-T segment and 'T' wave duration. The duration of Q-T interval depends on the heart rate. It is short if heart rate is fast and vice versa i.e. it is inversely related to the heart rate. 'Q-T' interval in isolation may not be of much diagnostic significance. As a thumb rule it is less than half the preceding 'R-R' interval when rhythm is sinus.

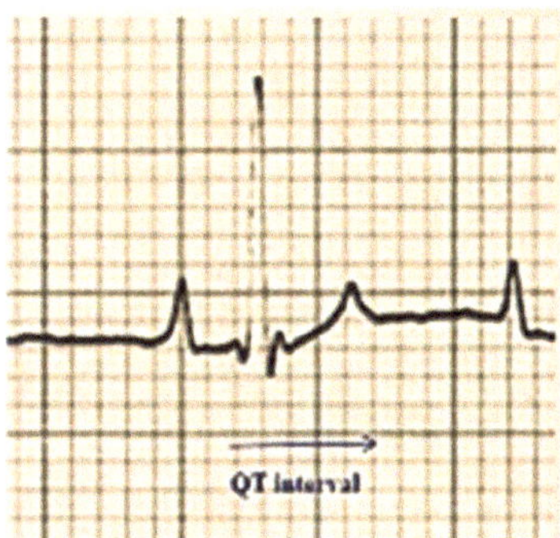

Fig. 80: Electrocardiogram of a dog is showing Q-T interval of 0.2 s. It comprises of 'QRS' duration, S-T segment and 'T' wave duration.

R-R Interval is the duration of time between two consecutive 'R' waves (Fig.81). Heart rate can be calculated by measuring R-R interval. If R-R interval is not uniform, it indicates arrhythmia.

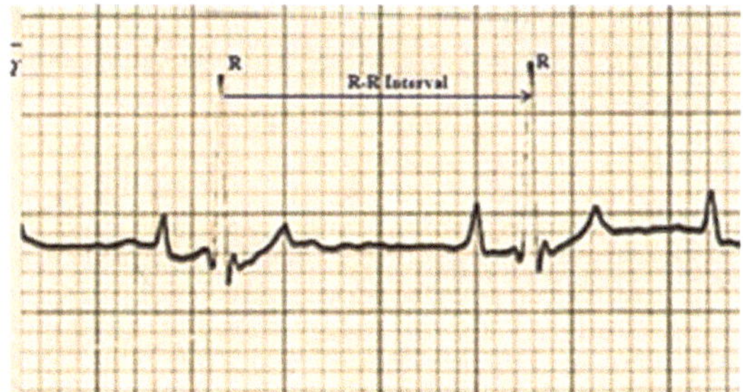

Fig.81. Electrocardiogram of a dog is showing R-R interval of 0.64 s. It is the duration of time between two consecutive waves.

4. *Configuration of the waves*

While reading an electrocardiogram, attention should also be paid to the configuration of the waves

'P' wave

Its configuration (as small, rounded, pointed, notched, or biphasic) and its positivity/ negativity should be noted (Fig.82). The 'P' wave is usually positive in lead I, II, III, and aVF. However, 'P' wave is normally negative in leads aVR and aVL (Fig.82).

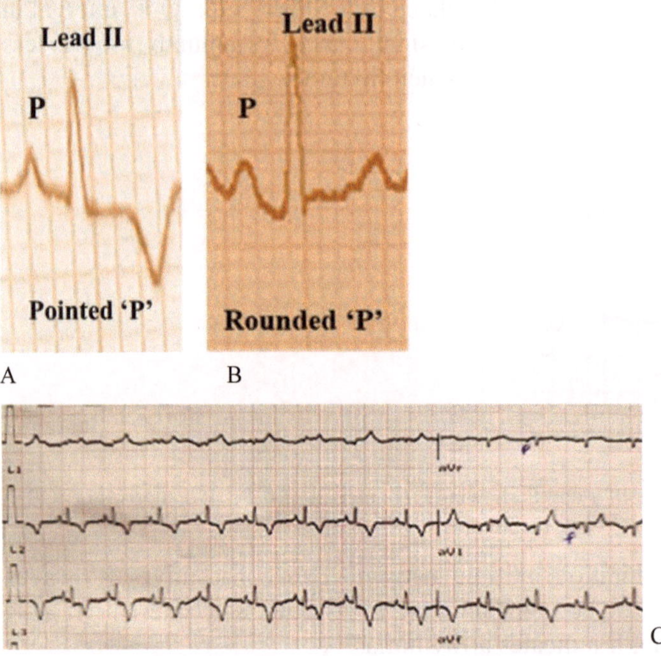

Fig. 82: Electrocardiograms of dogs are showing configuration of 'P' wave. It is small pointed (A) or rounded (B) wave. It is positive in lead II, III, and aVF and negative in lead aVR and aVL (C). It may not be very conspicuous in lead I. P wave is of 0.15 mV and 0.04 s in A and B electrocardiograms.

'Q' Wave

The presence / absence of the 'Q' wave and its amplitude is noted (Fig.83). It is usually a negative wave in lead I, II, III and aVF. Deep 'Q' wave is suggestive of right ventricular enlargement.

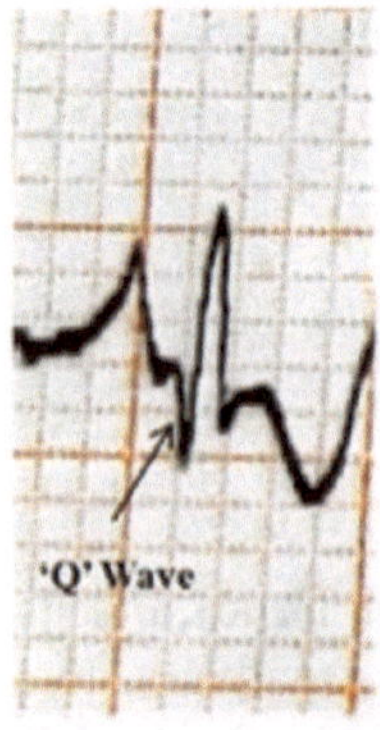

Fig. 83: Electrocardiogram of a dog is showing 'Q' wave (marked with arrow). It is of 0.2 mV.

'R' Wave

It is positive deflection (Fig.84) in lead I, II, III, and aVF and negative in lead aVR and aVL. Amplitude of 'R' wave is noted. Very large 'R' wave is suggestive of left ventricular enlargement. 'R' wave may have different configurations as described in Chapter 4.

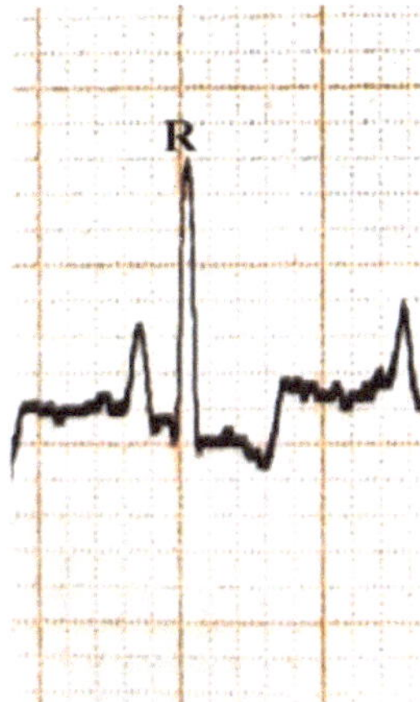

Fig. 84: Electrocardiogram of a dog is showing 'R' wave. It is of 0.7 mV amplitude.

'S' Wave

'S' wave (Fig.85) is the negative deflection after 'R' wave. Its presence/ absence and amplitude is noted. It is also due to depolarization of right ventricle. Deep 'S' wave is suggestive of right ventricular enlargement.

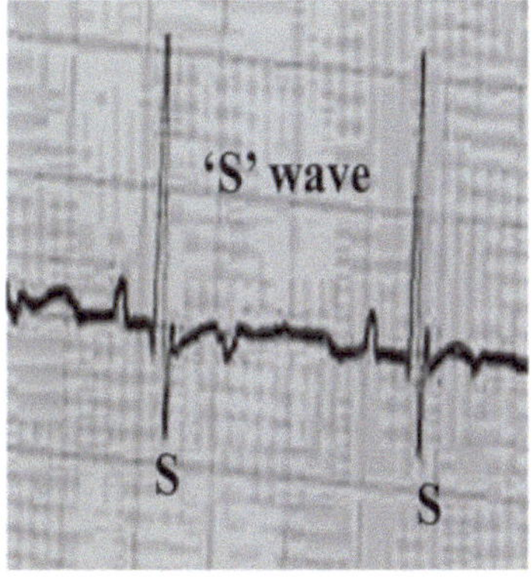

Fig. 85: Showing 'S' wave (marked as S). It is a negative deflection (below base line) that follows 'R 'wave and denotes right ventricle depolarization. S wave in this electrocardiogram is of 0.4 mV.

'QRS' complex

Its duration is noted. There are various forms of 'QRS' complex in limb leads as shown below (Fig.86). Broad 'QRS' alone is suggestive of left bundle branch block. While broad 'QRS' with increased amplitude of 'R' wave is suggestive of left ventricle enlargement.

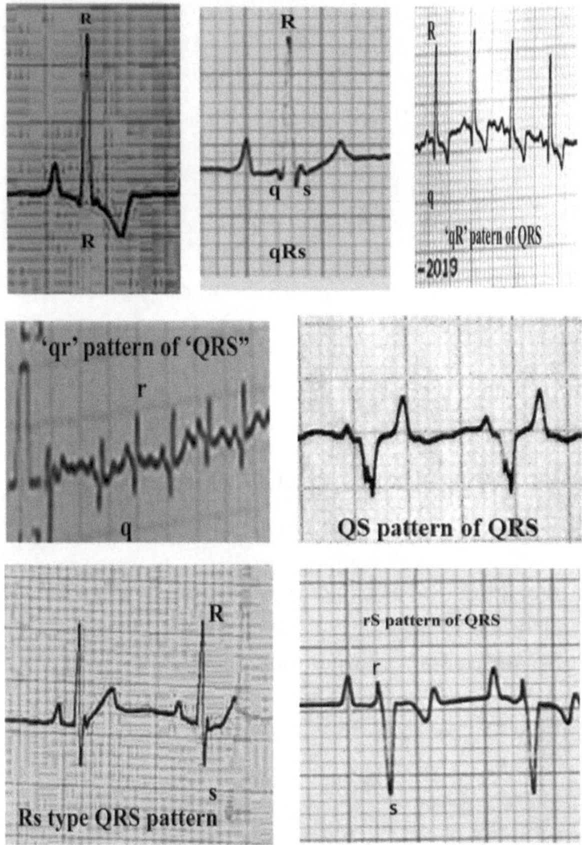

Fig. 86: Electrocardiograms of the dogs are showing different patterns of 'QRS' complex.

'T' wave

It is the first major positive or negative deflection after 'QRS' complex (Fig. 87). 'T' wave represents repolarization of ventricles. There are many configurations (positive, negative, notched, biphasic, flat) of the 'T' wave . Its height and width are to be noted.

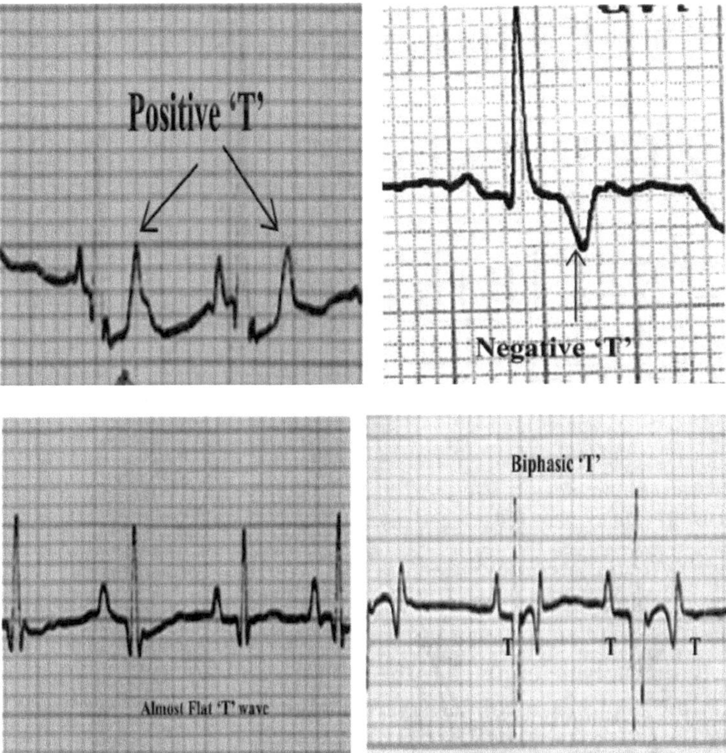

Fig. 87: Electrocardiograms of dogs are showing different types of 'T' wave. It is the first major deflection after 'QRS' and signifies ventricular repolarization. In humans 'T' wave is very important.

5. *Finding Mean Electrical Axis*

The mean electrical axis is the principal vector of ventricular depolarization. It represents the sum of all the waves of depolarization occurring simultaneously. It describes the net direction of cardiac depolarization across the frontal plane and denotes the direction of the movement of the electric potential generated by the heart during the cardiac cycle corresponding with cardiac physical axis. In other words it is the mean direction of the ventricular vectors generated during cardiac cycle. An idea about the cardiac topography in the thoracic cavity can be obtained through MEA. The concept of mean electrical activity of 'QRS' in the electrocardiogram was introduced for the first time by Einthoven in 1913. In healthy dogs mean electrical axis of the normal heart is between + 40 ^{0} to +100 ^{0}(Fig. 88 A). In healthy cats mean electrical axis of the normal heart is between 0 to +160 ^{0}(Fig.88 B).

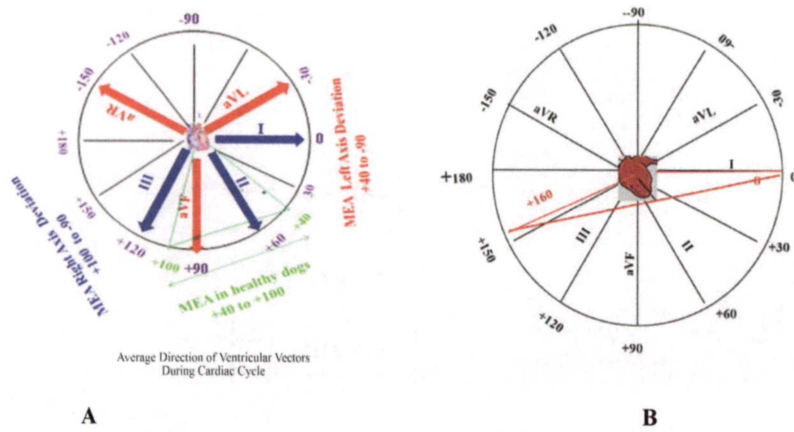

Fig. 88: Diagrammatic representation of an average direction of ventricular vectors during cardiac cycle. MEA in healthy dogs is +40 to +100^0 marked by green triangle **(A)**. MEA in healthy cats is +0 to +160^0 marked by red triangle **(B)**.

Determining MEA is recommended when cardiac enlargement and intraventricular conduction disorders are suspected as an abnormal MEA indicates defects in intraventricular conduction, ventricular size and/or cardiac axis deviation. It is usually determined in the frontal plane. MEA is determined using the observations of hex-axial lead system (standard bipolar limb leads I, II, III; and unipolar augmented leads aVR, aVL, aVF) on the electrocardiogram. There are four methods for determining the mean electrical axis.

The Method 1 (Finding Isoelectric Lead) -Electrocardiogram recorded in hex-axial lead system (leads I, II, III, aVR, aVL, aVF) is used to determine MEA in this method. Lead with smallest amplitude close to isoelectric line is chosen and a perpendicular line is drawn on the direction of this lead as shown in the Fig. 89. In case, the 'QRS' complex is predominantly positive in perpendicular lead, then the MEA is directed towards the positive pole. MEA is directed away from the positive pole if 'QRS' complex in negative in the perpendicular lead. If two leads are isoelectric, lead with smallest 'QRS' complex is chosen. If all leads are isoelectric, then it is difficult to determine MEA

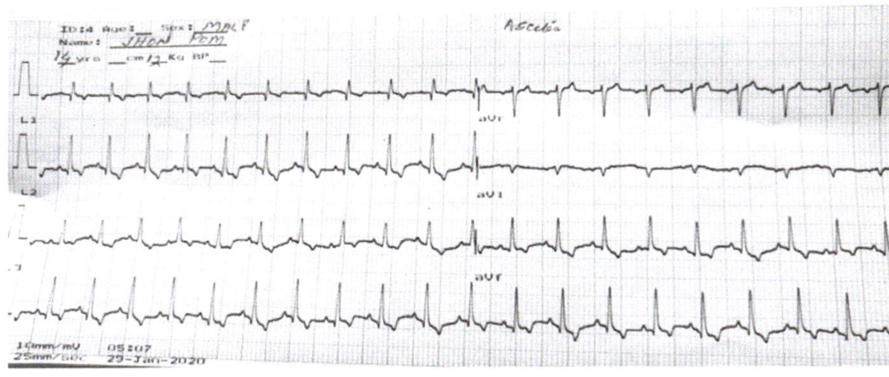

A

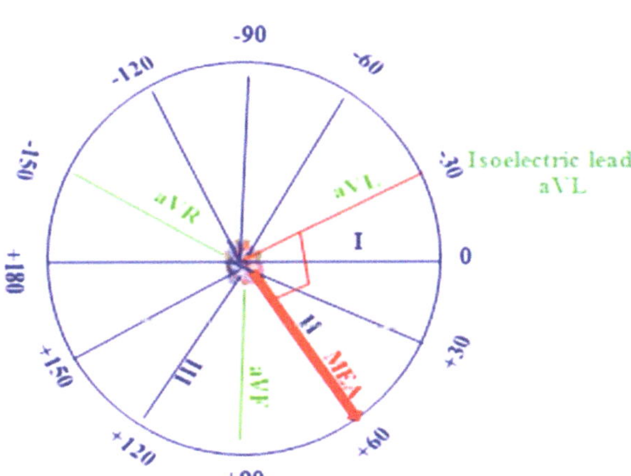

B

Fig. 89: Determining mean electrical axis (MEA) by choosing a lead close to iso-electric line in an electrocardiogram recorded with six leads (I, II, III, aVR, aVL, aVF). In the above electrocardiogram of a dog recorded at the sensitivity of 1 and speed of 25 mm/s (A), lead aVL is having smallest amplitude (close to isoelectric line). It is marked in the Fig. B as thin red line. A line perpendicular to aVL is drawn as shown in the Fig .B (marked as thick red line with arrow) indicating mean electrical axis of + 60^{0}.

The Method 2- Lead with tallest 'R' wave deflection is identified. The MEA is within 30 degrees of positive pole of tallest 'R' wave. This is less specific method. Tallest 'R' wave in the electrocardiogram (Fig.90) is in lead II. Therefore, MEA is +60 ^{0} as the direction of lead II is + 60 ^{0}.

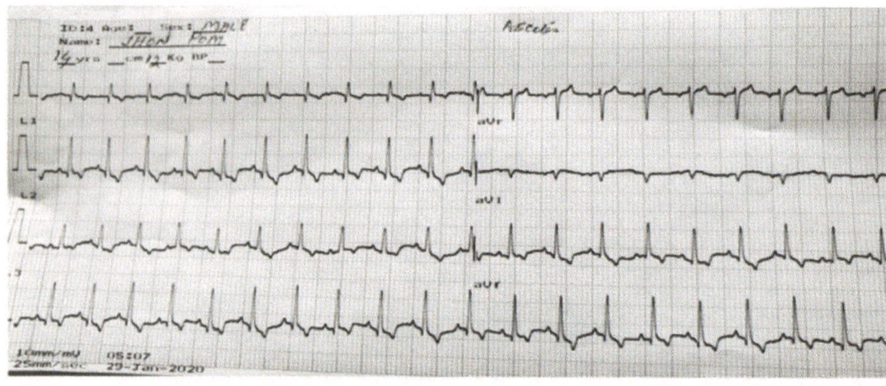

A

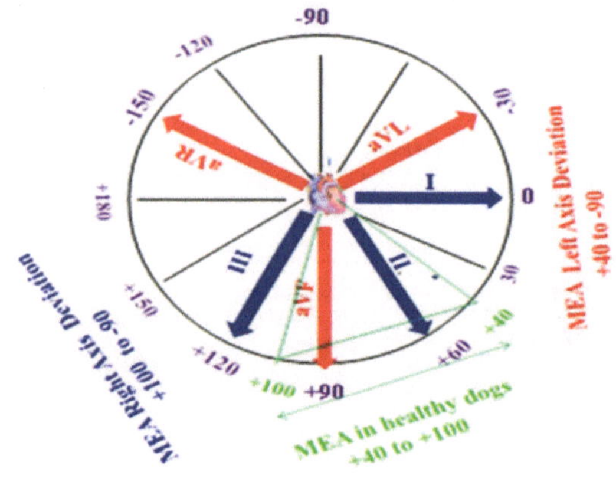

Average Direction of Ventricular Vectors
during cardiac Cycle

B

Fig. 90: Determining mean electrical axis (MEA) by choosing a lead with tallest 'R' wave in an electrocardiogram recorded with six leads (I, II, III, aVR, aVL, aVF). In the above electrocardiogram of a dog (A) recorded at the sensitivity of 1 and speed of 25 mm/s, lead II is having tallest 'R' wave. The direction of lead II is +60 ^{0} (B), hence mean electrical axis of the heart is +60 ^{0}.

The Method 3 (Lead graphic method) - Net amplitude of the QRS complexes (the difference between positive and negative waves i.e. 'R' amplitude and 'Q' or 'S' amplitude) in lead I and lead III is determined. Net deflections are plotted on each lead. Then perpendicular line is drawn through each of these points. The point where the lines from lead I and III intersect is the mean electrical axis (Fig.91) . Any two leads can be used for calculating MEA but generally lead I and III are used.

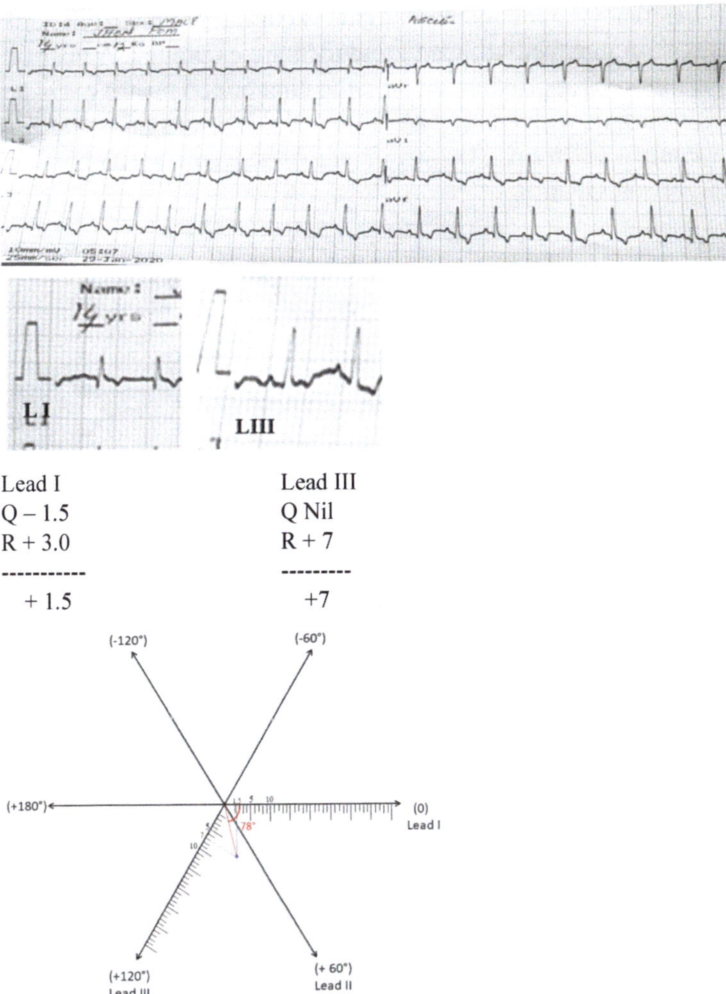

Fig. 91: Determining mean electrical axis (MEA) by lead graphic method plotting the values of lead I and Lead III. The sum of positive and negative deflections in lead I and lead III is calculated and marked on from zero point on lead I and lead III respectively. From these points perpendicular lines are drawn .Intersection point and center point are joined together by a line. The angle is read. This is the MEA. In the above example, the net sum of deflections in lead I and III is +1.5 and +7 respectively. It is marked on the respective lines of the leads. The angle of the line meeting the intersection point and center point comes to 78^0 approximately.

It is a little cumbersome procedure and not practical in routine clinical practice. Alternatively the net amplitudes of QRS in lead I and lead III are worked out and the value of MEA can be found out from the table given by Tilley (1992). As per table MEA in this case is 81^0.

The Method 4 (Quadrant Graphic method) - This is considered most efficient way to estimate axis. In this method, lead I and aVF are examined. A positve 'QRS' in lead I puts the axis approximately in same direction. A positive 'QRS' in lead 'aVF' aligns the axis with the lead aVF. Hexaxial lead system is divided by leads I and aVF into 4 quadrants. Arrows are drawn on lead I and aVF in the direction of predominant QRS.

Abnormal MEA

- In dogs MEA of more than $+100^0$ suggests right axis deviation.
- In dogs MEA of less than $+40\ ^0$ suggests left axis deviation.
- In cats, MEA of less than $0\ ^0$suggests left axis deviation.
- In cats, MEA of more than $+160\ ^0$suggests right axis deviation

Keeping ECG Record

Record of electrocardiogram and relevant information should be kept properly in digital form or hard copy for further reference. Electrocardiographic interpretations should be jotted down immediately after ECG tracing is completed. The information may be kept in the following format. It can be changed as per requirement.

Electrocardiographic Report

Reference Number.: Date.

Name of the Dog.:

Breed of the Dog.: Date of Birth/ Age.:

Male/Female:

Referred by Dr.

Electrocardiographic Observations in Lead II

Sensitivity 0.5/1/2 ECG Machine Speed 25/50 mm/s

Heart Rate: bpm, Rhythm: Sinus/Arrhythmic

Waves

‘P’ mV, s

‘Q’ mV

‘R’ mV

‘S’ mV

‘T’ mV, s

‘QRS’ s

Intervals

‘P-R’ s

‘R-R’ s

‘Q-T’ s

‘T-P’ s

Segments

P-R s

S-T s Normal / Elevated mV/ Depressed mV

Polarity of Waves

‘P’ Positive/Negative

‘T’ Positive/Negative/ Biphasic

Mean electrical axis on frontal plane (MEA):

Other Important Observations, if any:

Electrocardiographic Interpretations

Signature
Name and qualification of the
Veterinarian.

Reading and Analysis of an Electrocardiogram of a dog

An analysis of an electrocardiogram of a dog, taken at the speed of 25 mm/s and at sensitivity of 1, is given below in Fig. 92.

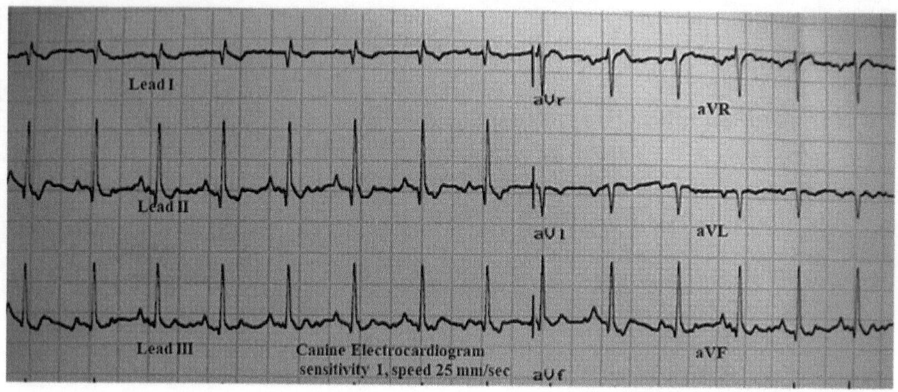

Fig. 92: Electrocardiogram (speed 25 mm/s, sensitivity 1) of a dog in standard and augmented limb leads. Lead I is near isoelectric in this electrocardiogram. Lead II analysis shows heart rate of 140 bpm with sinus rhythm; 'P' wave (small, pointed and positive) of 0.1 mV and 0.04 s duration; P-R segment of 0.08 s; P-R interval of 0.12 s; 'Q' wave of 0.2 mV; 'R' wave of 1.15 mV; 'QRS' 0.06 s; S-T slurring /0.04-0.05 s; 'T' wave of 0.1 mV and 0.04 s; R-R interval of 0.42 s: 'Q-T' interval of 0.14 s; 'T-P' segment of 0.12 - 0.14 s; and MEA of +90 ^{0} suggesting an normal electrocardiogram.

Reference

Tilley, LP. (1992).Generation of the electrocardiogram: basic principles. In: Essentials of canine and feline electrocardiography: interpretation and treatment. 3rd ed. Philadelphia, Pa: Lea & Fibiger; 1-18.

Further Reading

Varshney, J.P. (2020). Electrocardiography in Veterinary Medicine. Springer Nature, Singapore, Pte, Ltd.

6

Normal Values of Electrocardiographic Indices in Healthy Dogs and Cats

An understanding of normal values of electrocardiographic indices of healthy dogs and cats is utmost necessary for interpreting an abnormal electrocardiogram. The criteria for normal configuration and measurements of the waves, segments and intervals in an electrocardiogram of healthy subjects provides basis for detecting abnormalities in the electrocardiogram of the ailing animals. The electrocardiogram, like other diagnostic aids, is not an absolute indicator of health and disease and therefore it is required to be interpreted in conjunction with patient's history, clinical manifestations, and the results of other investigations. Any departure from normal electrocardiographic values may be suggestive of anomaly but do not confirm structural change or valvular abnormality in the heart. Undoubtedly an electrocardiogram is of immense diagnostic value in confirming arrhythmias and conduction disturbances. To some extent chamber enlargement in advanced stage can also be detected in the dogs. It is not always feasible to confirm chamber enlargement by electrocardiography in cats. It is important to remember that an electrocardiogram may be normal even in the face of advanced cardiovascular disease. Generally accepted values of electrocardiographic indices in healthy dogs and cats are given below.

Electrocardiographic Indices in Healthy Dogs

Heart Rate

It varies in different age groups as well as in different breeds. Nevertheless following values are considered normal.

Neonates and Puppies	< 220 bpm
Adult dogs (small breeds)	80 to 180 bpm
Adult dogs (large breeds)	70 to 160 bpm
Adult dogs (Giant breeds)	60 to 140 bpm

Heart Rhythm

Sinus Rhythm

Wandering Pace maker

Measurements of Waves, Segments and Intervals (Lead II)

'P' wave	
Amplitude (height of the 'P' wave)	up to 0.4 mV
Duration (width or duration of 'p' wave)	up to 0.04 s or 40 millisecond
'Q' Wave	
Amplitude (depth of the 'Q' wave)	< 0.5 mV
'R' Wave	
Amplitude (height of the 'R' wave)	up to 2.5 mV (small breeds)
	up to 3.0 mV (large or giant breeds))
'S' Wave	
Amplitude (depth of the 'S' wave)	<0.35 mV
'QRS' complex	
Duration (width of the 'QRS')	up to 0.05 second or 50 millisecond (small breeds)
	up to 0.06 second or 50 millisecond (giant breeds)
'P-R' Interval	
Duration	up to 0.13 second or 130 millisecond
'S-T' Segment	
Base line	No elevation or depression
Elevation	Not more than 0.15 mV
Depression	Not more than 0.20 mV
'T' wave	
Polarity	Positive, negative, biphasic
Amplitude	Less than 1/4th of the 'R' wave
Duration	0.02 to 0.08 second or 20 to 80 millisecond
'Q-T' Interval	
Duration	0.10 to 0.25 seconds (100- 250 millisecond)
	'Q-T' interval is influenced by heart rate.
'R-R' Interval	It depends on heart rate and rhythm.
Mean Electrical Axis on Frontal Plane (MEA)	+40^{0} to +100^{0}

Important Measurements in Chest Leads

CV_5RL	'T' wave positive
	'R' wave up to 3.0 mV
CV_6LL	'S' up to 0.8 mV
	'R' wave up to 2.5 mV
CV_6LU	'S' wave up to 0.7 mV
	'R' wave up to 3.0 mV
V_{10}	'QRS' negative
	T wave –ve in healthy dogs except in healthy Chihuahua (in them it is +ve).

Table 1: Values of Electrocardiographic indices in Healthy Pugs (Observed at our hospitals)

Parameter	MEAN±S.E	RANGE
P wave duration (sec)	0.03±0.003	0.02-0.04
P wave-amplitude (mV)	0.175±0.02	0.1-0.3
PR interval (sec)	0.09±0.008	0.05-0.12
R wave duration (sec)	0.03±0.004	0.02-0.04
R wave amplitude (mV)	1.34±0.132	0.9-2.2
QT Segment (sec)	0.17±0.005	0.15-0.2
ST Segment (sec)	0.11±0.007	0.1-0.15
T wave duration (sec)	0.03±0.006	0.02-0.06
T wave amplitude (mV)	0.16±0.027	0.1-0.3
MEA (^{0})		+50 -+90 ^{0}

Influence of Exercise on the Electrocardiogram

Physical activity and exercise influences the activity of the heart. The extent of change in the activity of heart depends on the nature and duration of physical activities or exercise. First effect of exercise is change in heart rate and related electrocardiographic indices followed by precipitation of arrhythmias and /or conduction disturbances if any. Therefore post exercise electrocardiography is recommended for detecting subtle arrhythmias which remain undetected in resting electrocardiography.

Electrocardiographic Indices in Healthy Cats

Heart Rate

It varies in different age groups as well as in different breeds. Nevertheless following values are considered normal.

Heart rate 140-220 bpm

Heart Rhythm

Sinus Rhythm

Wandering Pace maker

Measurements of Waves, segments and Intervals (Lead II)

'P 'Wave	
Amplitude (height of the 'P' wave)	up to 0.2 mV
Duration (width or duration of 'P' wave)	up to 0.03 s or 30 millisecond
'Q' Wave	
Generally Q wave is not seen in healthy cats	
'R' Wave	
Amplitude (height of the 'R' wave)	up to 0.9 mV
'S' Wave	
Generally S wave is not seen in healthy cats.	
'QRS' complex	
Duration (width of the 'QRS')	up to 0.04 second or 40 millisecond
'P-R' Interval	
Duration	up to 0.09 second or 90 millisecond
'S-T' Segment	
Base line	No elevation or depression
'T' wave	
Polarity	Positive, negative, biphasic. It is mostly +ve
Amplitude	up to 0.3 mV
Duration variable and may be	up to 0.04 s
'Q-T' Interval	
Duration	up to 0.18 seconds (180 millisecond)
	'Q-T' interval is influenced by heart rate.
Mean Electrical Axis on Frontal Plane (MEA)	Varies from 0 to + 160 ^{0}

Chest Leads

Information is not well documented.

Table 2: Values of Electrocardiographic indices in Healthy Cats (Observed at our hospitals).

Parameter	Mean ±S.E	Range
P wave duration (sec)	0.02±0.002	0.02-0.03
P wave-amplitude (mV)	0.1±0.023	0.05-0.25
PR segment (sec)	0.04±0.002	0.03-0.05
PR interval (sec)	0.06±0.004	0.06-0.09
R wave duration (sec)	0.03±0.003	0.02-0.04
R wave amplitude (mV)	0.40±0.07	0.1-0.7
QT Interval (sec)	0.11±0.007	0.08-0.14
ST Segment (sec)	0.04±0.004	0.03-0.06
T wave duration (sec)	0.035±0.005	0.02-0.05
T wave amplitude (mV)	0.08±0.008	0.05-0.1
MEA (^{0})		+ 40 to +100 ^{0}

Further Reading

Varshney, J.P. (2020). Electrocardiography in Veterinary Medicine. Springer Nature, Singapore, Pte, Ltd.

7

Electrocardiographic Peculiarities in Different Species of Animals

Electrocardiogram is a visual record of electrical activities going on in the heart during depolarization and repolarization (cardiac cycle). It is one of the simplest and fasted non-invasive diagnostic test available to evaluate cardiac function. Though the heart of large mammals have many similarities, difference in shape, size, positioning in thoracic cavity and innervation of Purkinje fibers exists in different species of the animals making the electrocardiogram peculiar for that species of animal. Peculiar characteristics that distinguish the electrocardiograms of different species of animals are given in this chapter.

Dogs

- Electrocardiogram is recorded in hex-axial lead system (bipolar and unipolar limb leads)
- Analysis of waves and intervals is done in Lead II.
- Electrocardiogram of dogs (Fig.93) shows predominantly positive 'QRS' in lead II.
- Electrocardiogram is a very good diagnostic tool for detecting arrhythmias and conduction disturbances.
- Heart chamber enlargement can also be detected when amplitude of 'Q', 'R' and/or 'S' waves increased beyond the prescribed height.
- Mean electrical axis of the normal heart on frontal plane varies from +40 to +100 ^{0} in healthy dogs.

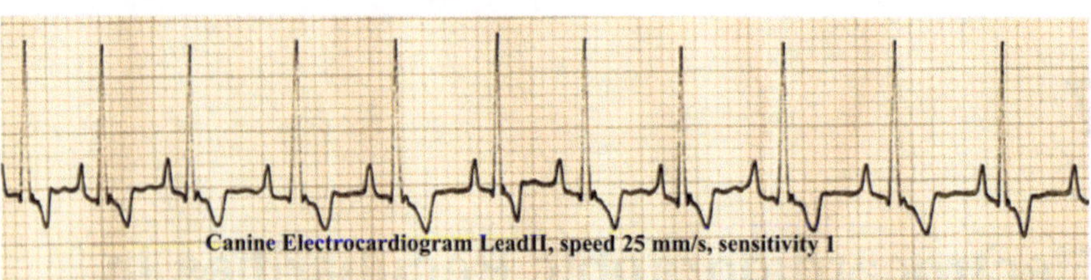

Fig. 93: Canine Electrocardiogram recorded in Lead II, Paper speed 25 mm/s and Sensitivity 1.

Cats

- Electrocardiography in cats is limited to the diagnosis of arrhythmias and conduction abnormalities.
- Cats with auscultative arrhythmias are excellent candidate for electrocardiography.
- Holter electrocardiography is not very much successful in cats.
- Electrocardiography is not a good tool to screen cats for subtle cardiac diseases.
- Electrocardiogram in cats is insensitive to detect chamber enlargement due to concentric hypertrophy.
- Deviations in MEA can be detected.
- Electrocardiography can be used to detect left atrial enlargement. It has good specificity but poor sensitivity.
- Electrocardiogram in cats (Fig.94) is recorded in hex-axial lead system (bipolar and unipolar limb leads) as in case of dogs.
- Analysis of waves and intervals is done in Lead II.
- Electrocardiographic complexes in cats (Fig.94) are small in comparison of dogs.
- Heart rate in cats is high as compared to dogs.
- Electrocardiographic intervals (P-R interval, R-R interval , Q-T interval) in cats are short as compared to dogs
- Many healthy cats may show low voltage QRS.
- Mean electrical axis of the normal healthy cat lies between + 0^0 to + 160^0.

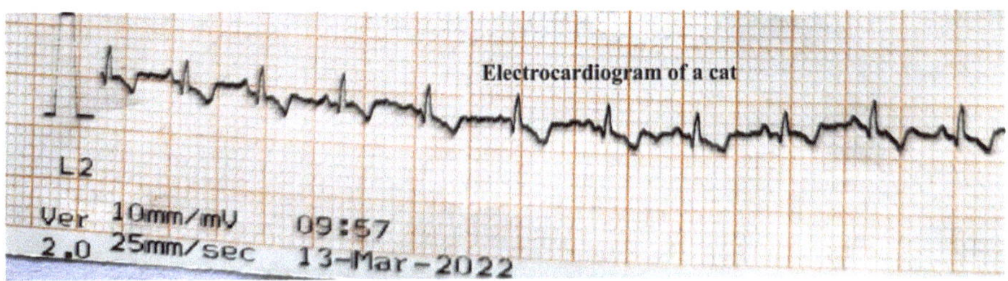

Fig. 94: Feline Electrocardiogram recorded in Lead II, Paper speed 25 mm/s and Sensitivity 1.

Exotic Pets

- Because of delicate skin of the exotic pets, alligator clips are not attached directly on the skin. Small gauge hypodermic needles are pierced subcutaneously and alligator clips are attached to the needles or stainless steel sutures are applied and clips are attached to them.
- In small mammals, adhesive patches or button electrodes can be applied on foot pads.
- Electrocardiogram is recorded in hex-axial lead system (bipolar and unipolar limb leads)
- Analysis of waves and intervals is done in Lead II.
- Normal electrocardiogram in healthy birds (Fig.95) is negative because of predominant 'S' wave. It may give illusion of ventricular tachycardia because of higher heart rate.
- Lead I in birds is nearly isoelectric.
- In birds' electrocardiogram, depression of the initial part of the PR segment is related to large atrial repolarization.
- In racing pigeons and parrots, S-T segment is very short, slurring or absent.
- Mean electrical axis in birds is generally negative because of inverted 'QRS' in lead II.

  Deviation of MEA in birds is confusing because of negative heart axis in healthy birds.

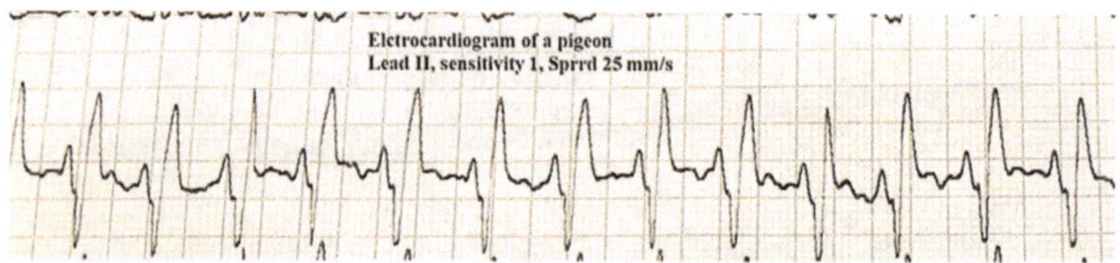

Fig. 95: Pigeon Electrocardiogram recorded in Lead II, Paper speed 25 mm/s and Sensitivity 1.

Rabbits

- Electrocardiogram of rabbits (Fig.96) is recorded in hex-axial lead system (bipolar and unipolar limb leads) as in case of dogs and cats.
- Analysis of waves and intervals is done in Lead II.
- Electrocardiogram of rabbits shows variability of QRS complexes (Fig.96).
- Great variability in the vector of frontal plane.
- Many times 'P' and 'T' waves are isoelectric.

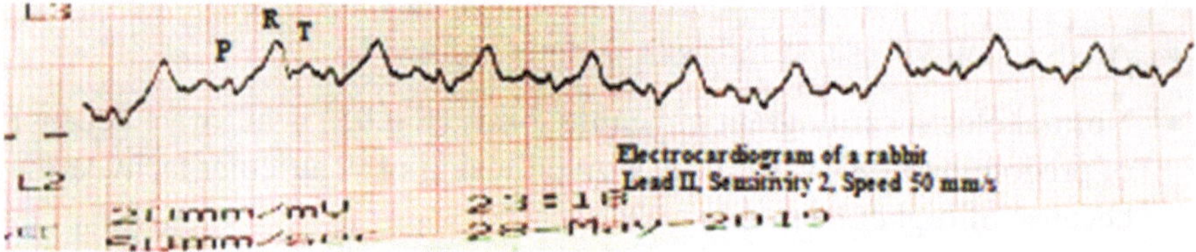

Fig. 96: Rabbit Electrocardiogram recorded in Lead II, Paper speed 50 mm/s and Sensitivity 2

Tortoises/Turtles

- Electrocardiogram of turtles/tortoises is recorded in hex-axial lead system (bipolar and unipolar limb leads)
- Analysis of waves and intervals is done in lead II.
- Heart rate in turtles/tortoises is low.
- Electrocardiogram of chelonians shows small waves (Fig.97) i.e. low voltage.
- 'Q' and 'S' waves generally absent (Fig. 97).
- 'P' and 'T' waves are very small (sometimes imperceptible)

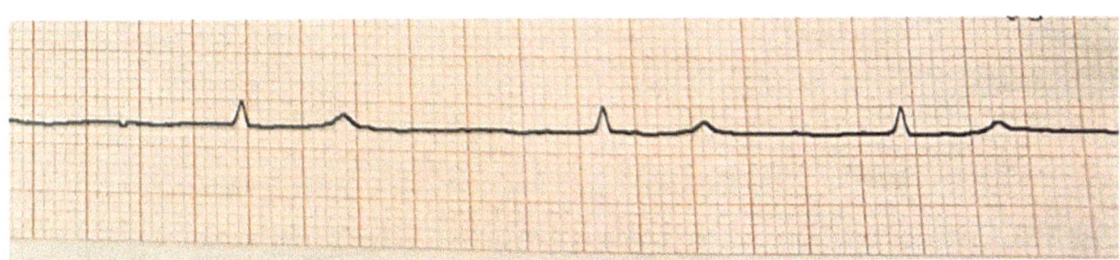

Fig. 97: Turtle Electrocardiogram recorded in Lead II, Paper speed 25 mm/s and Sensitivity 1. Note 'P' wave is imperceptible. There is no q or s waves. 'R' wave is of low voltage.

Ruminants (Cattle, Buffaloes, Sheep , Goat and Mithun)

- Perkinjee fibers are deeply penetrating.
- Explosive depolarization from ventricular endocardium to pericardium in many directions at a time. Therefore, setting criteria for chamber enlargement in ruminants is difficult.
- Base –apex lead system is more appropriate for recording electrocardiogram of ruminants.
- Electrocardiograms of buffalo calf, cow calf and goat are given in Fig.98, 99 and 100 respectively.
- Analysis of waves and intervals in ruminants' electrocardiogram is done in Lead I.
- Heart rate is lower than dogs and cats
- 'QRS' (as 'rS' or 'QS' type) is predominantly negative.
- 'R' wave is generally absent. If present it is of very low amplitude (r)

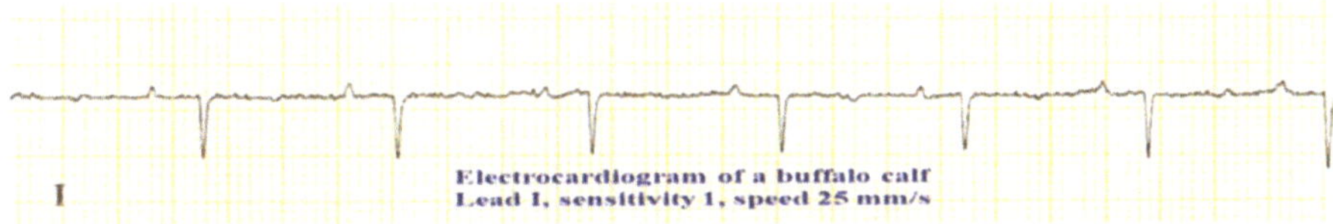

Fig. 98: Buffalo calf Electrocardiogram recorded in Lead I (Base-apex lead system), Paper speed 25 mm/s and Sensitivity 1.

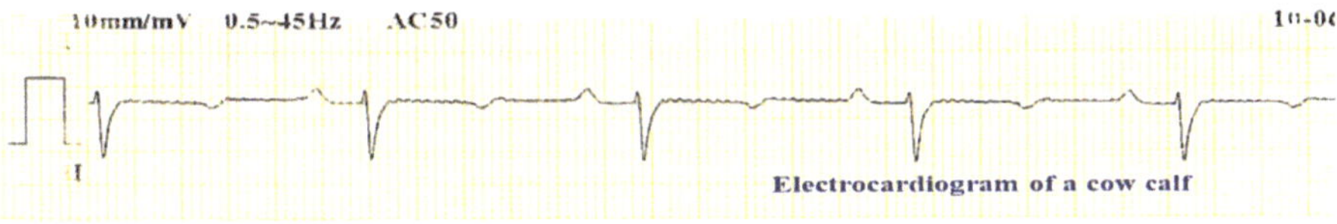

Fig. 99: Cow calf Electrocardiogram recorded in Lead I (Base-apex lead system), Paper speed 25 mm/s and Sensitivity 1.

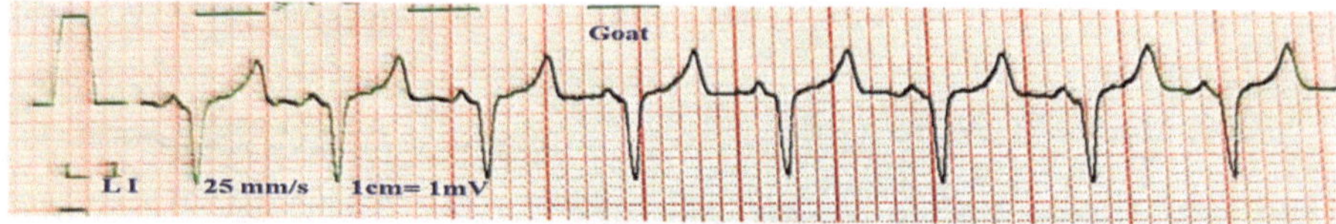

Fig. 100: Goat Electrocardiogram recorded in Lead I (Base-apex lead system), Paper speed 25 mm/s and Sensitivity 1.

Equines (Horses and Donkeys)

- Base –apex lead system is more appropriate for recording electrocardiogram in equines as in case of ruminants.
- Electrocardiogram of a horse is illustrated in Fig.101.
- Analysis of waves and intervals is done in Lead I.
- ECG of equines is similar to ruminants.
- ECG of equines is predominantly negative.
- ‘P’ wave is monophasic or biphasic.
- Duration of ‘P’ wave in equines is more as compared to canines.
- ‘R’ wave in equines is very small (r)
- ‘T’ wave in equines may be monophasic or biphasic.
- Artifacts and muscle tremors are common in electrocardiogram of equines.

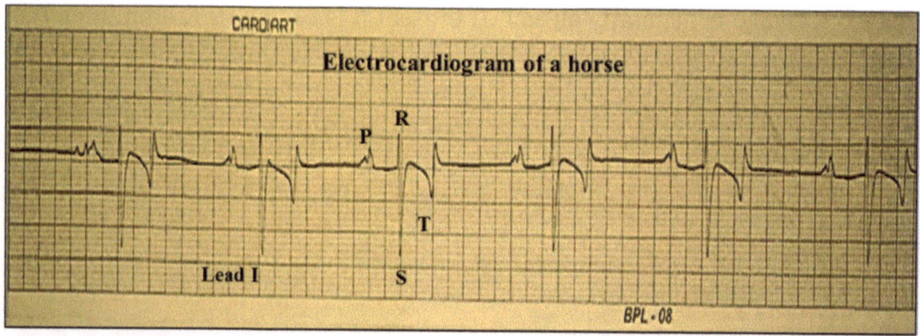

Fig. 101: Horse Electrocardiogram recorded in Lead I (Base-apex lead system), Paper speed 25 mm/s and Sensitivity 1.The electrocardiogram is showing M shaped ‘P’ wave, small “R’ wave , deep ‘S’ wave and biphasic ‘T’ wave.

Further Readings

Varshney, J.P. (2020). Electrocardiography in Veterinary Medicine. Springer Nature, Singapore, Pte, Ltd.

8

Abnormalities of Waves, Intervals and Segments

Departure of waves (P,Q,R,S, T), segments (P-R, S-T and T-P) and /or intervals (P-R, Q-T, R-R) from their normal values (configuration, morphology, amplitude and duration of wave; prolonging /shortening of intervals : elevation /depression of segments from their isoelectric line) is said to be abnormal feature of the electrocardiogram. These abnormalities are suggestive of specific cardiac abnormalities such as a defect in the current generation, its conduction or both; or change in the size of the chambers (atria / ventricles/both.).

Abnormalities of Waves

'P' Wave

- Abnormalities of 'P' wave include change in configuration, amplitude (height), duration (width), polarity (positive /negative in lead II), and presence/ absence of the wave.
- Change in the configuration and amplitude of the 'P' wave from wave to wave (Fig.102) indicates wandering pacemaker in the SA node.

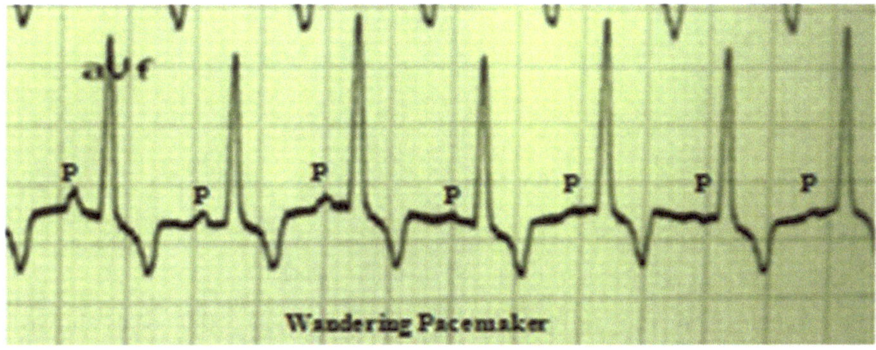

Fig. 102: Electrocardiogram (Lead II, speed 25 mm/s, sensitivity 1) of a dog is showing varying amplitude of 'P' wave suggesting wandering pacemaker.

- Increased amplitude or height (>0.4 mV) of 'P' waves (Fig.103) is suggestive of right atrium enlargement. It is also termed as P-pulmonale.

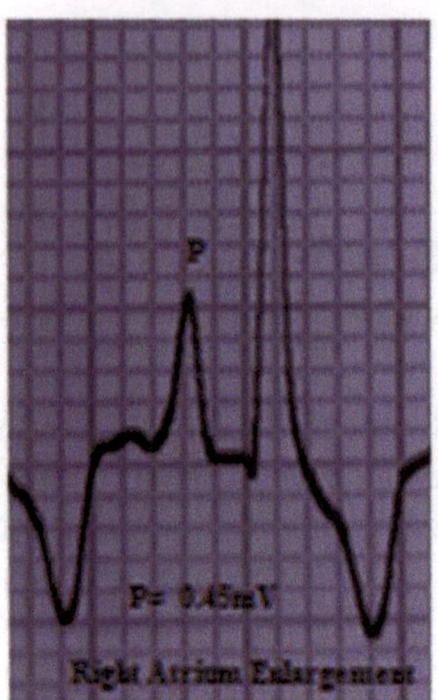

Fig. 103: Electrocardiogram (Lead II, sensitivity 1, speed 25 mm/s) of a dog is showing 'P' wave of increased amplitude (>0.4 mV) suggesting right atrial enlargement.

- Broad 'P' or increased duration (>0.04 s) of 'P' wave (Fig.104) is suggestive of left atrial enlargement. It is also termed as P-mitrale.

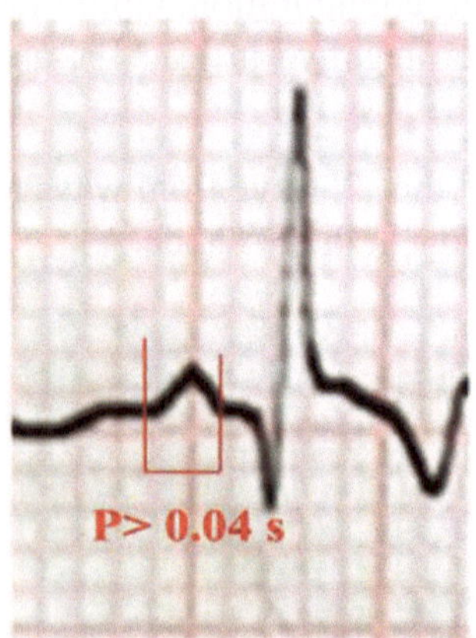

Fig. 104: Electrocardiogram (Lead II, sensitivity 1, speed 25 mm/s) of a dog is showing wide 'P' wave of 0.07 s (> 0.04 s) suggestive of left atrial enlargement.

- When 'P' wave is tall (>0.4 mV) as well as wide (>0.04 s) as shown in Fig. 105, it is suggestive of biatrial enlargement.

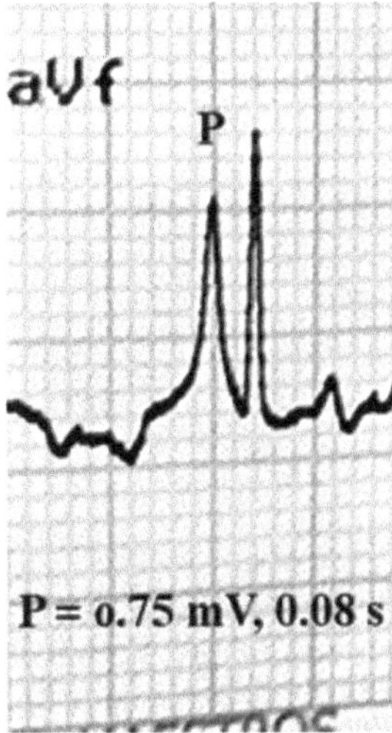

Fig. 105: Electrocardiogram (Lead II, sensitivity 1, speed 25 mm/s) of a dog is showing tall (0.75 mV) and broad (0.08 s) 'P' wave suggestive of biatrial enlargement.

- 'P' wave is usually positive in lead II in healthy dogs and cats. When 'P' wave is negative (Fig.106) in lead II, it is suggestive of supraventricular ectopic focus (AV junctional) and a single focus is termed as AV-junctional premature complex (Fig.106).

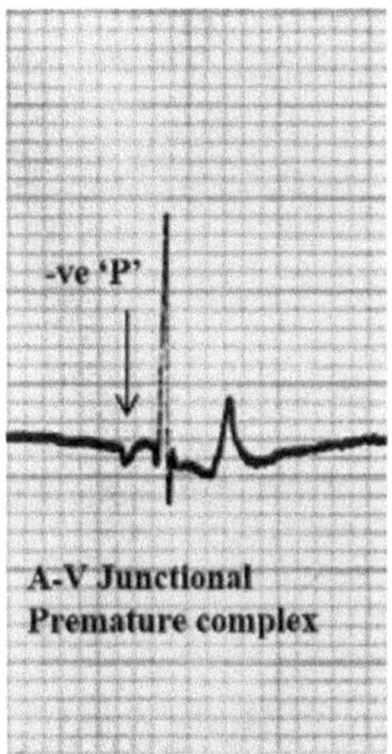

Fig. 106: Electrocardiogram (Lead II, sensitivity 1, speed 25 mm/s) of a dog is showing negative 'P' wave suggestive of supraventricular ectopic focus (AV junctional) aptly known as A-V junctional premature complex.

- Absence of 'P' wave (Fig.107) in an electrocardiogram is termed as atrial standstill or silent atrium.

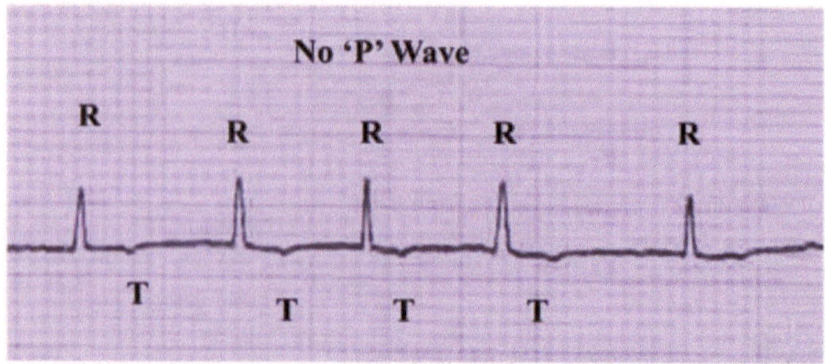

Fig. 107: Electrocardiogram (lead II, sensitivity 1, speed 25 mm/s) of a dog is showing an absence of 'P' wave in the electrocardiogram suggesting atrial standstill.

- Sometimes a slight depression of the base line following 'P' wave (Fig.108) is seen. It is termed as 'Ta' wave. It can be seen in right atrial enlargement. 'Ta 'wave denotes atrial repolarization.

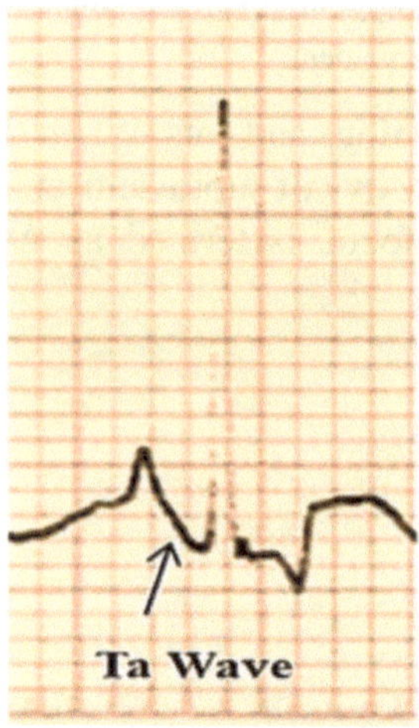

Fig. 108: Electrocardiogram (Lead II, sensitivity 1, speed 25 mm/s) of a dog is showing 'Ta' Wave. It is slight depression of the base line following the 'P' wave. It denotes atrial repolarization and can be seen in cases of right atrial enlargement.

'Q' Wave

- A small 'Q' wave in the electrocardiograms is normal. But a deep 'Q' wave (in lead I,II,III and aVF; > 0.5 mV in lead II and aVF) is abnormal and is suggestive of right ventricular enlargement (RVE). A deep Q wave in lead II is shown in Fig. 109.

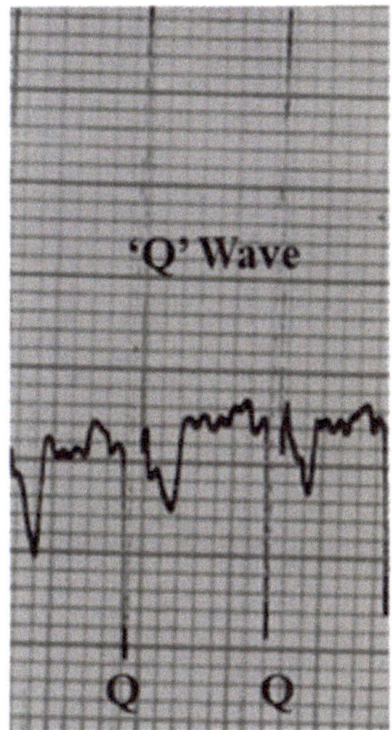

Fig. 109: Electrocardiogram (Lead II, sensitivity 1, speed 25 mm/s) of a dog is showing deep 'Q' wave (1.1 mV) in lead II . It is one of the criteria of right ventricular enlargement.

'R' Wave

- 'R' wave in the electrocardiogram represents depolarization of the left ventricle. It is the largest wave in normal electrocardiograms. When its amplitude (height) exceeds 2.5 mV in small breeds and 3.0 mV in large breeds of dogs, it is said to be Tall 'R' wave (Fig. 110). A tall 'R' wave is indicative of left ventricular enlargement (LVE).

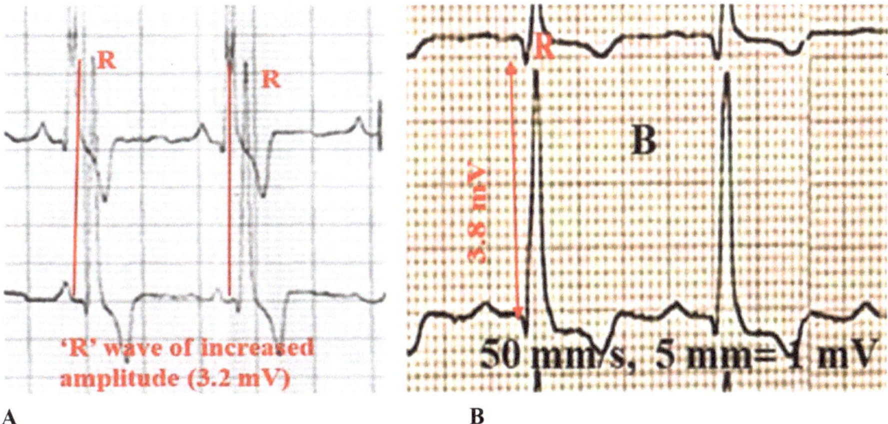

Fig. 110: Electrocardiograms (A - lead II, sensitivity 1, speed 25 mm/s ; B – lead II, sensitivity 0.5 , speed 50 mm/s) of dogs are showing 'R' waves of increased amplitude (A 3.2 mV ; B 3.8 mV) suggestive of left ventricular enlargement.

- Small amplitude 'R' wave (<0.5 mV in lead II, III and aVF) is called as low voltage 'QRS' (Fig.111) and is seen in cases of pericardial effusion, pleural effusion, pneumothorax, hypothyroidism, poor skin –lead contact, obesity or cardiomyopathy.

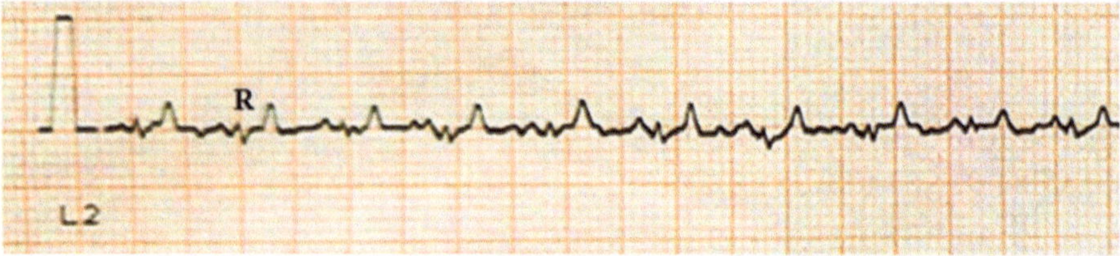

A

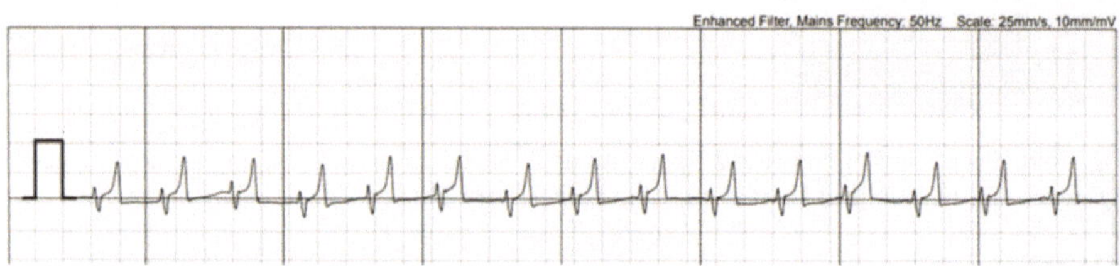

B

Fig. 111: Electrocardiograms (Lead II, sensitivity 1, speed 25 mm/s) of dogs are showing low voltage complexes. The voltage of 'R' wave is 0.1 mV in both electrocardiograms.

- Varying amplitude of 'R' wave is termed as 'R' alternans (Fig.112). It is seen in cases of pericardial effusion, alternating bundle branch block or supraventricular tachycardia.

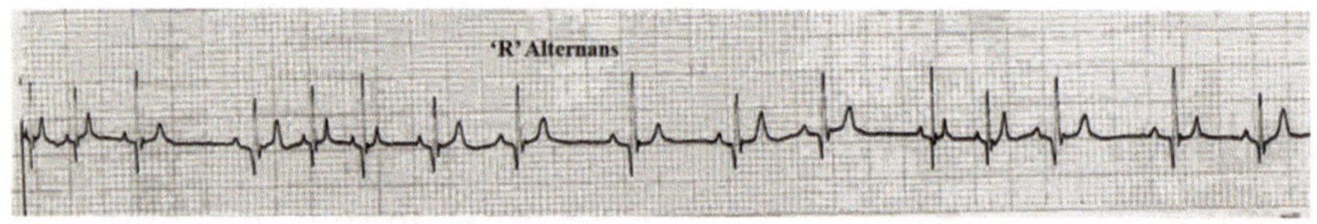

Fig. 112: Electrocardiogram (Lead II, sensitivity 1, sped 25 mm/s) of a dog is showing varying amplitude of 'R' waves indicative of 'R' alternans.

'QRS' Complex

- 'QRS' complex of > 0.05 s in small breeds or >0.06 s in large breeds of dog is termed as broad or wide 'QRS' (Fig.113) . It is seen in cases of left ventricular enlargement (LVE) or left bundle branch block (LBBB).

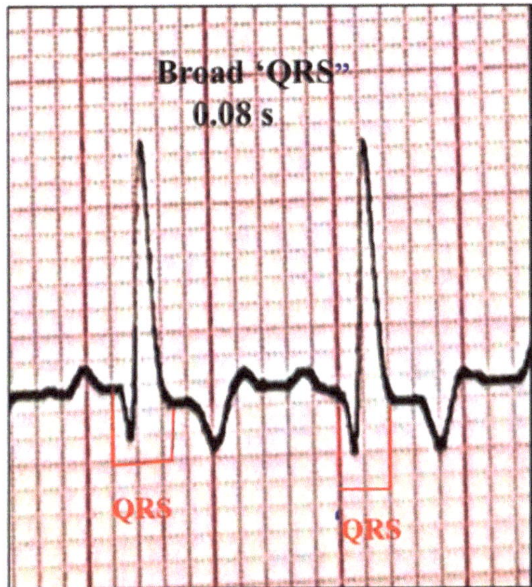

Fig. 113: Electrocardiogram (Lead II, sensitivity 1, speed 25 mm/s) of a dog is showing broad 'QRS' of 0.08 s.

- Notched 'QRS' with normal width or duration (Fig.114) is seen in healthy dogs or dogs with minor atrio-ventricular defect.

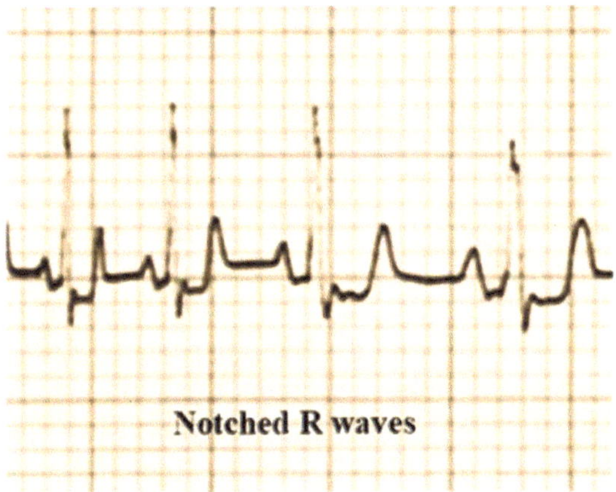

Fig. 114: Electrocardiogram (Lead II, sensitivity 1, speed 25 mm/s) of a dog is showing notched 'QRS'.

'S' Wave

- A small 'S' wave in an electrocardiogram is normal. However, presence of 'S' wave in lead I,II,III and aVF; deep 'S' wave in lead I (> 0.05 mV), lead II (>0.35 mV Fig.115), lead CV_6LL (0.8 mV), lead CV_6LU (>0.7 mV); and ratio of R:S (<0.87) have been considered indicative of right ventricle enlargement (RVE) .

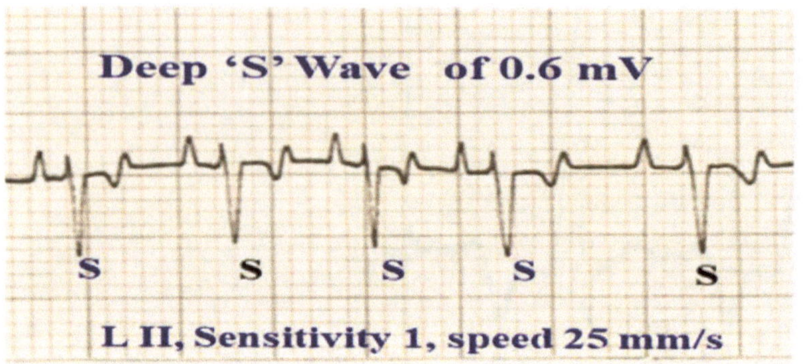

A

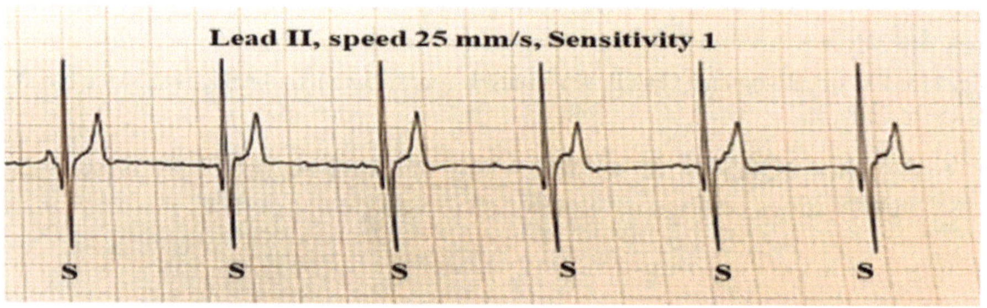

B

Fig. 115: Electrocardiograms (Lead II, sensitivity 1, speed 25 mm/s) of dogs are showing deep 'S' wave (A 0.6 mV , B 1.1 mV) suggestive of right ventricular enlargement.

'J' Wave

- A small positive deflection at 'R'- 'ST' junction ('J' point) is known as 'J' wave or Osborn wave (Fig.116). 'J' point is the point where 'QRS' complex joins the 'S-T' segment. 'J' point represents the approximate end of depolarization and the beginning of repolarization. This wave can partially or completely be buried in the 'QRS' complex. In humans the presence of 'J' wave can represent a "current of injury" and seem to be indicative of severe ischemia (Yan and Antzelevitch, 1996). It is seen in many healthy humans and dogs as well as in hypothermic dogs (Varshney, 2016). It has also been seen in humans with hypercalcemia, brain injury, subarachnoid hemorrhage, sepsis, Chagas disease, vasospastic angina, Brugada syndrome, acute myocardial ischemia, Prinzmetal angina, left ventricular hypertrophy or ventricular fibrillation.

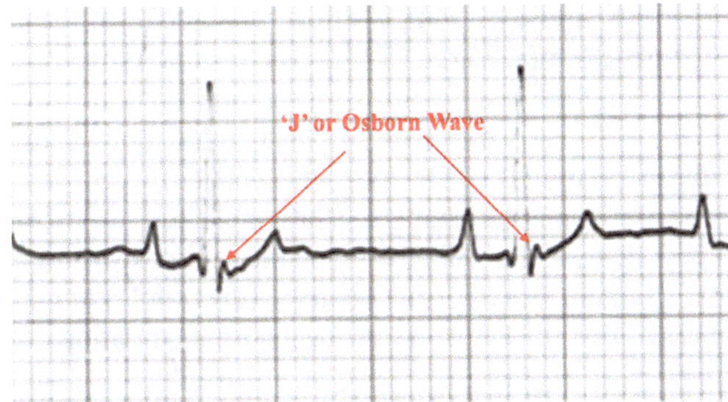

Fig. 116: Electrocardiogram (lead II, speed 25 mm/s, sensitivity 1) of a dog is showing 'J' or 'Osborn' wave (marked with red arrows). It is a small positive deflection at 'J' point. It is commonly related with hypothermia and is also seen in healthy subjects.

'T' wave

- T' wave represents repolarization of the heart. Changes in 'T' wave morphology are mostly nonspecific in dogs and cats. Nevertheless, sudden change in polarity, increased height in relation to 'R' wave, small biphasic morphology, tented 'T' and 'T' alternans have some significance.
- If 'T' wave changes its polarity suddenly i.e. from positive to negative or negative to positive (Fig.117), it is pathological. It has been associated with hypoxia, abnormal conduction, ventricular enlargement or metabolic disorders.

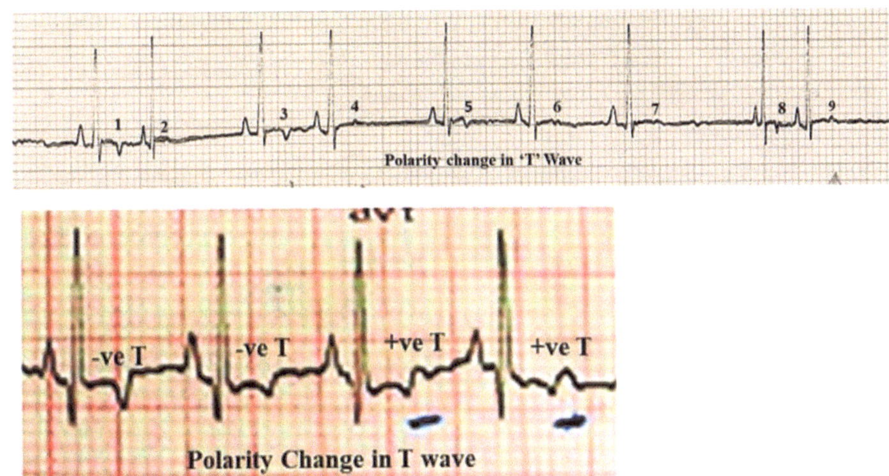

Fig. 117: Electrocardiograms (Lead II, sensitivity 1, speed 25 mm/s) of dogs are showing change in the polarity of 'T' wave.

- Increased amplitude of 'T' wave > 25% of 'R' wave (Fig.118 A) is seen in cases of hyperkalemia. Large 'T' wave (Fig.118 B) has also been associated with myocardial hypoxia, anesthetic complications, hyperventilation in heat stroke, heart disease with bradycardia, myocardial infarction (large T with polarity change), ventricular enlargement, intraventricular conduction abnormalities, electrolyte imbalances (hyperkalemia), metabolic (anemia, shock, uremia, ketoacidosis, hypoglycemia, fever), drug toxicity (digitalis, quinidine, procainamide) or respiratory diseases. It may be a normal variation also.

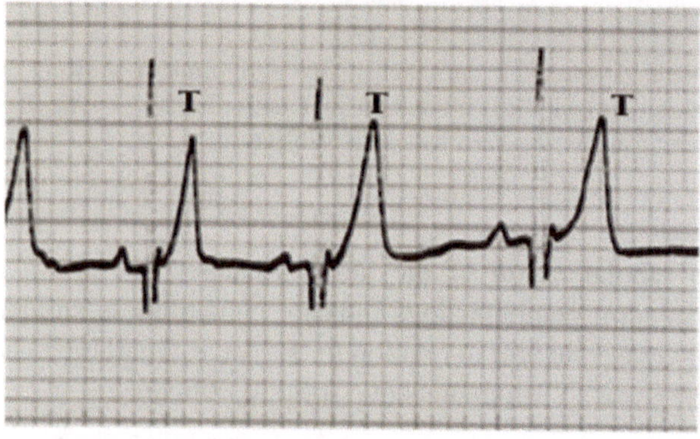

A

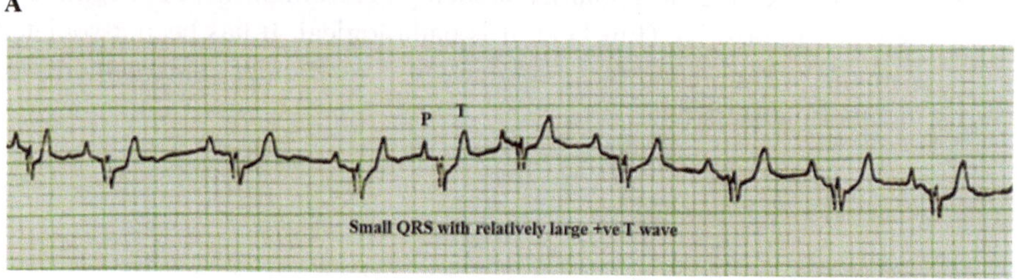

B

Fig. 118: Electrocardiograms (Lead II, sensitivity 1, speed 25 mm/s) of dogs are showing large + ve 'T' waves of 0.7 mV in relation to 'R' wave of 1.0 mV (A) ; and 'T' wave of 0.25 mV in relation of very small QRS (B) .The electrocardiogram at B is suggestive of pericardial effusion because of very small QRS and relatively large T wave.

- Tented 'T' is also associated with hyperkalemia.
- A small biphasic 'T' (Fig.119) has been associated with hypokalemia.

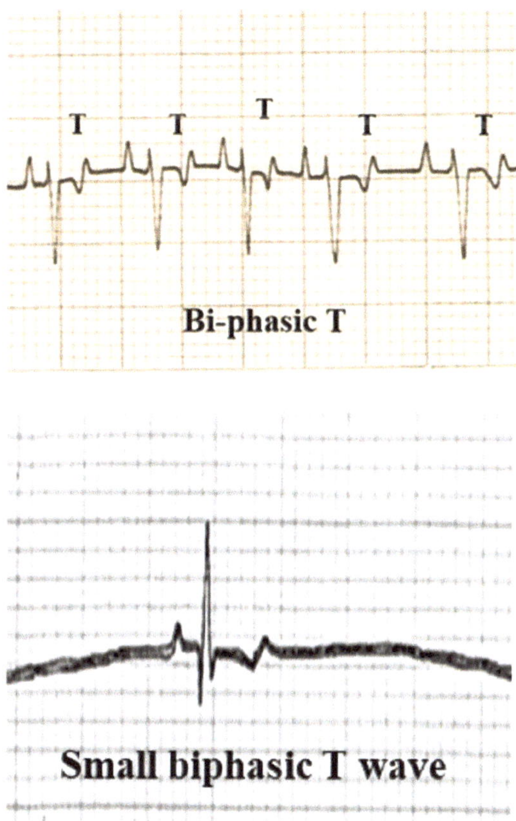

Fig. 119: Electrocardiograms (Lead II, sensitivity 1, speed 25 mm/s) of dogs are showing biphasic 'T' Wave

- 'T' wave in lead V_{10} is usually negative in dogs of all breeds except Chihuahua. Therefore a positive T wave in lead V_{10} (Fig.120 A and B) is abnormal in dogs of all breeds except Chihuahua.

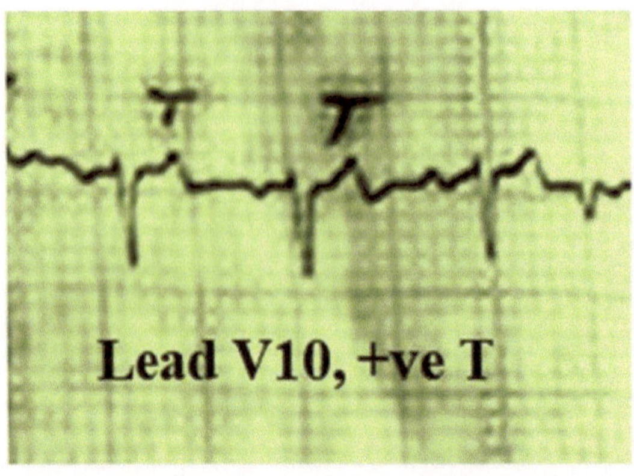

A

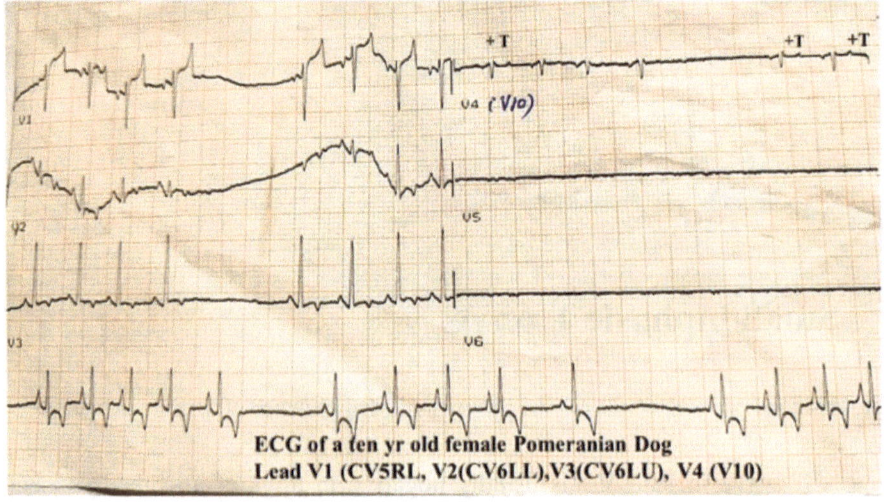

B

Fig.120: A. Electrocardiogram of an adult male German Shepherd dog (Lead V_{10}, sensitivity 1, speed 25 mm/s) is showing a positive T wave in lead V_{10}. B. Electrocardiogram of an eight year old Pomeranian dog (in all four chest leads, sensitivity 1, speed 25 mm/s) is showing a positive T wave in lead V_{10}. T wave is negative in lead II, CV_6LL and CV_6LU and is positive in CV_5RL and V_{10}.

Electrical Alternans

- Usually alteration in configuration and amplitude of 'QRS' complex (Fig.121) in any or all leads with no additional changes in the conduction pathway of the heart on the electrocardiogram is termed as electrical alternans.

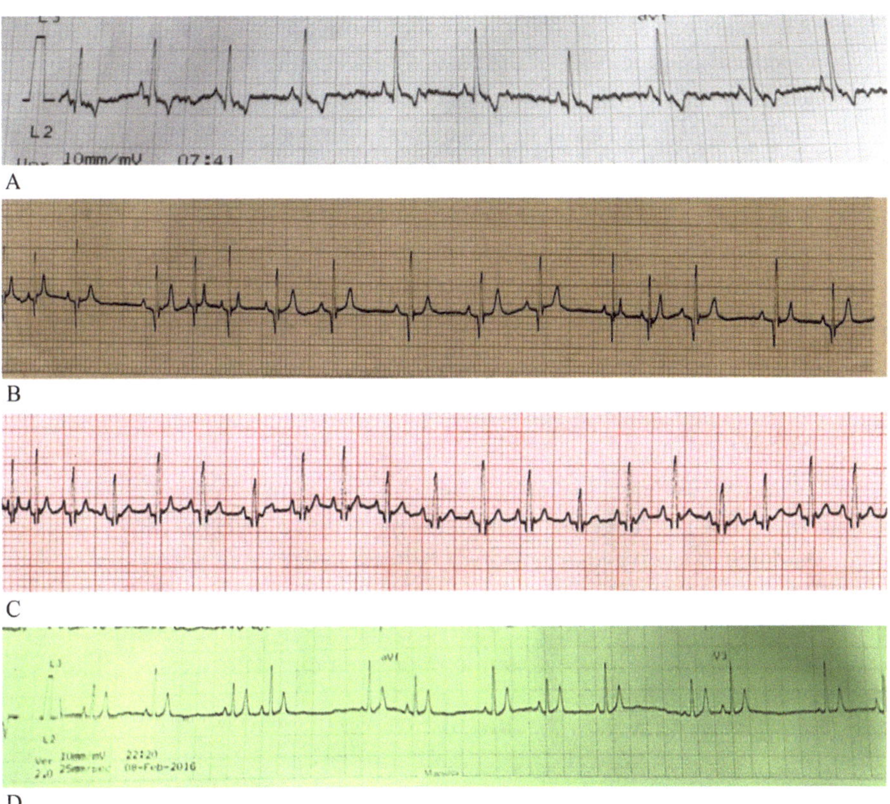

Fig. 121: Electrocardiograms (Lead II, sensitivity 1, speed 25 mm/s) of dogs are showing alteration in the amplitude of many 'R' waves suggestive of R alternans.

- The alteration in configuration may be on every other complex, every 3rd complex, every 4th complex etc. but each complex originates from same focus. Alteration in the configuration of every other complex is quite common.
- Variations in the amplitude of 'QRS' complex are because of swinging motion of the heart with each beat in the fluid-filled pericardial sac causing electric signals to travel varying distances through fluid resulting in variation in the amplitude of the waves.
- Electrical alternans is generally associated with severe pericardial effusion or cardiac tamponade. It can also be associated with ventricular tachycardia, Wolf-Parkinson-white syndrome, accelerated idioventricular rhythm, supraventricular tachycardia, AV nodal reentrant tachycardia or bundle branch block.

- Alternans can also be seen in pneumothorax or emphysema wherein the electrical conductivity of the tissues between the heart and the electrodes are affected causing variations in the QRS amplitudes. Recently atypical electrical alternans due to left pleural effusion (Shekar *et al.,* 2022) or pregnancy (Alp *et al*., 2018) have been reported in humans.
- Electrical alternans with sinus tachycardia (Fig.121 C) is a specific sign for large pericardial effusion . The Fig.121 C is showing sinus tachycardia (heart rate 220 bpm, almost uniform R-R interval) along with electrical alternans suggestive of large pericardial effusion.
- The diagnostic feature of electrical alternans, on the electrocardiogram of dogs, is the alterations in the amplitude of 'QRS' complex from beat to beat.
- 'T' wave alternans (Fig.122) can also be seen on many electrocardiograms. Wave to wave variation in amplitude of 'T' wave is termed as 'T' alternans. Isolated 'T' wave alternans may be seen in severe hypocalcaemia. Such changes have been associated with pericardial effusion, alternating bundle branch block, supraventricular tachycardia, occlusion of a coronary artery, hypocalcaemia, increased circulatory catecholamine or long Q-T syndrome.

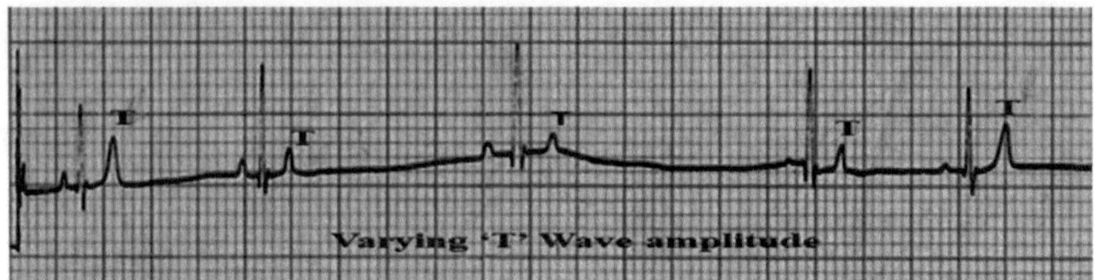

Fig. 122: Electrocardiogram (Lead II, sensitivity 1, speed 25 mm/s) of a dog is showing alteration in the amplitude of 'T' waves suggestive of T alternans.

Abnormalities of Intervals

P-R interval

- P-R interval includes the time from the depolarization of the SA node to the onset of ventricular depolarization. It is inversely correlated to the heart rate. If P-R interval is > 0.12-0.13 second (Fig.123), it is considered as prolonged. Prolonged P-R interval indicates 1st degree heart block.

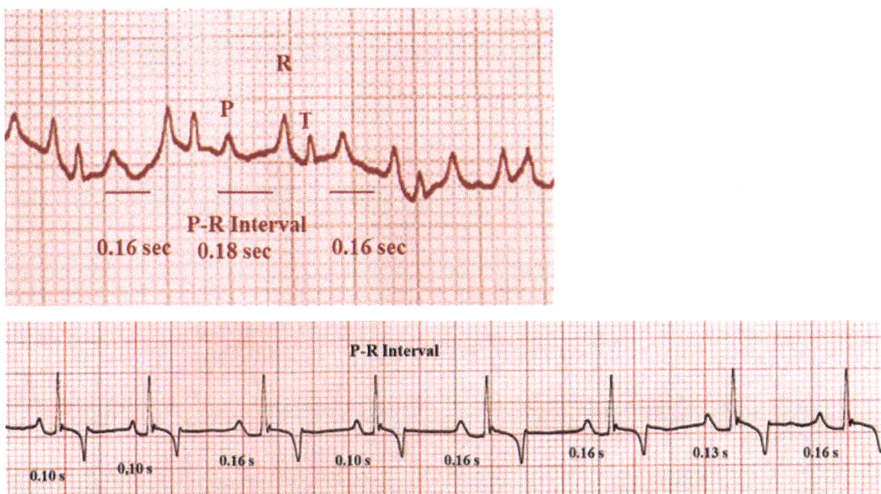

Fig. 123: Electrocardiograms (Lead II, sensitivity 1, speed 25 mm/s) of dogs are showing variable and prolonged 'P-R' interval (> 0.12- 0.13 s) suggesting 1st degree heart block (AV block).

Q-T interval

- 'Q-T' interval represents the total time of ventricular depolarization and repolarization on an electrocardiogram. It is influenced by fluctuations in the heart rate. 'Q-T' interval abnormalities include its prolongation (>0.25 second) or shortening (<0.15 second).
- 'Q-T' interval of >0.25 second (Fig.124) is termed as 'Prolonged Q-T' interval. It has been observed in cases of hypocalcaemia, hypothermia, hypokalemia, CNS disorders, ventricular hypertrophy, conduction disorders, strenuous exercise, quinidine toxicity, ethylene glycol poisoning, or secondary to prolonged QRS.

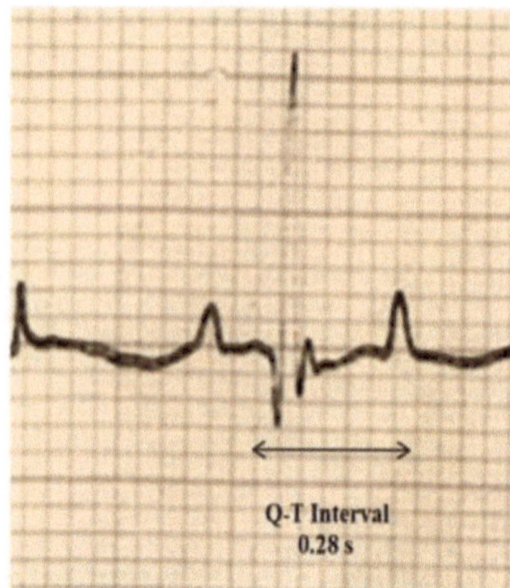

Fig.124: Electrocardiogram (Lead II, sensitivity 1, speed 25 mm/s) of a dog is showing prolonged 'Q-T' interval of 0.28 s (>0.25 s) .

- Abnormally prolonged 'Q-T' interval predisposes to potentially fatal ventricular arrhythmias. Some drugs and conditions that alter ion channel function can lead to acquired prolongation of 'Q-T' interval.
- 'Q-T' interval of < 0.15 second (Fig. 125) is termed as 'Shortened Q-T' interval. It may be seen in cases of hypercalcemia, hyperkalemia or digitalis toxicity.

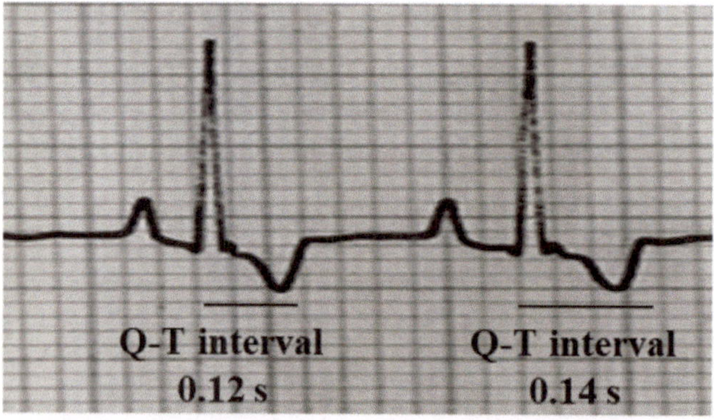

Fig. 125: Electrocardiogram (Lead II, sensitivity 1, speed 25 mm/s) of a dog is showing shortened 'Q-T' intervals of 0.12 – 0.14 s < 0.15 s) .

'R-R' Interval

- 'R-R' interval is the time period elapsed between two successive 'R' waves of the 'QRS' complex on an electrocardiogram.

- If the R-R interval is uniform, the rhythm is said to be sinus.
- 'R-R' interval may be regular, irregular or regularly irregular.
- Variable 'R-R' interval (Fig.126) is suggestive of arrhythmia.

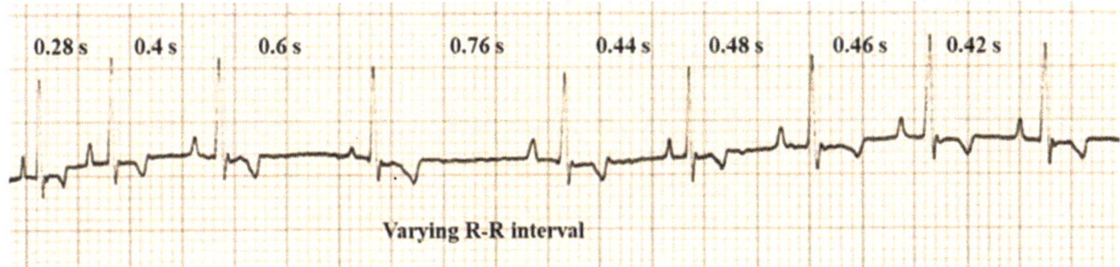

Fig. 126: Electrocardiogram (Lead II, sensitivity 1, speed 25 mm/s) of a dog is showing varying 'R-R' interval (from 0.28 to 0.76 s) suggesting arrhythmia.

- If time period (pause) between two 'R' waves is < twice of normal 'R-R' interval, it is said to be sinus block (Fig.127).

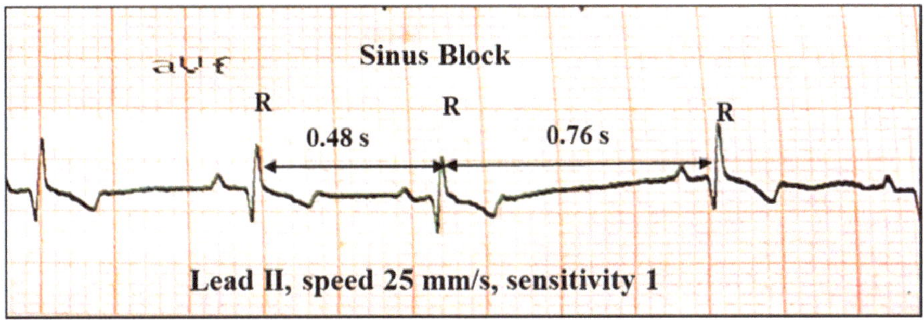

Fig. 127: Electrocardiogram (Lead II, sensitivity 1, speed 25 mm/s) of a dog is showing sinus block. The maximum pause between two 'R' waves (0.76 s) is < than twice of normal minimum 'R-R' interval' (0.48 s).

- When time period (pause) between two 'R' waves is > twice of the normal 'R-R' interval it is termed as sinus arrest (Fig.128).

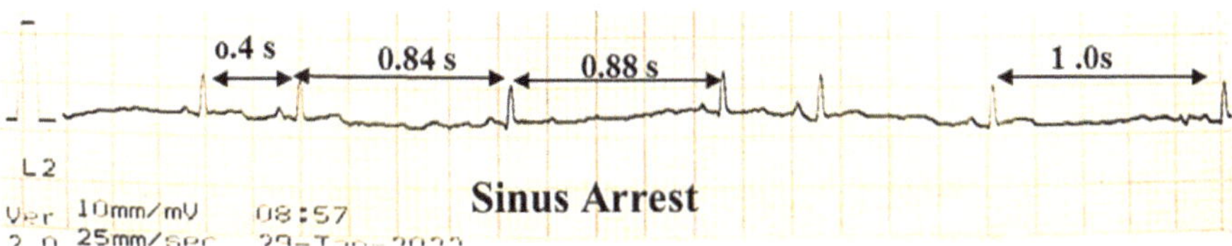

Fig. 128: Electrocardiogram (Lead II, sensitivity 1, speed 25 mm/s) of a dog is showing sinus arrest. The maximum pause between two 'R' waves (1.0 s) is > than twice of normal minimum 'R-R' interval' (0.4 s).

Abnormalities of Segments

S-T segment

- 'S-T 'segment is an isoelectric line from the end of 'QRS' complex to the beginning of 'T' wave. Its significant deviation from the isoelectric base line is pathological.
- Elevation of 'S-T' segment > 0.15 mV or depression > 0.2 mV is considered abnormal.
- Elevation of S-T segment (>0.15 mV) is termed as S-T segment elevation (Fig.129) and it has been observed in cases of hypoxia, infarction, pericarditis, secondary change (ventricular hypertrophy, ventricular premature complexes, conduction disturbances), left ventricular epicardial injury, transmural myocardial infarction or digoxin intoxication.

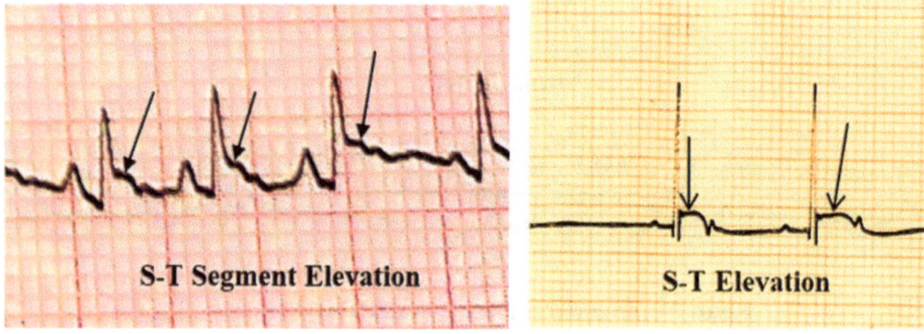

Fig. 129: Electrocardiograms (lead II, sensitivity 1, speed 25 mm/s) of dogs are showing elevated 'S-T' segment .

- Depression of 'S-T' segment (> 0.2 mV) is termed as S-T segment depression (Fig.130) and it has been associated with infarction; ischemia; conduction disturbances; cardiac trauma; hyperkalemia; hypokalemia; secondary changes to conduction disturbances, ventricular premature complexes, ventricular hypertrophy; digitalization; or subendocardial myocardial infarction/ injury. Sometimes it may be a pseudo- depression.

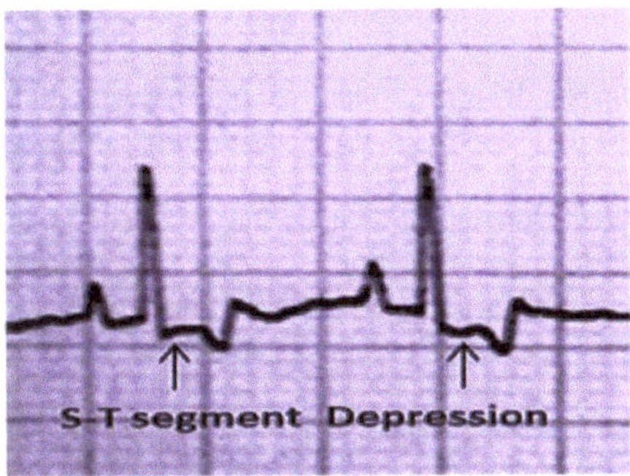

A

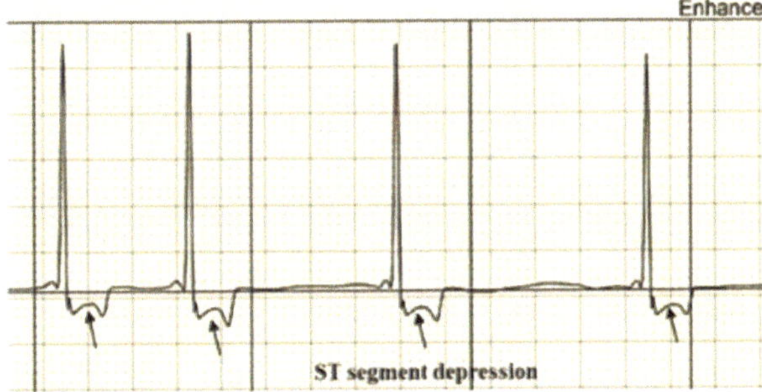

B

Fig. 130: Electrocardiograms (Lead II, sensitivity 1, speed 25 mm/s) of dogs are showing depression of S-T segment (A 0.2 mV, B .25 mV) suggesting 'S-T' depression

- Slurring or coving of 'S-T' segment (Fig.131) is associated with left ventricular hypertrophy/ ventricular enlargement.

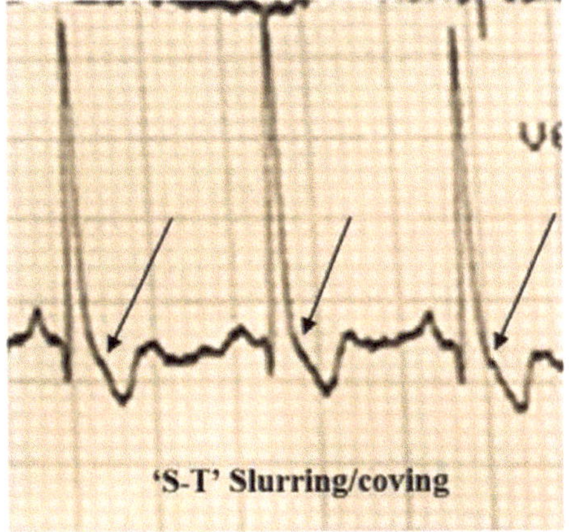

Fig. 131: Electrocardiogram (Lead II, sensitivity 1, speed 25 mm/s) of a dog is showing 'S-T' segment slurring/coving. (marked by the arrows) .

References

Alps, C., Ekinozu, I., Karaarslan, O., Dogan, T., Yetim, M., Bekar, L., Kalcik, M. and Karavelioglu, Y. (2018). Pregnancy as a rare cause of electrical alternans on electrocardiography. J. Cardiol. Current Res.11: 76-77.

Shekar, P.V. and Rangaswamy, V.V. (2022). Atypical electrical alternans due to left pleural effusion. IHJ Cardiovascular case Report (CVCR) 6: 94-96. https:// doi. Org/ 10.1016/j. ihjccr.2022.05.002

Varshney, J.P. (2016). 'J' wave syndrome in dogs-An Electrocardiographic study. Indian. J. Vet. Med. 36:120-121.

Yan, G.X. and Antzelevitch, C. (1996). Cellular basis of the electrocardiograpraphic J wave. Circulation 93:372-379. doi: 10.1161/01.cir.93.2.372.

Further Reading

Varshney, J.P. (2020). Electrocardiography in Veterinary Medicine. Springer Nature, Singapore, Pte, Ltd.

9

ECG Patterns Associated with Chamber Enlargement

Apart from the heart rate and rhythm, the electrocardiogram also provides information pertaining to the chamber size, i.e. the presence of chamber enlargement in dogs. It can more precisely be evaluated if the P QRS and T complexes are clearly visible without any artifacts. Further, the measurement of the chamber enlargements is only possible when all the segments of the ECG are clearly visible. When the impulse is conducted uninterruptedly from sino-atrial node (SA node) to AV node to the ventricles, the measurement of the amplitude of the complexes (P, QRS, T) is more precise in providing information regarding the presence of chamber enlargement. Broadly changes in the amplitude and width of 'P' are associated with atrial enlargement and changes in the amplitude of 'Q', 'R' and 'S', and duration of 'QRS' are associated with ventricular enlargement. In general, the common ECG patterns associated with chamber enlargement are detailed below:

Changes in 'P' Wave

'P' wave in dogs is usually < 0.4 mV in height < 0.04 s in width. It represents depolarization of atria. Change in height and /or duration of 'P' wave is considered abnormal.

Tall P wave: The presence of a tall P wave with an amplitude of more than 0.4 mV (Fig.132) is suggestive of right atrial enlargement which is also termed as P-pulmonale.

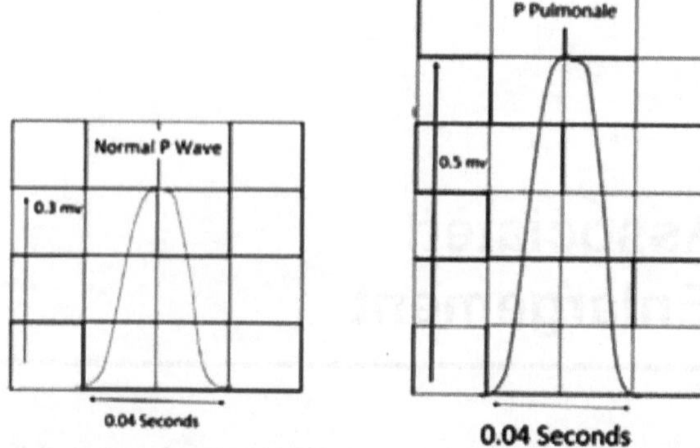

Fig. 132: Drawing showing normal 'P' wave and tall 'P' wave (> 0.4 mV). The distance between two horizontal lines represents 0.1 mV and between two vertical lines represents 0.02 second.

Wide P wave: The presence of a wide P wave with a duration of more than 0.04 second (Fig.133) is suggestive of left atrial enlargement which is also termed as P-mitrale.

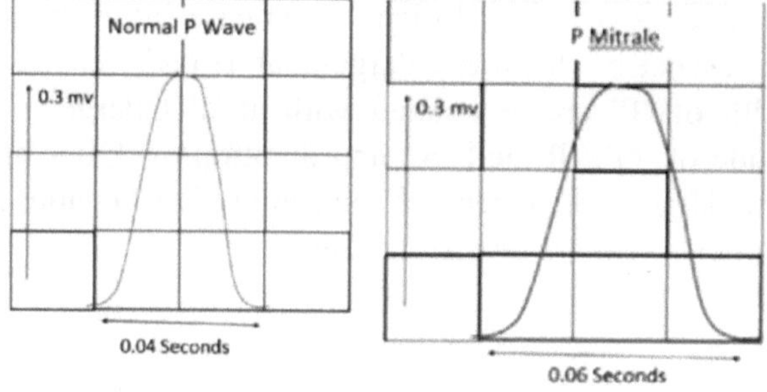

Fig. 133: Drawing showing normal 'P' wave and wide 'P' wave (0.06 second). The distance between two horizontal lines represents 0.1 mV and between two vertical lines represents 0.02 second.

Changes in 'QRS' Complex

'R' wave in dogs is usually < 2.5 mV in height in small breeds and geriatric dogs; and < 3.0 mV height in large breed of dogs.

Tall R wave: The presence of a tall R wave (Fig.134) > 2.5 mV in dogs of small breeds and geriatric dogs and > 3.0 mV in dogs of large breeds, is suggestive of left ventricle enlargement. Sometimes a wide QRS complexes may also be associated with it.

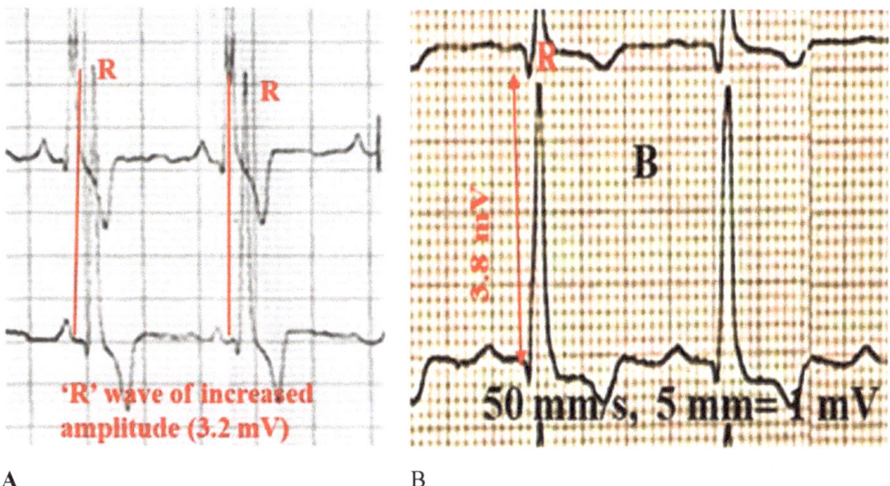

A B

Fig.134: Electrocardiograms of dogs (A- Lead II, speed 25 mm/s, sensitivity 1; B- Lead II, speed 50 mm/s, sensitivity 0.5) are showing tall 'R' wave (A 3.2 mV, B 3.8 mV.) suggestive of left ventricular enlargement.

Deep Q and / or S waves: The presence of a deep Q and / or deep S wave of more than 0.5 mV (Fig. 135) is suggestive of right ventricle enlargement .

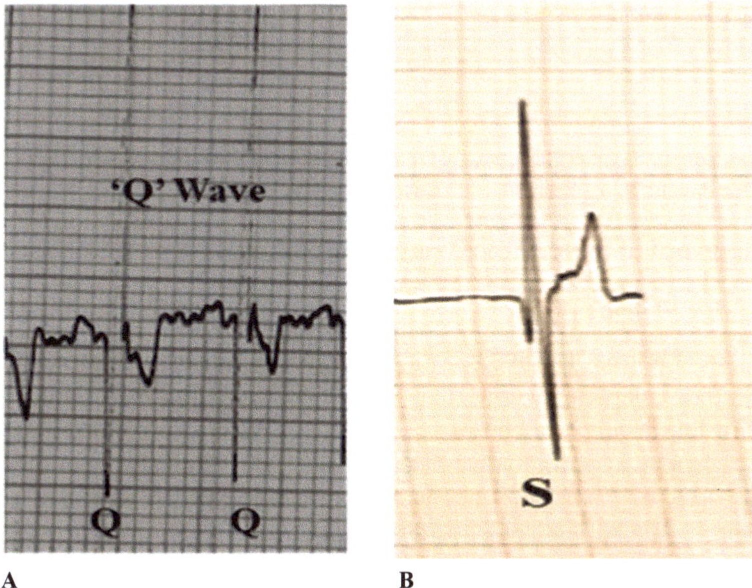

A B

Fig. 135: Electrocardiograms of dogs (Lead II, speed 25 mm/s, sensitivity 1) are showing deep 'Q' wave of 1.1 mV (A) and deep 'S' wave of 1.4 mV (B).

However, chamber enlargement cannot be diagnosed solely on the basis of an electrocardiogram as there is a possible overlap between normal animals and those affected by chamber dilatation. Hence interpretation of chamber enlargement needs to be done in the light of other available information such as, chest x-ray and echocardiography (Boswood, 2007). Certain factors such as the distance between the electrode and the left atrium, electrode contact with the skin, obesity, heart rate, autonomic tone and cardiac position have been found to influence the amplitude of electrocardiographic deflections on the body surface (Tilley, 1992).

Changes in 'QRS': Broad 'QRS' (Fig.136) associated with increased amplitude of 'R' wave is also suggestive of left ventricular enlargement.

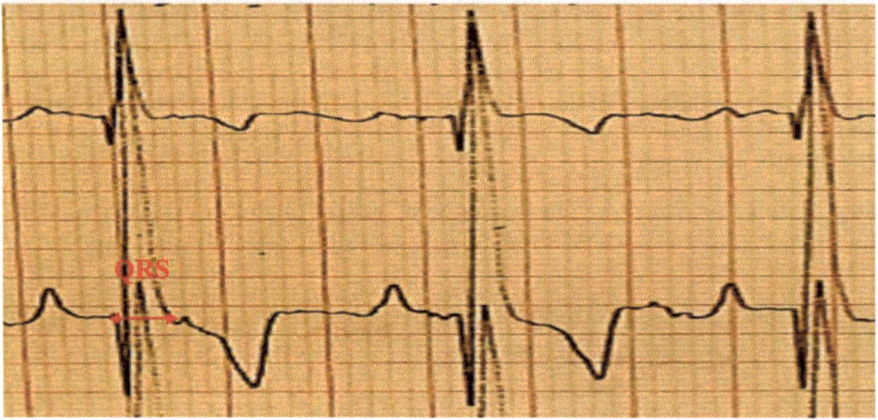

Fig. 136 : Electrocardiogram of a Cocker Spaniel dog (Lead II, speed 25 mm/s, sensitivity 1) showing broad / wide 'QRS' (0.1 s) and tall 'R' wave (4.5 mV).

Electrocardiographic Pattern of Atrial Enlargement

Left Atrial Enlargement

Even though, an abnormal P wave duration (Fig.137) indicates dilated left atrium or left atrial enlargement, a normal P wave does not always exclude it. Enlargement of left atrium is a chronic outcome of several cardiac diseases, of which the degenerative mitral valve disease (DMVD) is the most common cardiac disease (Oslen *et al*., 2010). The assessment of the left atrium size is an important prognostic indicator for therapeutic response as it is strongly correlated to the development of left side heart failure and associated complications like fibrillations and arrhythmias (Boswood *et. al*. 2016 ; Cote, 2010 ;Oslen *et al*., 2010). Though the left atrial enlargement can be diagnosed by various procedures, electrocardiography is a simple, non-invasive and cost-effective technique.

Documented evidence suggests that the atrial muscle activation reflects the 'P' wave duration primarily depending on the atrial tissue mass excited and prolonged duration of the 'P' wave could represent a criterion for the left atrial enlargement in both human (Mirvis and Goldberger,2007) and veterinary medicine (Tilley, 1992). In veterinary medicine, electrocardiographic parameters related to left atrial enlargement are prolonged duration of the 'P' wave and its electrical axis (Cote, 2010). Normally the duration or width of the 'P' wave increases in left atrial enlargement as the time taken for the cardiac action potential to travel through the increased mass of the enlarged chamber is increased. It is termed as P- mitrale. The presence of a notched 'P' (Fig.138) wave is also suggestive of enlarged left atrium and is the result of depolarization of both left and right atria (visible in the 'P' wave). However, the presence of atrial fibrillation, an erratic atrial activity with no clear 'P' waves, interferes with the diagnosis of the left atrial chamber dilation/enlargement. The most common electrocardiographic parameter suggestive for left atrial enlargement in dogs is the increased duration or wide 'P' wave. There are many more parameters in human medicine that suggest left atrial mass and chamber size abnormalities or reflect conduction delays within the atria (Cote, 2010) viz. increased 'P' wave amplitude, notched 'P' wave (Lee *et al.*, 2007), left axis deviation, increased 'P' wave area (Zing *et al.*, 2003), increase in the ratio of the 'P' wave duration to the PR segment (Macruz Index) (Macruz *et al.*,1958) and increased 'P'wave duration and P-R interval ratio (Mirvis and Goldberger, 2007).These criteria are yet to be established in veterinary medicine. To the authors' knowledge, these patterns have not yet been studied prospectively in dogs. However, the recent documentation puts on record about the diagnostic accuracy of electrocardiogram and thoracic radiography in the assessment of left chamber (atrium) enlargement in cats (Schober *et al.*, 2007). In some dogs, despite mitral regurgitation with left atrium volume overload, electrocardiographic abnormalities do not prevail until left atrial chamber enlargement is detected. Similarly, in geriatric dogs remodeling and fibrosis of cardiac muscle interfere with occurrence of altered P wave-related electrocardiographic features (Scott *et al.*, 1983). The complex sequential phenomenon involved in the genesis of the abnormal atrial electrical forces is related with the size of left atrium and cardiac disease. Myocardial changes (such as ischemia, infarction or inflammation); left atrial dilatation, stretch and hypertension; extent and severity of left atrial fibrosis; and progression and periodicity of the disease are associated with intra-atrial conduction abnormalities.

For all practical purposes a prolonged P wave duration (wide 'P' wave), especially the prolongation of the terminal portion of the P wave, should be indicative of left atrial involvement (most commonly dilatation). Drugs such as digitalis glycosides, other antiarrhythmic and vagal stimulation can prolong intra-atrial conduction (Waggoner *et al.*, 1976).

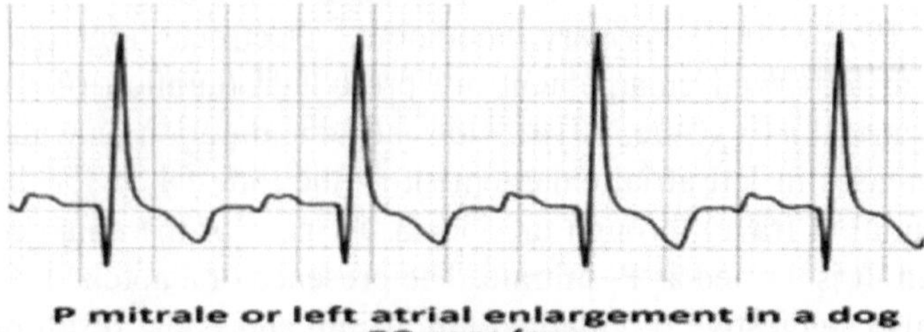

Fig. 137: Electrocardiogram of a dog is showing wide 'P' wave of > 0.04 s suggesting left atrial enlargement.

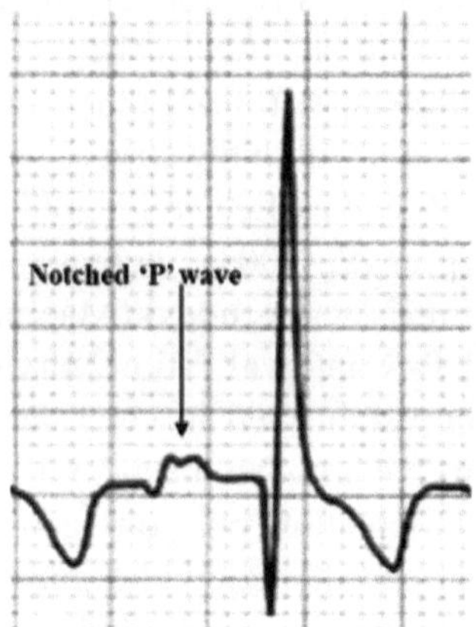

Fig. 138: Electrocardiogram of a dog is showing notched 'P' wave suggestive of left atrial enlargement.

Right Atrial Enlargement

Unlike left atrial enlargement, right atrial enlargement does not take longer travel for cardiac action potential through the atrial myocardium, but the direction of the same is diverted away from the positive dipole i.e. the apex of the heart. Thus the amplitude of the 'P'wave is increased (Fig.139). It is also referred to as P-pulmonale, as most of the lung diseases may cause severe stress on right atrial myocardium and hence, may lead to its enlargement.

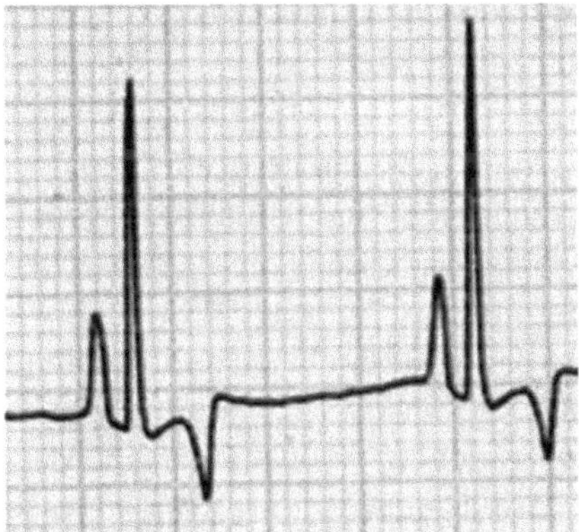

Fig. 139: Electrocardiogram (Lead II, sensitivity 1, speed 25 mm/s) of a dog is showing tall 'P' wave or increased amplitude of 'P' wave (>0.4 mV) suggesting right atrial enlargement.

Biatrial Enlargement

Biatrial (left and right atrium) chamber enlargement is reflected as substantially wide and tall 'P' wave on the same electrocardiogram (Fig.140).

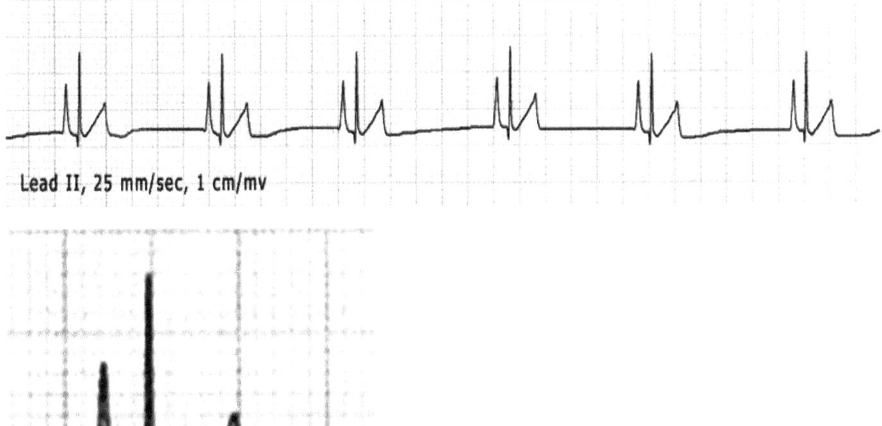

Fig.140. Electrocardiogram (Lead II, sensitivity 1, speed 25 mm/s) of a dog is showing tall (>0.4 mV) and wide (> 0.04 s) 'P' wave suggesting biatrial enlargement.

Electrocardiographic Pattern of Ventricular Enlargement

Left Ventricular Enlargement

When the left ventricular chamber is dilated (DCM), the myocardial mass or area increases resulting into an increased electrical impulse to pass through leading to an increased positive deflection of the 'QRS' complex (Fig.141). QRS' also widens along with increased amplitude of 'R' wave (Fig. 141) with left ventricular enlargement. Simply a broad 'QRS' without increased amplitude of 'R' wave may indicate left bundle branch block (Fig.142). Similarly, when there is thickened or hypertrophied left ventricular myocardium (HCM), it takes a longer period to traverse the entire cardiac mass leading to an increased duration/widening of the 'QRS' complex (Fig.142).

It further affects the repolarization via the similar mechanism resulting into certain abnormalities in the 'S-T' segment (Fig.142) or 'T' wave (LVH with strain or LVH with repolarization abnormality). The common repolarization abnormalities include discordance of 'ST' and 'QRS' complex i.e. deviation of 'ST' segment against the direction of 'QRS' complex along with negative deflection of the 'T' wave.

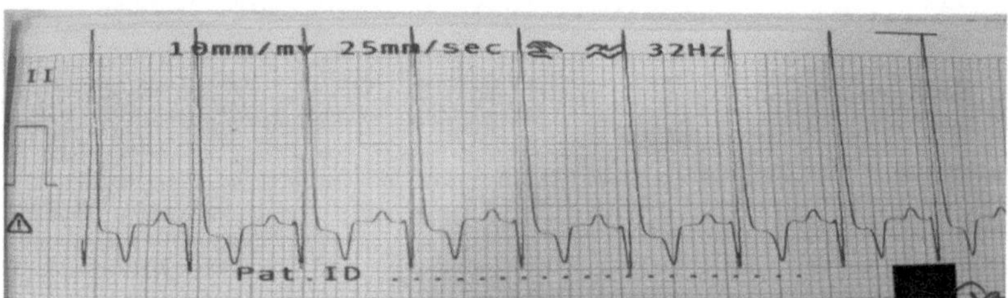

Fig. 141: Electrocardiogram (lead II, sensitivity 1, speed 25 mm/s) of a dog is showing increased amplitude of the 'R' wave (> 3.0 mV) as well as wide 'QRS (0.08 s) suggesting left ventricular enlargement.

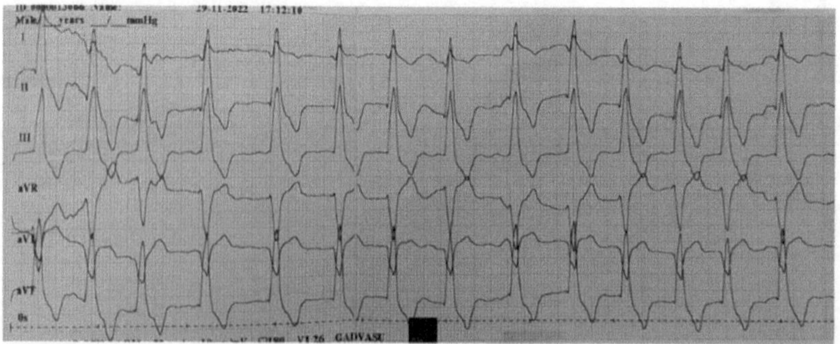

Fig. 142: Electrocardiogram (lead I, II,III, aVR, aVL, aVF; sensitivity 1, speed 50 mm/s) of a seven year old Rottweiler is showing only wide (0.08 s) and positive 'QRS' of normal amplitude (2.0 mV); and 'S-T' coving or slurring suggestive of left bundle branch block (LBBB).

Criteria Suggestive of Left Ventricular Enlargement in Dogs

- ‘R’ wave Amplitude

>3.0 mV in lead II, aVF in large and giant breeds of dogs (Fig.143).

>2.5 mV in lead II, aVF in toy and small breeds of dogs.

>2.5 mV in lead II, III and aVF in old dogs.

>3.0 mV in lead CV_6LU or >2.5 in lead CV_6LL (Fig.144).

Greater amplitude of the ‘R’ wave in lead I than that of lead III or aVF is suggestive of concentric hypertrophy.

Increased amplitude of the ‘R’ wave in lead I, II,III has also been observed in eccentric hypertrophy and dilation.

- Width of the ‘QRS

  ‘QRS’ of > 0.05 s in lead II in small and medium breeds of dogs.

  ‘QRS’ of > 0.06 s in lead II in large and giant breeds of dogs (Fig.143).

- ‘S-T’ Segment Changes

  Sagging or coving

- ‘T’ wave Changes

  Increased amplitude (>25% of the amplitude of ‘R’ wave)

- Mean Electrical Axis (MEA) on frontal plane

  $< 40^{0}$

- Associated broad ‘P’ wave (left atrium enlargement)
- If ‘R’ wave amplitude in lead I is > lead III and aVF, it is indicative of concentric hypertrophy.

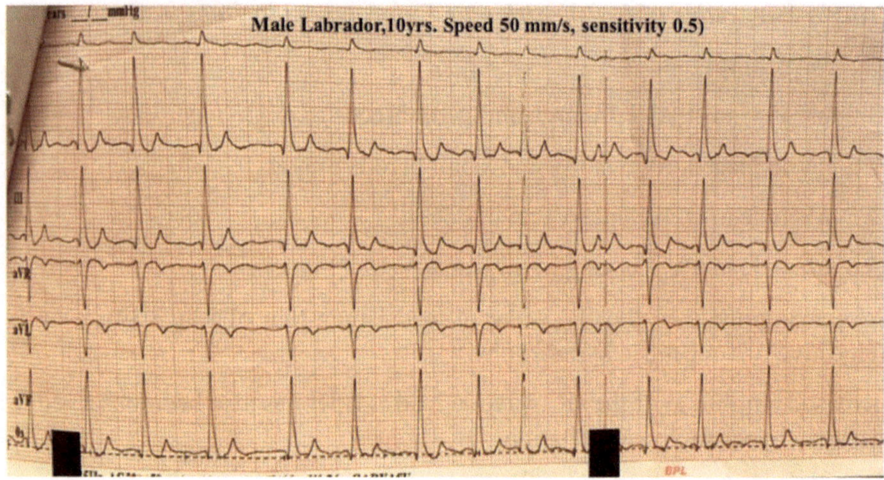

Fig. 143: Electrocardiogram (Lead I,II, III, aVR, aVL, aVF ; sensitivity 0.5, speed 50 mm/s) of a male 10 year old Labrador with dilated cardiomyopathy (confirmed on echocardiographic evaluation) is showing tachycardia (H.R. 180 bpm); abnormally high amplitude of 'R' wave in lead II (3.4 mV), III (3.1 mV), and aVF (3.1 mV); broad 'QRS' (0.08 s); and mean electrical axis (MEA) of +84^0.

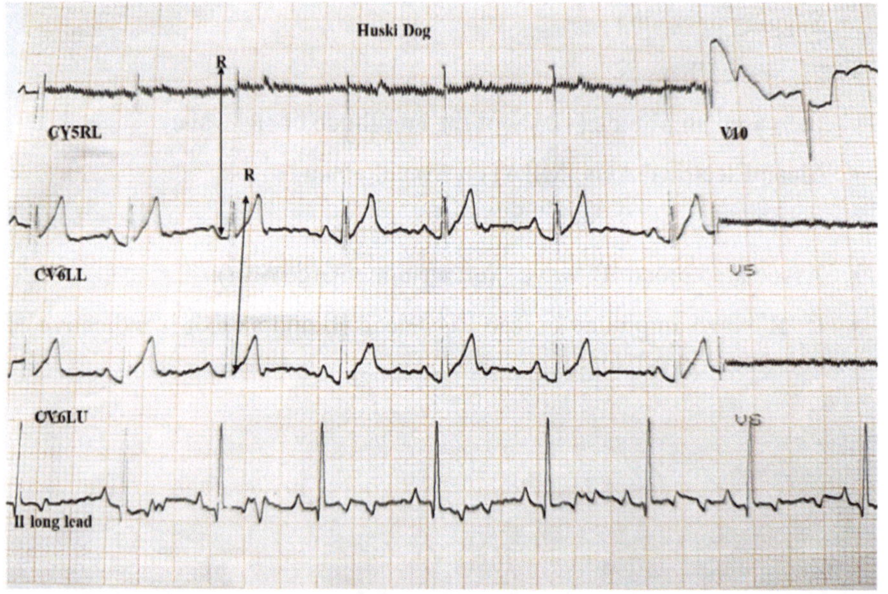

Fig. 144: Electrocardiogram (Lead $CV_5RL,CV_6LL,CV_6LU,V_{10}$; sensitivity 1.0, speed 25 mm/s) of a male 7 year old Huskie is showing tall 'R' wave in lead CV6LL (2.7 mV greater than 2.5 mV) and in lead CV6LU (2.75 mV).

Though not practiced in canine, various other criteria have been followed in humans to evaluate the left ventricle hypertrophy

- *Cornell criteria*: If the sum of R wave in lead aVL and S wave in lead V3 is more than 20 in females and 28 in males, left ventricular hypertrophy is suggested.
- *Modified Cornell Criteria*: Left ventricular hypertrophy is present if the R wave in aVL is more than 12 mm.
- *Sokolow-Lyon Criteria*: Left ventricular hypertrophy is present if the sum of S wave in V1 plus and the R wave in V5 or V6 is greater than 35 mm.
- Romhilt-Estes LVH Point Score System: This is more specific to diagnose left ventricular hypertrophy (LVH) based on ECG. This method of evaluation depends on the score values. LVH is present if the score value is 4-5.
    - Amplitude of largest R or S in limb leads ≥ 20 mm = 3 points
    - Amplitude of S in V1 or V2 ≥ 30 mm = 3 points
    - Amplitude of R in V5 or V6 ≥ 30 mm = 3 points
    - ST and T wave changes opposite QRS without digoxin = 3 points
    - ST and T wave changes opposite QRS with digoxin = 1 point
    - Left Atrial Enlargement = 3 points
    - Left Axis Deviation = 2 points
    - QRS duration ≥ 90 ms = 1 point
    - Intrinsicoid deflection in V5 or V6 > 50 ms = 1 point.

Criteria Suggestive of Left Ventricular Enlargement in Cats

- R' wave Amplitude

  >0.9 mV in lead II

  > 1.0 mV in lead CV6LU
- Width of 'QRS'

  >0.04 second in lead II
- S-T segment Changes

  Sagging or coving

- 'T' wave Changes

  >0.3 mV in lead II

- Mean Electrical Axis (MEA) on frontal Plane

  < 0 ^{0}

- Associated left atrium enlargement and/or right atrial enlargement

  Deep 'Q' in lead I, aVL (0.5 mV) is suggestive of asymmetric hypertrophy of the septum

Right Ventricular Enlargement

Enlargement of right ventricular chamber is most commonly associated with lung diseases, as they cause pulmonary hypertension. The American Heart Association criteria for right ventricle enlargement include deep Q and S wave on lead II. Further, it can also be diagnosed with a low incidence of false-positive results in dogs when at least 3 of the following criteria are present:

Criteria suggestive of Right Ventricular Enlargement in Dogs

- 'S' wave

  'S' wave in lead I, II (Fig.145), III and aVF

  'S' wave > 0.05 mV in lead I

  'S' wave > 0.35 mV in lead II

  'S' wave > 0.8 mV in lead CV6 LL (Fig. 147)

  'S' wave > 0.7 mV in lead CV6 LU (Fig.147)

- R:S Ratio

  <0.87

- Width of 'QRS'

  W-shaped 'QRS' in lead V10

- 'T' Wave

  Positive in lead V10 (Fig. 147) in all dogs except in Chihuahua

- Mean Electrical Axis in Frontal Plane

  103^{0} and clockwise

- 'Q' Wave

>0.5 mV in lead I, II, III, and aVF (Fig.146)

'Q' wave of 0.5 mV in lead II and aVF thin certain chested dogs may be normal.

- 'P' Wave

  >0.4 mV 'P' wave (right atrial enlargement) may also be associated with right ventricular enlargement

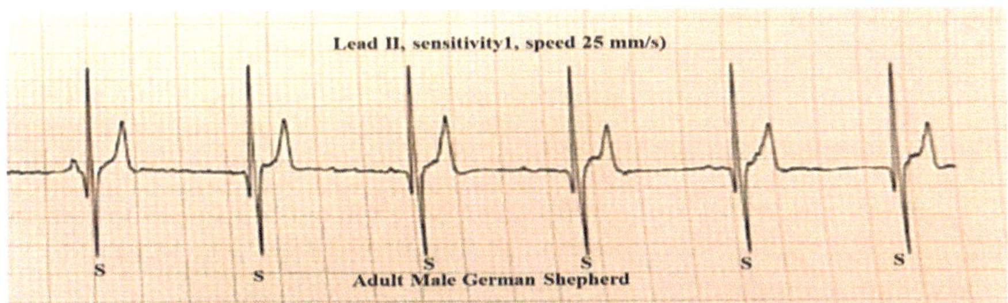

Fig. 145: Electrocardiogram (Lead II, sensitivity 1, speed 25 mm/s) of an adult male German Shepherd showing deep 'S' wave (1.5 mV) and wide QRS (0.08 s) suggesting right ventricle enlargement

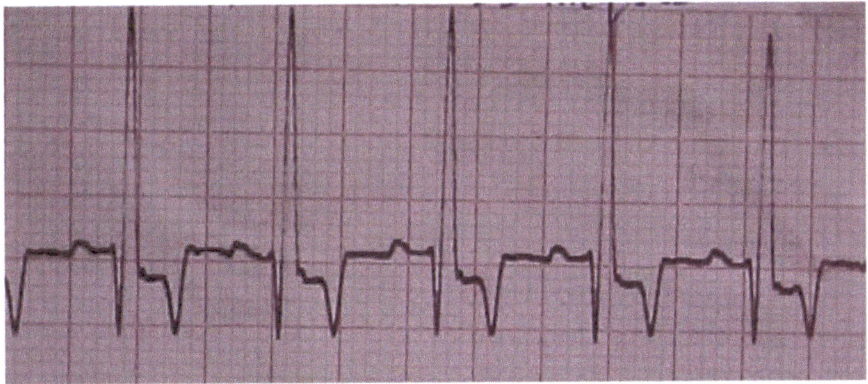

Fig. 146: Electrocardiogram (Lead II, sensitivity 1, speed 25 mm/s) of a dog showing deep 'Q' wave (0.6 mV) and wide QRS (0.08 s) suggesting right ventricle enlargement.

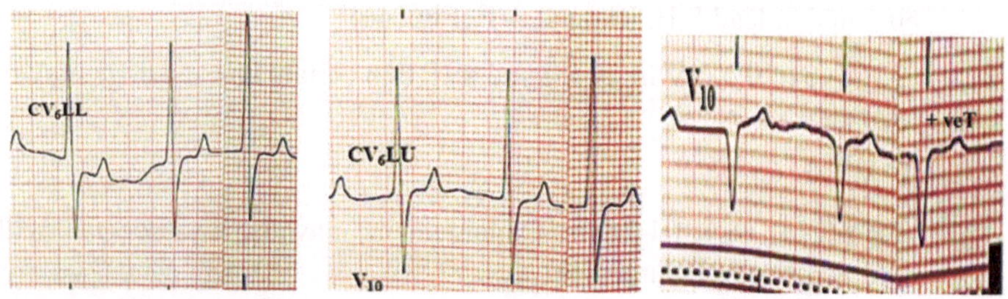

Fig. 147: Electrocardiogram (Lead CV6LL, CV6LU and V10, sensitivity 1, speed 50 mm/s) of an eight year old Labrador showing deep 'S' wave (1.3 mV in CV6LL, 1.1 mV in CV6LU ; and +ve T in lead V10) suggesting right ventricle enlargement.

Criteria suggestive of Right Ventricular Enlargement in Cats

Criteria suggestive for right ventricular enlargement are not well defined. Nevertheless, the following criteria , as observed in dogs, may be observed in cats with severe right ventricular enlargement .

- 'S' wave

  'S' wave of> 0.5 mV in amplitude in lead I, II, III and aVF

  'S' wave of> 0.7 mV in lead CV6 LL and CV6LU

- 'T' Wave

  Positive in lead V10

- Mean Electrical Axis in Frontal Plane

  $+160^0$ and clockwise

- 'P' Wave

  >0.4 mV 'P' wave (right atrial enlargement) may also be associated with right ventricular enlargement

- Differentiation of right bundle branch block and right ventricular enlargement is difficult

Biatrial and Biventricular Enlargement Pattern

Enlargement of total heart (both atrium and ventricles) is electrocardiographically characterized by enlargement of left atrium (P > 0.04 s), left ventricle ('R'> 2.5 to 3.0 mV as per breeds, QRS > 0.06 s), right atrium ('P'> 0.4 mV) and right ventricle (deep 'Q' or S' waves) as shown in Fig.148.

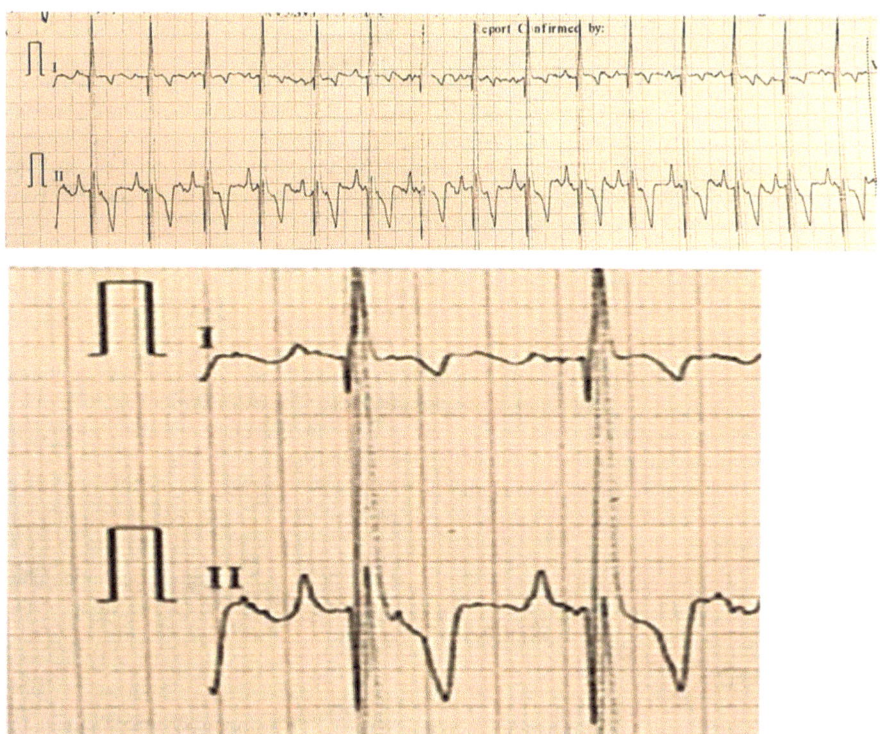

Fig. 148: Electrocardiogram (Lead II, speed 25 mm/s, sensitivity 1) of a Cocker Spaniel dog with dilated cardiomyopathy is showing increased amplitude of 'P' wave (0.5 mV), 'Q' (1.2 mV), 'R' wave (3.5 mV), broad 'P' wave (0.08 s), and broad 'QRS' (>0.08 s) suggesting biatrial and biventricular enlargement.

References

Boswood, A., Häggström, J., Gordon, S. G., Wess, G., Stepien, R. L., Oyama, M. A., Keene, B. W., Bonagura, J., MacDonald, K. A., Patteson, M., Smith, S., Fox, P. R., Sanderson, K., Woolley, R., Szatmári, V., Menaut, P., Church, W. M., O'Sullivan, M. L., Jaudon, J. P., Kresken, J. G., Rush, J., Barrett, K. A., Rosenthal, S. L., Saunders, A. B., Ljungvall, I., Deinert, M., Bomassi, E., Estrada, A. H., Fernandez Del Palacio, M. J., Moise, N. S., Abbott, J. A., Fujii, Y., Spier, A., Luethy, M. W., Santilli, R. A., Uechi, M., Tidholm, A. and Watson, P. (2016). Effect of Pimobendan in Dogs with Preclinical Myxomatous Mitral Valve Disease and Cardiomegaly: The EPIC Study-A Randomized Clinical Trial. J. Vet. Intern. Med. 30: 1765–1779.

Boswood, A.M.A. (2007). ECG Interpretation. Proceedings, WSAVA world congress.

Côté, E.(2010). Electrocardiography and Cardiac Arrhythmias. pp. 1159–1187. In: Textbook of Veterinary Internal Medicine, 7th ed. (Ettinger, S.J. and Feldman, E. eds.) WB Saunders, Philadelphia.

Lee, K. S., Appleton, C. P., Lester, S. J., Adam, T. J., Hurst, R. T., Moreno, C. A. and Altemose, G. T. (2007). Relation of electrocardiographic criteria for left atrial enlargement to two-dimensional echocardiographic left atrial volume measurements. Am. J. Cardiol. 99: 113–118

Macruz, R., Perloff, J. K. and Case, R. B. (1958). A method for the electrocardiographic recognition of atrial enlargement. Circulation 17: 882–889.

Mirvis, D. M. and Goldberger, A. L. (2007). Electrocardiography. In: Braunwald's Heart Disease: A Textbook of Cardiovascular Medicine. 8th ed., WB Saunders Co., Philadelphia. pp 167-172.

Olsen, L. H., Häaggström, J. and Petersen, H. D. (2010). Acquired valvular heart disease. In: Textbook of Veterinary Internal Medicine. Ettinger, S. J. and Feldman, E. (eds.) 7th edn. WB Saunders, Philadelphia. pp 1299-1319.

Schober, K.E., Maerz, I., Ludewig, E. and Stern, J.A. (2007). Diagnostic accuracy of electrocardiography and thoracic radiography in the assessment of left atrial size in cats: comparison with transthoracic 2-dimensional echocardiography. J. Vet. Intern. Med. 21: 709–718.

Scott, C.C., Leier, C.V., Kilman, J.W., Vasko, J. S. and Unverferth, D. V. (1983). The effect of left atrial histology and dimension on P wave morphology. J. Electrocardiol. 16: 363–366.

Tilley, L. P. (1992). Analysis of canine P-QRS-S deflections. In: Essentials of Canine and Feline Electrocardiography. 3rd ed., Lea and Febiger, Philadelphia. pp 59-99.

Waggoner, A. D., Adyanthaya, A. V., Quinones, M. A. and Alexander, J. K. (1976). Left atrial enlargement. Echocardiographic assessment of electrocardiographic criteria. Circulation 54: 553–557.

Zeng, C., Wei, T., Zhao, R., Wang, C., Chen, L. and Wang, L. (2003). Electrocardiographic diagnosis of left atrial enlargement in patients with mitral stenosis: the value of the P-wave area. Acta. Cardiol. 58: 139–141.

Further Readings

Varshney, J.P. (2020). Electrocardiography in Veterinary Medicine. Springer Nature, Singapore, Pte, Ltd.

10

Arrhythmias and Conduction Abnormalities

The word “arrhythmia” has been derived from ancient Greek ἄρρυθμος (arruthmos) via new Latin “arrhythmia”. Arruthmos is made up of ‘a ‘(without) and ‘rruthmos’ (rhythm) means without rhythm. By definition as per dictionary, arrhythmia is defined as any disturbance in the rhythm of the heartbeat. In fact in medical sense arrhythmias are the disturbances not only in cardiac rhythm but also in cardiac rate or both. The seat of generating impulse in the heart is the pacemaker, of highest automaticity, in the SA node. If any impulse is generated outside the SA node pacemaker it leads to arrhythmias. The abnormal or ectopic impulses are referred on the basis of their seat of origin (pacemaker) as atrial, junctional or ventricular. The abnormal impulses are further classified as premature if impulses are occurring earlier than the next expected sinus impulse or escape if the impulses are occurring late. Premature impulses may occur as single impulse or in multiple.

Classification of Arrhythmias

There are many ways to classify or categorize arrhythmias and conduction disturbances (Fig.149) such as on the basis of cardiac rhythm, cardiac rate, cardiac rhythm and rate both , abnormality of impulse formation , abnormality of impulse conduction or both impulse generation as well as conduction as follows.

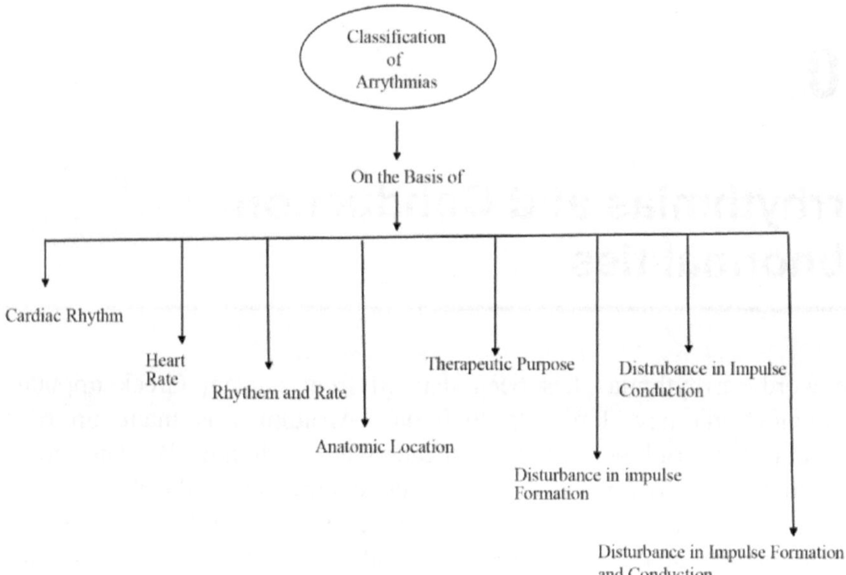

Fig. 149: Diagrammatic representation of classifying arrhythmias.

1. Arrhythmias Classified on the Basis of Cardiac Rhythm

(a) *Normal or Sinus Rhythm*

This type of arrhythmia have regular or sinus rhythm but decreased or increased heart rate than the normal specified limit.

- Sinus tachycardia (heart rate more than the normal specified for the species of the animal but the rhythm is regular)
- Sinus bradycardia (heart rate less than the normal specified for the species of the animal but the rhythm is regular)
- Wandering sinus pacemaker (varying amplitude of P wave) also falls under this category.

(b) *Irregular rhythm*

This type of arrhythmia has heart rate within specified limits but rhythm is irregular.

- Sinus arrhythmia (heart rate within normal range but irregular cardiac rhythm).

2. Arrhythmias Classified on the Basis of Heart Rate

This type of arrhythmias have either increased or decreased heart rate with or without alteration in the cardiac rhythm.

- Sinus Arrhythmia (heart rate normal but rhythm is irregular). Atrial premature beat, sinus arrest/sinus block, junctional (nodal) premature beat, junctional tachycardia, ventricular premature beat, heart block (1st and 2nd degree), bundle branch block and Wolf-Parkinson-White Syndrome fall in this category.
- Sinus Tachycardia (heart rate more than the normal specified for the species of the animal but the rhythm is regular). Sinus tachycardia, atrial tachycardia, atrial fibrillation/atrial flutter, junctional tachycardia and ventricular tachycardia fall in this category.
- Sinus bradycardia (heart rate less than the normal specified for the species of the animal but the rhythm is regular). Sinoatrial standstill (No 'P' wave). ventricular escape rhythm, 3rd degree heart block, sinus arrest with decreased heart rate and junctional escape rhythm fall in this category.
- Tachyarrhythmia (heart rate more than the normal specified for the species of the animal with irregular cardiac rhythm)
- Bradyarrhythmia (heart rate less than the normal specified for the species of the animal with irregular cardiac rhythm).

3. Arrhythmias Classified on the Basis of Variations in Heart Rate and Rhythm

This type of arrhythmias have changes in both heart rate and heart rhythm.

- Slow heart rate and regular rhythm - Sinus bradycardia, complete AV block with ventricular escape rhythm and atrial standstill with ventricular escape rhythm fall under this category.
- Slow heart rate and irregular rhythm - Sinus bradyarrhythmia, sinus arrest, sick sinus syndrome and high grade 2nd degree heart blocks fall under this category.
- Fast heart rate and regular rhythm - Sinus tachycardia, sustained supraventricular tachycardia and sustained ventricular tachycardia are the arrhythmias in this category.
- Fast heart rate and irregular rhythm - Atrial or supraventricular premature contractions, paroxysmal atrial or supraventricular tachycardia, atrial

flutter/fibrillation, ventricular premature contractions and paroxysmal ventricular tachycardia are the arrhythmias in this category.

4. Arrhythmias Classified on the Basis of Anatomical Location

This type of classification of arrhythmias is based on the seat of origin of arrhythmia such as SA node, pacemaker other than SA node (ectopic foci), pacemaker from bundle of His, bundle branches, or Purkinje fibers (Fig.150).

- Arrhythmias arising from abnormal functioning of pacemaker located in the SA node – Sinus arrhythmia , sinus arrest/block, wandering pacemaker, sinus tachycardia and sinus bradycardia fall in this category.
- Arrhythmias arising from the activation of the pacemaker lying at a site/ focus other than SA node. It may be supraventricular foci lying above the ventricle, or ventricular foci lying within the ventricular mass (but such pacemakers reside, usually, in the main bundle of His,the left or right bundle branches, or in Purkinje fibers) or escape rhythm. Such arrhythmias are termed as ectopic beats.

Atrial premature beats / complexes, junctional premature beats/complexes, atrial tachycardia, atrial fibrillation/flutter and junctional tachycardia are arrhythmias in this group.These ectopic beats arise from supraventricular foci lying above the ventricles at a site/focus definitely other than SA node.

Ventricular premature beats/complexes, ventricular fibrillations/flutters, ventricular tachycardia and atrioventricular dissociation are the arrhythmias which arise from a ventricular foci lying within ventricular mass but pacemakers reside in the bundle of His, bundle branches (left or right) or in Purkinje fibers.

The 3rd type of arrhythmias which arise from activation of pacemaker lying at places other than SA node are junctional escape beats and rhythms; and ventricular escape beats and rhythms. The junctional escape beat/rhythm is due to failure/ slowing of SA node pacemaker and the pacemaker located at AV junction rescues the heartbeat. When a single spontaneous impulse is rescued by a pacemaker lying in the ventricle (bundle of His, bundle branches or Purkinje fibers), it is termed as ventricular escape complex. When subsidiary pacemaker (AV junction or ventricular) takes over the role of SA node pacemaker, it is termed as junctional escape rhythm.

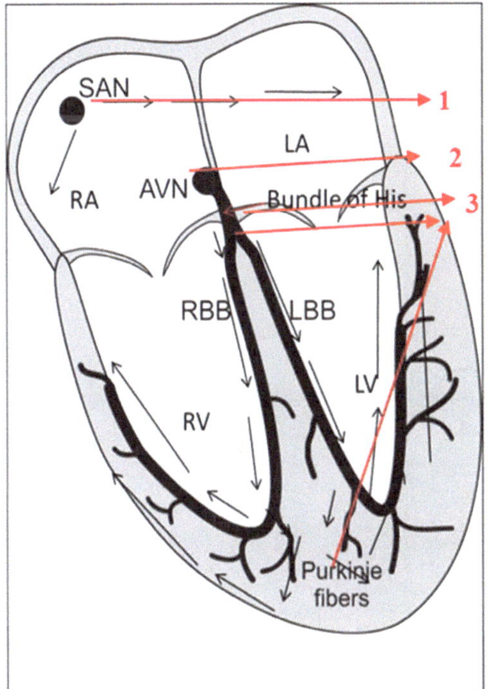

1. Arrhythmias arising from abnormal functioning of SAnode pace maker
2. Arrhythmias arising from pacemaker in AV junction
3. Arrhythmias arising from pace maker in Bundle of His, bundle branches or Purkinje fibers

Fig. 150: Diagram is showing location of arrhythmias as per their anatomical origin.

5. Arrhythmias Classified for Therapeutic Purposes

For the sake of convenience and ease of treatment, arrhythmias can also be classified as supraventricular, ventricular and escape beats (Fig.151).

- Supraventricular arrhythmias are sinus bradycardia, sinus tachycardia, wandering pacemaker, SA block/SA arrest, atrial premature complex, atrial flutter/atrial fibrillation, atrial tachycardia, junctional tachycardia.
- Ventricular arrhythmias are ventricular premature complex, ventricular tachycardia, ventricular fibrillations/flutters and atrioventricular dissociation.
- Escape beats are junctional escape beat or ventricular escape beat. These are single spontaneous beats rescued by pacemaker located at AV-junction or ventricle respectively.

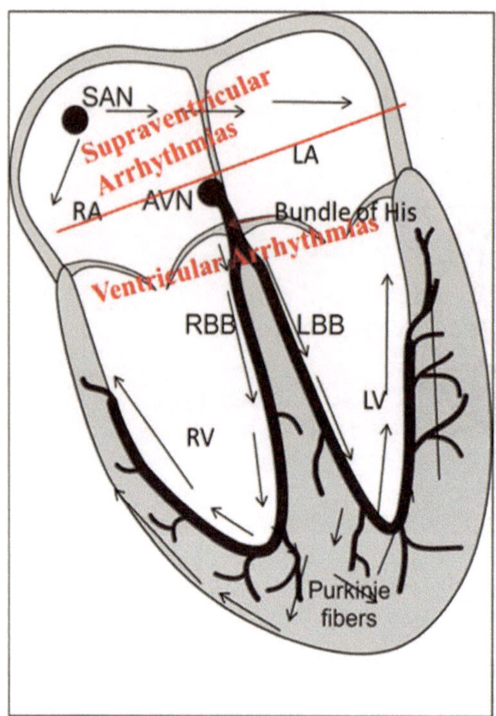

Fig. 151: Diagram is showing arrhythmias classified for therapeutic purpose. Arrhythmias arising from locations above the red line are called supraventricular arrhythmias and those arising from locations below the red line are called ventricular arrhythmias.

6. Arrhythmias Classified on the Basis of Abnormalities of Impulse Formation

These type of arrhythmias arise due to abnormalities/disturbance in impulse formation in SA node and are grouped as supraventricular, junctional and ventricular.

- Supraventricular arrhythmias are sinus arrest, atrial premature complex, atrial tachycardia, atrial fibrillation, and atrial flutter.
- Atrio-ventricular junctional arrhythmias are AV junctional beat, A-V junctional tachycardia and A-V junctional escape beat /rhythm.
- Ventricular arrhythmias are ventricular premature complexes, ventricular tachycardia, ventricular fibrillation/ flutter, ventricular asystole and ventricular escape beat/rhythm.

7. Arrhythmias Classified on the Basis of Abnormalities of Impulse Conduction

These type of arrhythmias arise due to abnormalities/disturbances in impulse conduction.

- Arrhythmias in this category are SA block/ SA arrest, atrial standstill, bundle branch blocks (RBBB and LBBB) and AV blocks or heart blocks (1st degree, 2nd degree and 3rd degree).

8. Arrhythmias Classified on the Basis of Abnormalities of Impulse Formation and Impulse Conduction

Arrhythmias in this category arise due to abnormalities in impulse formation as well as impulse conduction.

- Parasystole and Wolf-Parkinson-White syndrome are classical example of this type of arrhythmia .

Electrocardiographic Diagnosis of Arrhythmias and Conduction Abnormalities

Electrocardiogram is of diagnostic value in cases of arrhythmias and conduction abnormalities.

Normal Sinus Rhythm

Normal sinus rhythm is electrocardiographically characterized by heart rate within the range (70-160 bpm), almost the same R-R interval, all QRS complexes having P wave, P-R interval of <0.12 sec and almost constant P-R interval in all complexes (Fig. 152).

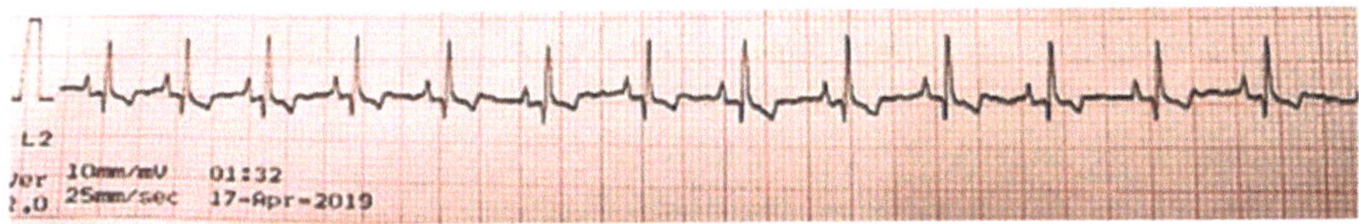

Fig. 152: Electrocardiogram of a Pomeranian dog (Lead II, sensitivity 1, speed 25 mm/second) is showing heart rate of 130 bpm , constant P-R interval (0.12 second) , 'P' wave for every 'QRS' complex and almost same R-R interval (0.44-0.47 second) suggesting normal sinus rhythm.

Arrhythmias

Sinus Arrhythmia

Sinus arrhythmia is electrocardiographically characterized by heart rate within normal range, 'P' wave for every QRS complex, almost same P-R interval and variations in R-R interval are > ± 10% (Fig.153) .Wandering pacemaker (changing configuration of P wave) may also be seen.

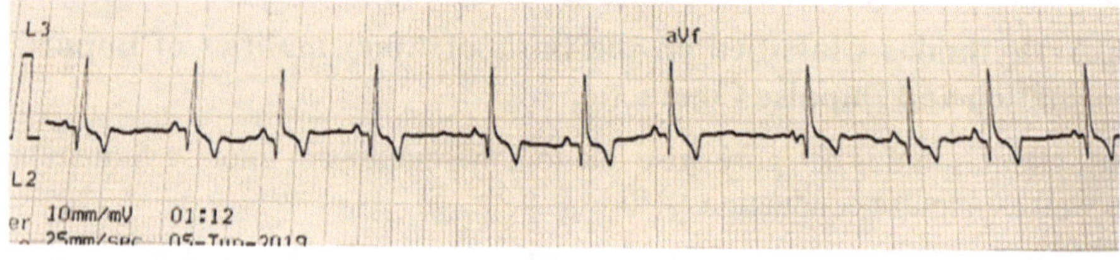

Fig. 153: Electrocardiogram (Lead II, sensitivity 1 , speed 25 mm/second) of a 4 year old dog is showing heart rate of 100 bpm (within range) , 'P wave for every 'QRS' and P-R interval varying from 0.08 to 0.10 s, R-R interval varying from 0.56 to 0.8 s and wandering pacemaker (configuration of 'P' wave varying) suggesting sinus arrhythmia.

Sino- atrial Arrest (SA Arrest) / Sino-atrial Block (SA Block)

Sinus arrest relates to failure of impulse generation within SA node due to a decrease in SA node automaticity. While sinus block relates to disturbance of conduction from regularly fired SA node. Differentiation of sinus arrest and sinus block is difficult. Failure of SA node to transmit impulse on time may sometime be fatal or lead to syncope.

Electrocardiographic characteristics of the SA node abnormality include variable heart rate, regularly irregular rhythm, pauses with the absence of electrocardiographic complexes (P, QRS, T), normal configuration of the P wave (amplitude may vary due to wandering pacemaker), normal configuration of QRS, and constant PR interval. If pauses are more than twice the normal R-R interval it is termed as Sinus arrest (Fig.154). Intermittent sinus arrest (Fig.155) may be an incidental finding in dogs of brachycephalic breeds. It may be associated with vagal nerve irritation (surgical handling, thoracic or cervical tumors); atrial dilatation, atrial fibrosis; cardiomyopathy; electrolyte imbalances; toxicity of digitalis, propranolol, or quinidine; sick sinus syndrome. When pauses are less than twice the normal R-R interval, it is termed as Sinus block (Fig. 156). Similar criteria are also applicable for cats (Fig. 157 and 158).

Usually no treatment is done in non-symptomatic cases. Symptomatic cases may be treated with atropine, glycopyrrolate or isoproterenol. Non-responding severe symptomatic cases require pacemaker implantation.

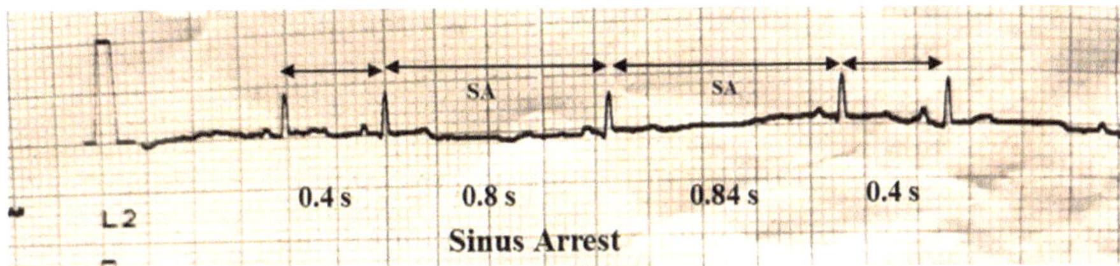

Fig. 154: Electrocardiogram(Lead II, sensitivity 1, speed 25 mm/second) of a dog is showing heart rate of 100 bpm and variable R-R intervals (0.4 to 0.84 s) with pauses greater than twice of the normal R-R interval (0.4 s) suggesting Sinus Arrest.

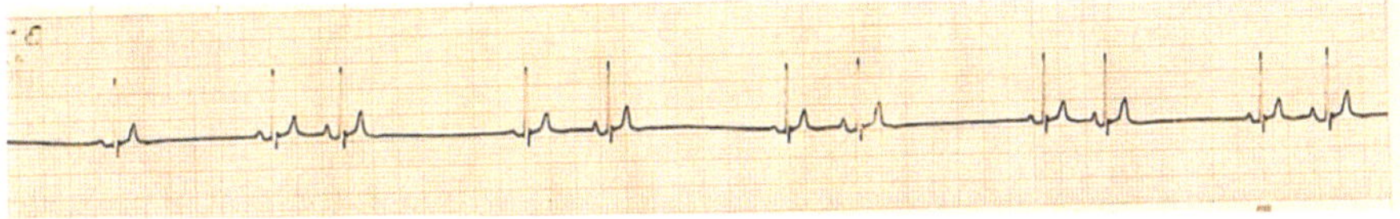

Fig. 155: Electrocardiogram of a dog (Lead II, speed 25 mm/s, sensitivity 1) is showing an intermittent sinus arrest regularly after two normal beats. The pauses 1.24 to 1.44 second is more than twice the normal R-R interval (0.48-0.6 second).

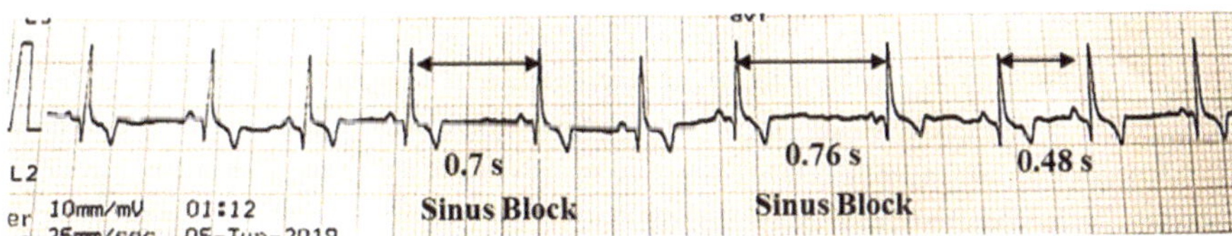

Fig. 156: Electrocardiogram (Lead II, sensitivity 1, speed 25 mm/second) of dog is showing heart rate of 100 bpm and variable R-R intervals (0.48 to 0.76 s) with pauses less than twice of the normal R-R interval (0.48 s) suggesting Sino-atrial Block.

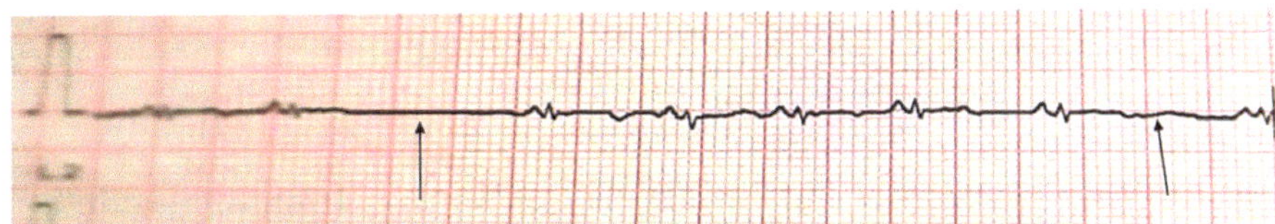

Fig. 157: Electrocardiogram (Lead II ; sensitivity 1, speed 25 mm/second) of a kitten is showing pauses less than or more than twice of the normal R-R interval (0.42 s) suggesting sino-atrial arrest /sinus block.

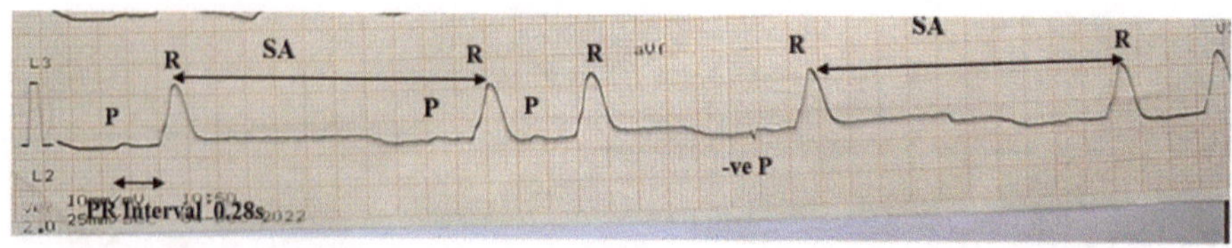

Fig . 158: Electrocardiogram (Lead II, sensitivity 1, speed 25 mm/second) of a cat is showing long pauses (2.08 s marked as SA) more than twice of the normal R-R interval (0.68 s) suggesting sino-atrial arrest .

Sick Sinus Syndrome

Sick sinus syndrome is popularly known as "bradycardia-tachycardia syndrome". It is due to abnormalities of SA node. Abnormalities of AV junction and/or bundle branches can also coexist with sick sinus syndrome. Clinical manifestations of sick sinus syndrome are related with hypo perfusion of the vital organs leading to marked weakness and syncope. Sick sinus syndrome is electrocardiographically (Fig.159) characterized by bradycardia, short or long SA blocks, atrial fibrillation, and sinus bradycardia alternating with supraventricular tachycardia (atrial tachycardia, atrial flutter or atrial fibrillation), AV junctional escape rhythm or any combination of these abnormalities. Sick sinus syndrome has been associated with disease affecting SA node artery, SA node fibrosis, digitalis toxicity and genetic inheritance. Treatment in asymptomatic cases is not required. Drug therapy alone is generally not rewarding. Permanent artificial pacemaker is the treatment of choice.

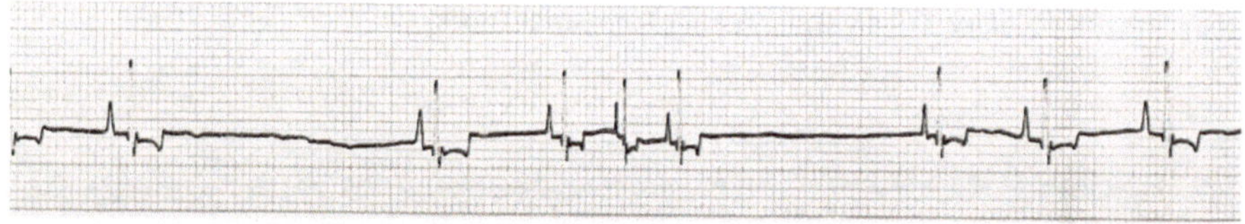

Fig. 159: Electrocardiogram (lead II, speed 25 mm/s and sensitivity 1) is showing bradycardia-tachycardia pattern suggesting sick sinus syndrome.

Wandering Pacemaker

Wandering pacemaker (Fig.160) is electrocardiographically characterized by variable amplitude of 'P' wave. 'P' wave may even become negative. 'P-R' interval is either normal or short.

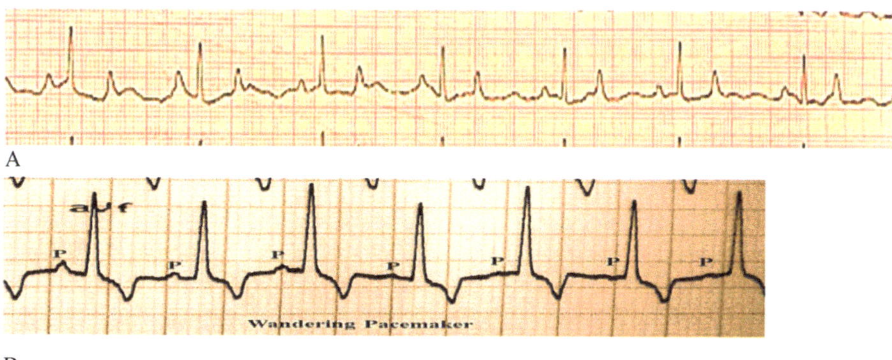

Fig. 160: Electrocardiograms (Lead II, sensitivity 1, speed 25 mm/second) of dogs (A and B) are showing varying amplitude of 'P' waves suggesting wandering pace maker.

Sinus Tachycardia

Sinus tachycardia (Fig.161) is electrocardiographically characterized by increased heart rate (> 160 bpm in large breeds; > 180 bpm in small breeds), sinus rhythm (almost constant R-R interval), 'P' wave for every 'QRS', almost constant' P-R ' interval, and normal configuration of 'P' and 'QRS' complexes. When the heart rate is too much increased, 'P' wave may not be clearly visible as it may be hidden in the preceding 'T' wave. When the heart rate is increased with variations in R-R interval, it is termed as tachyarrhythmia. In cats sinus tachycardia is electrocardiographically characterized by sinus rhythm but an increased heart rate (> 240 bpm), P wave for every QRS, and almost constant PR interval.

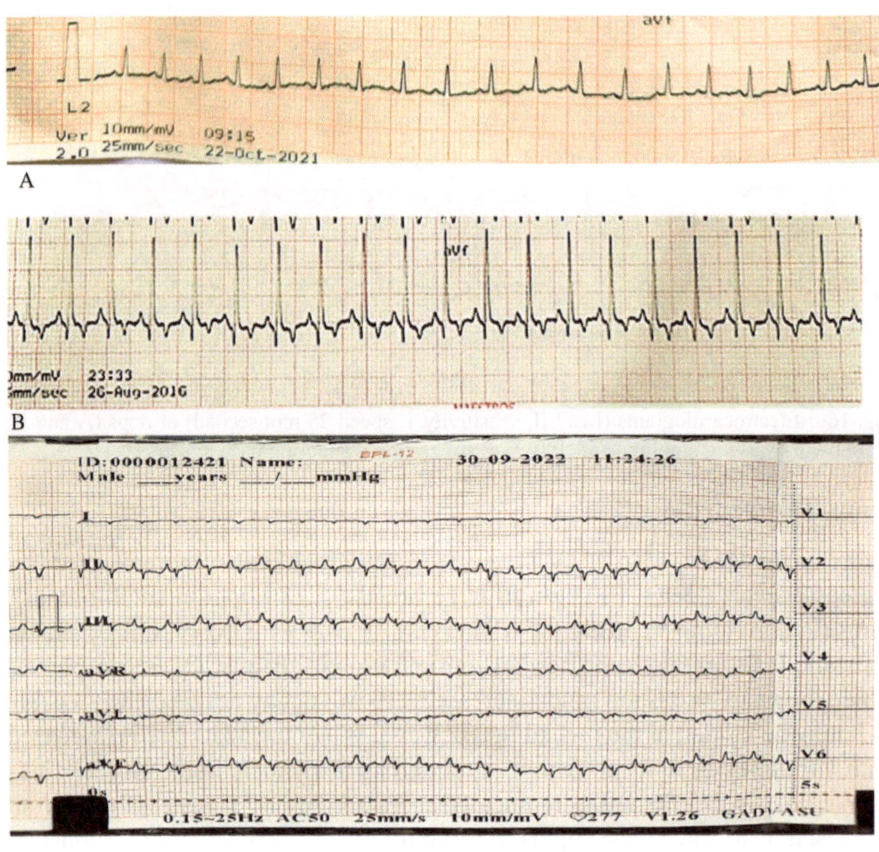

C

Fig. 161: Electrocardiograms (Lead II, sensitivity 1, speed 25 mm/second) of adult dogs (A. Pomeranian; B Labrador) are showing increased heart rate (A. 195 bpm ; B 180 bpm), sinus rhythm, 'P' for every 'QRS', almost constant P-R interval (0.08 second) and normal configuration of 'P' and 'QRS' suggesting sinus tachycardia. Electrocardiogram (Leads I,II,III, aVR ,aVL, aVF; sensitivity 1, speed 25 mm/s) of an adult cat (C) is showing sinus rhythm (R-R interval 0.21 s), increased heart rate (280 bpm >240 bpm), 'P' wave for every 'QRS', almost constant P-R interval (0.08 s), normal configuration of 'P' and 'QRS' suggesting sinus tachycardia.

Sinus Bradycardia

Sinus bradycardia in dogs (Fig. 162 and 163) is electrocardiographically characterized by decreased heart rate (< 80 bpm in small breeds; < 70 bpm in large breeds ; < 60 bpm in giant breeds), sinus rhythm (regular R-R interval), 'P' wave for every 'QRS', prolonged 'P-R' interval, and normal configuration of 'P' and 'QRS' complexes. There may be wandering pacemaker. When heart rate is slow with variation in 'R-R' interval, it is termed as bradyarrhythmia (Fig.164). In cats sinus bradycardia is electrocardiographically characterized by sinus rhythm but decreased heart rate (<160 bpm), 'P' wave for every 'QRS' and almost constant 'P-R' interval (Fig.165).

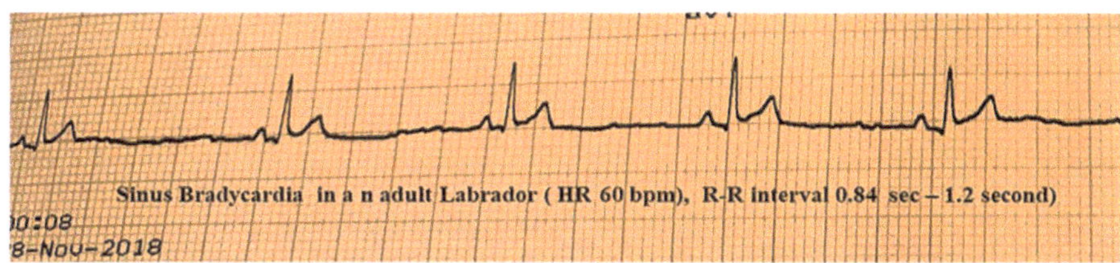

Fig. 162: Electrocardiogram (Lead II, sensitivity 1, speed 25 mm/second) of a seven year old male Labrador dog is showing heart rate of 60 bpm , sinus rhythm ,'P' for every 'QRS', almost constant P-R interval (0.10 second) , normal and similar configuration of 'QRS' suggesting sinus bradycardia.

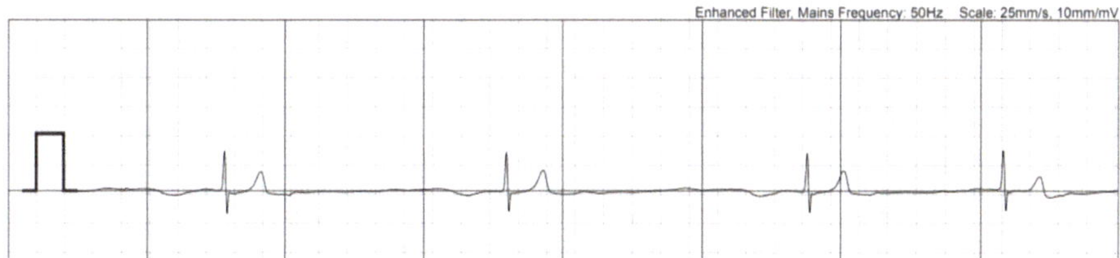

Fig. 163: Electrocardiogram (Lead II, sensitivity 1, speed 25 mm/second) of dog is showing heart rate of 30 bpm , sinus rhythm (R-R interval 2 s), normal and similar configuration of 'QRS' suggesting severe sinus bradycardia.

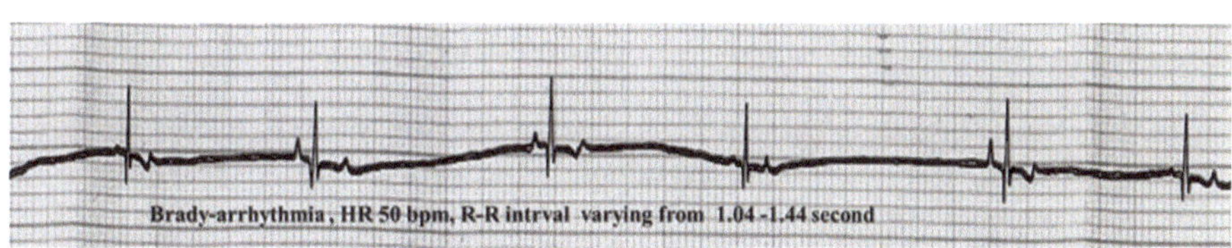

Fig. 164: Electrocardiogram (Lead II, sensitivity 1, speed 25 mm/second) of an adult large breed dog is showing heart rate of 50 bpm , varying R-R interval (1.04 to 1.44 s) ,'P' for every 'QRS', almost constant P-R interval (0.10 second) , normal configuration of 'QRS' and wandering pacemaker suggesting Sinus bradyarrhythmia.

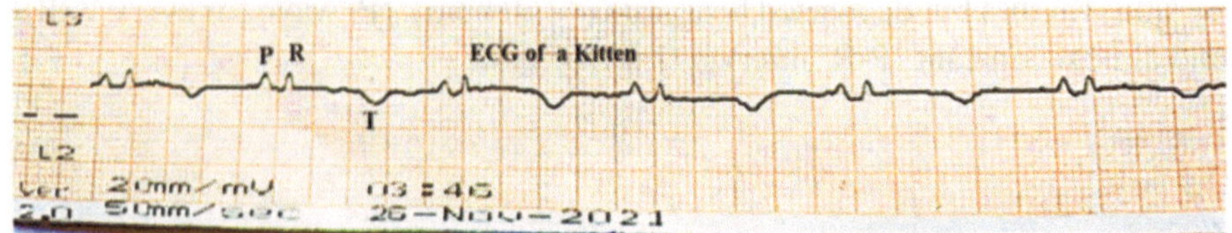

Fig. 165: Electrocardiogram (Lead II, speed 50 mm/s, sensitivity 2) of a kitten is showing heart rate of 120 bpm with regular R-R interval suggesting sinus bradycardia.

Supraventricular Premature Complex

Supraventricular premature complexes have their origin above the AV node (either atrium or AV junction area) with normal heart rate. The rhythm is broken by premature P, QRS complex followed by a pause. P-R interval is slightly shorter or longer. There is P wave for every QRS. P wave of premature beat is altered in configuration and may be hidden in the preceding T wave. The atrial premature beat is positive P wave but differs in configuration from that of normal P wave. While the junctional premature beat is an inverted P wave (Fig.166).

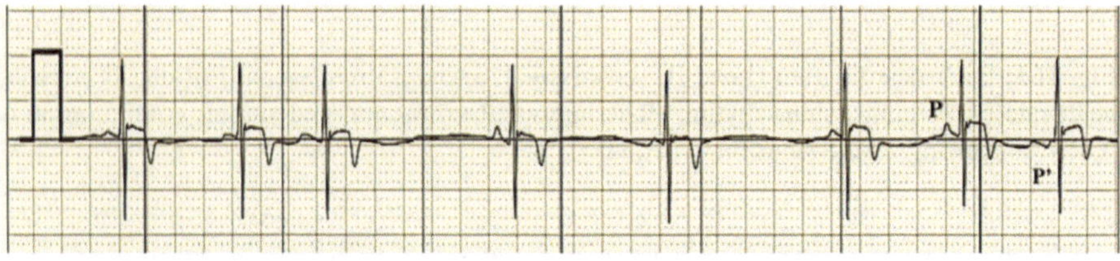

Fig. 166: Electrocardiogram of an adult dog is showing supraventricular premature complex of AV junction origin. The P' wave in the last complex is negative while in all other complexes it is positive. It is aptly known as AV junctional premature complex.

Atrial Premature Beat or Contractions (APC)

Atrial premature beats or contractions have P wave of different configuration (Fig.167). Normal beats have normal P-QRS-T complexes but atrial premature beats have no 'QRS-T' complex. P-R interval of atrial premature beat is prolonged with altered morphology of QRS.

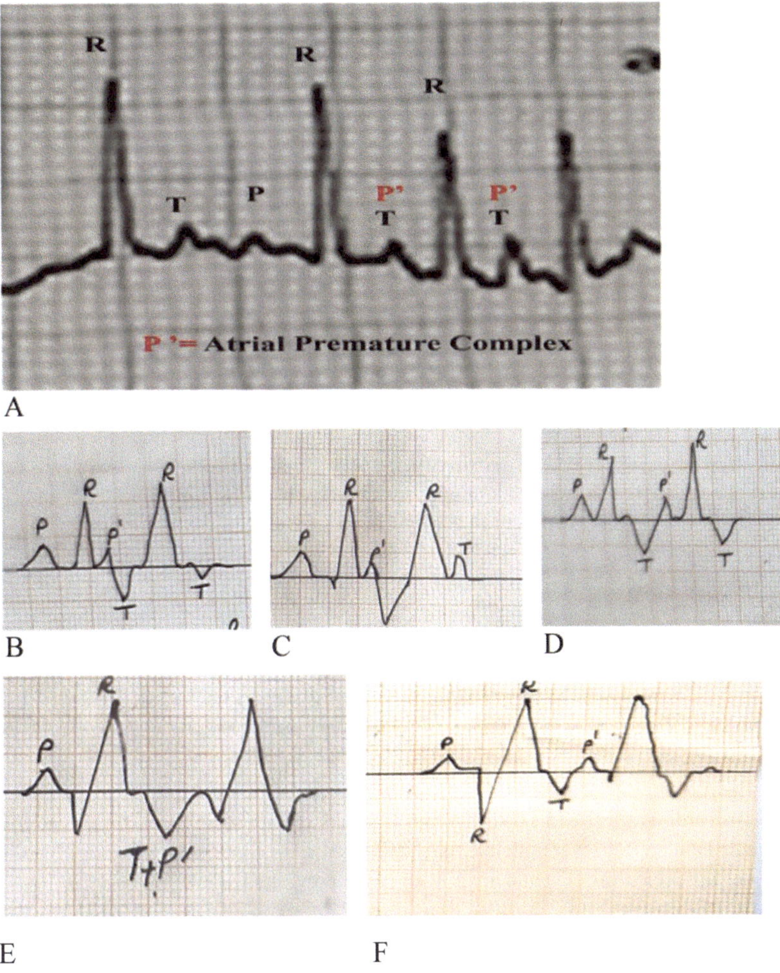

Fig. 167: Electrocardiogram (Lead II, sensitivity 1, speed 25 mm/second) of a dog (A) is showing atrial premature complex (APC) marked as P' (in red colour). The upright P' wave is superimposed on the previous 'T' wave. B, C, D, E, and F are hand drawings showing different patterns of atrial premature complex.

Atrial Tachycardia or Paroxysmal Atrial Tachycardia

Atrial tachycardia is a fast regular rhythm having origin in atria away from SA node. Three or more consecutive APCs are termed as atrial tachycardia. It may be intermittent (paroxysmal) or continuous. Heart rate in such cases is more than 160 bpm in large breeds or more than 180 in small breeds. Heart rhythm is slightly irregular. Premature waves (P') in lead II are positive with regular P'-P' interval. P' wave may be hidden in preceding T wave (Fig.168

and 169). The configuration of P' wave is different from that of sinus P wave. Premature atrial waves (P') of varying configuration associated with irregular atrial rhythm are termed as multifocal atrial tachycardia. The configuration of QRS is almost similar to sinus QRS. QRS may be wide and bizarre if there is a bundle branch block also.

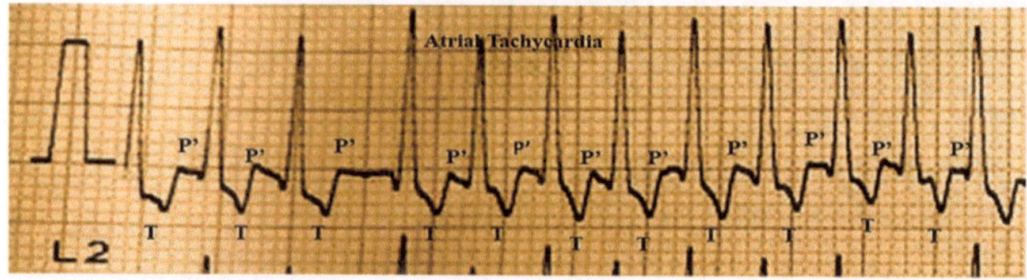

Fig. 168: Electrocardiogram (Lead II, sensitivity 1, speed 25 mm/second) of three years two month old French Mastiff is showing continuous atrial tachycardia. The atrial rate (P and P') averages 260 bpm with P' wave different in configuration from that of Sinus P waves.

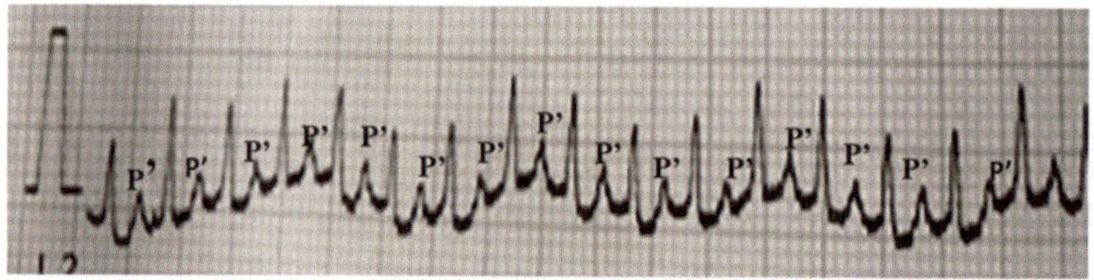

Fig. 169: Electrocardiogram (Lead II, sensitivity 1, speed 25 mm/second) of a six year four month old female Golden Retriever with liver cirrhosis is showing continuous atrial tachycardia. Note all P waves are premature (P') and are hidden in the previous T wave.

Atrial Fibrillation

Atrial fibrillation is commonly associated with underlying severe heart disease. Heart rate (atrial and ventricular both) are rapid and the rhythm is irregular. As compared to ventricular rhythm, atrial rhythm is more irregular. P wave is not visible and there is no P-R interval but 'P' is replaced by fine base line undulations (Fig. 170). QRS complexes are of normal configuration but without P wave. When heart rate is rapid, amplitude of R wave may vary. Electrocardiographic features of atrial fibrillation in cats (Fig.171) are similar to that of dogs.

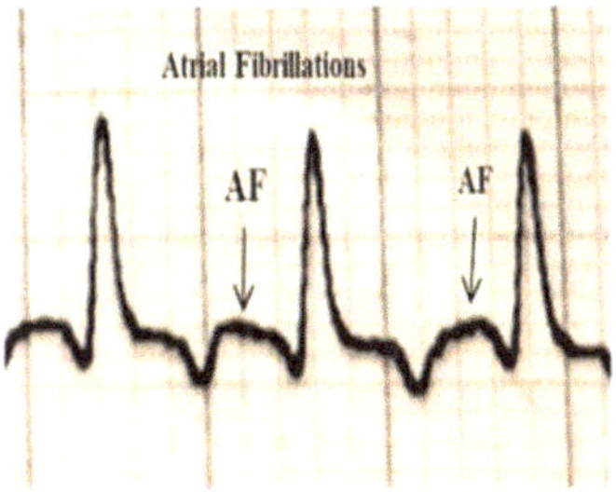

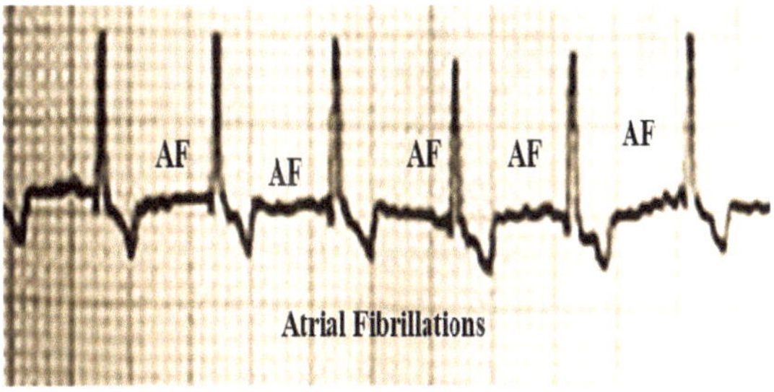

A B

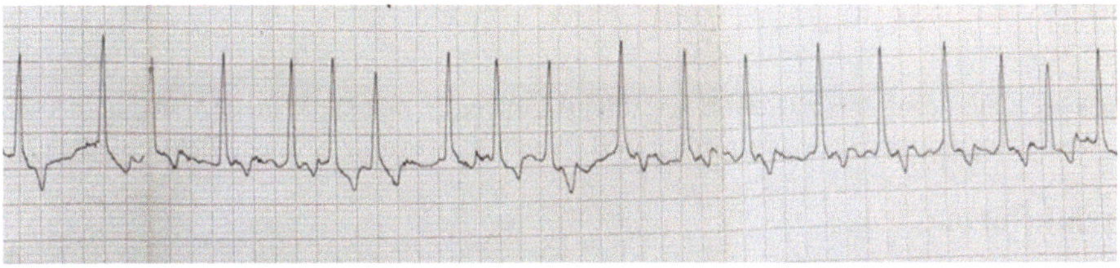

C

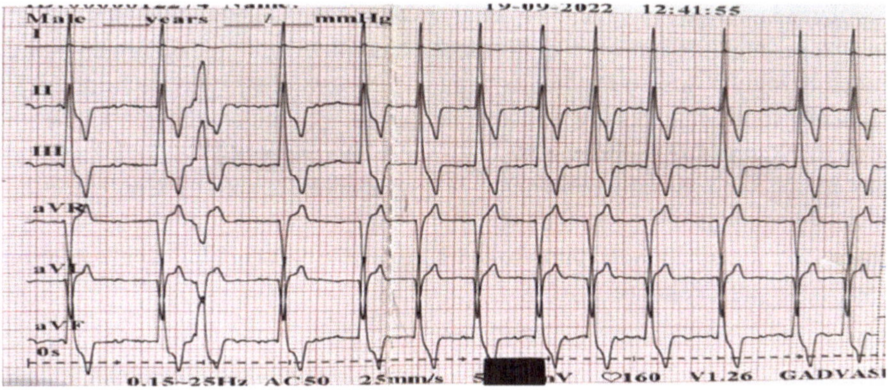

D

Fig. 170: Electrocardiograms (A ,B , D Lead II, sensitivity 1, speed 25 mm/s ; C Lead II, sensitivity 1 speed 50 mm/s) of dogs are showing fine oscillations replacing well formed 'P' wave suggesting Atrial Fibrillation .

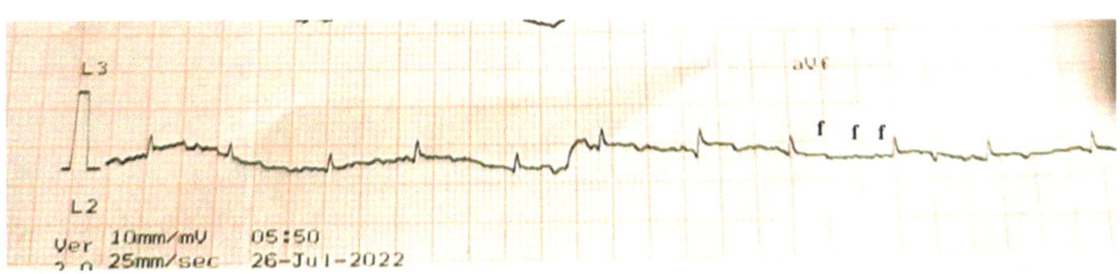

A

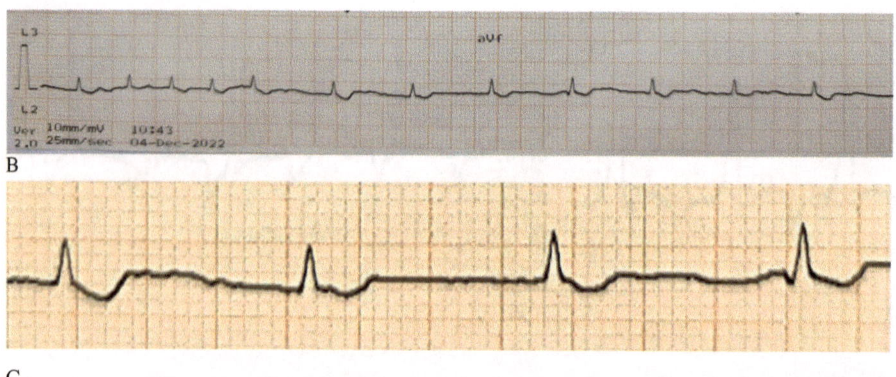

Fig. 171: Electrocardiogram (Lead II, sensitivity 1, speed 25 mm/s) of kitten (A,B) and of a cat (C) is showing fine oscillations replacing well formed 'P' wave suggesting atrial fibrillation.

Atrial flutter

P wave is not visible in atrial flutter but is replaced by saw tooth wave (Fig. 172) popularly known as F wave. The atrial rhythm is rapid and regular at a higher rate exceeding 300 bpm . Atrial flutter can be typical or atypical. Typical atrial flutter is regular where P wave is replaced by saw tooth waves. In atypical form saw tooth changes are not seen making it difficult to differentiate from atrial tachycardia. The flutters are commonly seen in lead II and CV5RL and may not be seen in some other leads. There is no P-R interval. Configuration of QRS is almost similar to that of sinus complex or may be wide and bizarre if associated with bundle branch block, irregular ventricular conduction or ventricular pre-excitation .

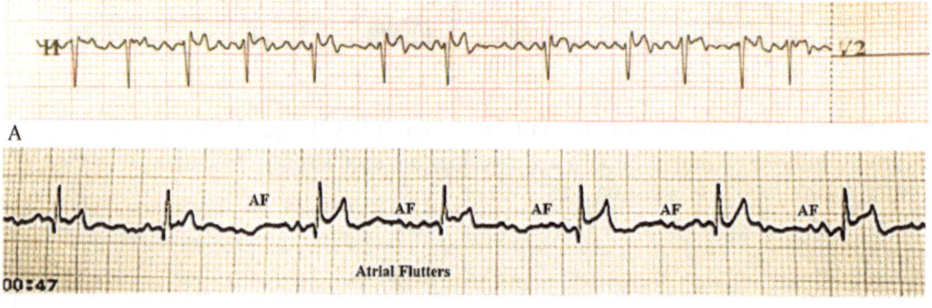

B

Fig. 172: Electrocardiograms of dogs (A. Lead II, sensitivity 0.5 speed 25 mm/s; B. Lead II, sensitivity 1, speed 25 mm/s) are showing coarse saw tooth wave ('F' wave) suggesting atrial flutter. The QRS complexes are of normal configuration in both cases. The electrocardiogram of the dog at B is also showing S-T segment elevation.

Sinoatrial Standstill or Silent Atrium

Atrial Stand still is electrocardiographically characterized by slow heart rate, regular or irregular rhythm, absence of 'P' wave (Fig.173) , 'QRS' without 'P' wave, no P-R interval, normal QRS (arise near Bundle of His) or bizarre 'QRS' arise in ventricular muscle mass. Atrial stand still may be temporary, persistent or terminal. It is reported in English Springer Spaniels.

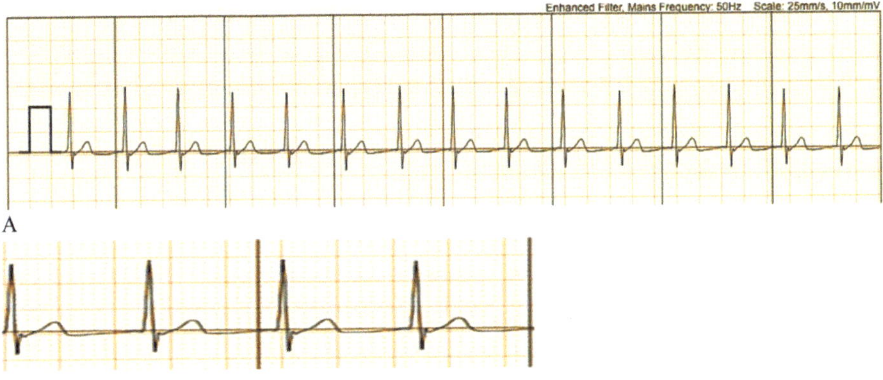

B

Fig.173: Electrocardiogram (sensitivity 1, speed 25 mm/second) of a dog is showing absence of 'P' wave in all complexes (A) suggesting atrial stand still . B. is the magnified view of few complexes showing clear cut absence of P wave.

Atrioventricular Junctional (Nodal) Premature Complex or Beat

AV junctional premature complexes are also known as AV nodal premature contractions or AV nodal extra systole. These complexes arise from the premature firing of an ectopic AV junctional focus. Heart rate may be normal or slow. The rhythm becomes irregular due to the presence of the premature complex. P' wave is negative in lead II (Fig.174) and it is a diagnostic criterion for AV junctional premature complex. Configuration of the 'QRS' complex is generally normal. It becomes wide and bizarre when AV junctional premature complex is associated with bundle branch block. The electrocardiographic feature of AV junctional premature beat in cat (Fig. 175) is similar to that of dog.

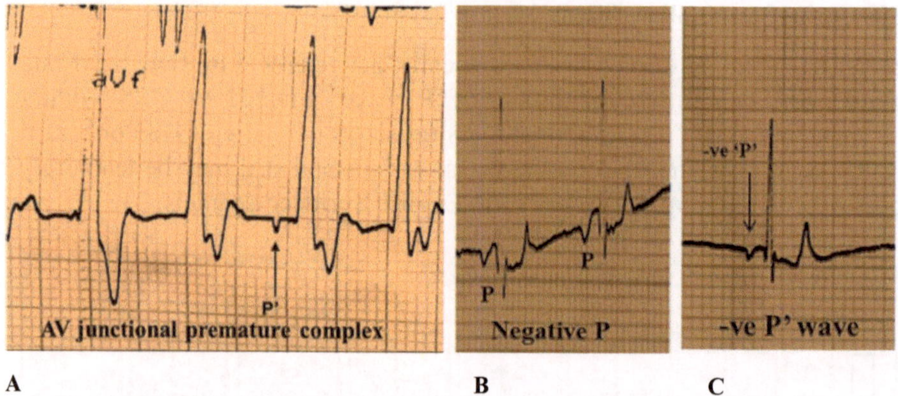

Fig. 174: Electrocardiographic strips (A,B,C; sensitivity 1, speed 25 mm/second) of dogs are showing negative 'P' wave (arrow) suggesting AV junctional premature complex .

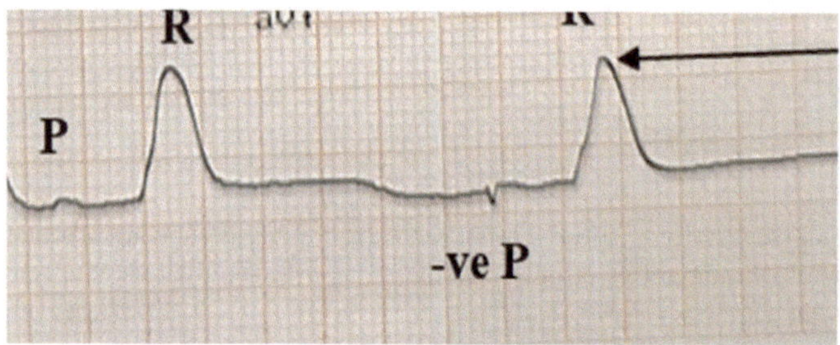

Fig. 175: Electrocardiographic strip (sensitivity 1, speed 25 mm/second) of a cat is showing negative 'P' wave suggesting AV junctional premature complex .

A V Junctional Tachycardia

In AV junctional tachycardia, the wave (P) does not originate from primary pacemaker located in the SA node but the ectopic focus in the AV junction assumes the role of primary focus (pacemaker in SA node) and P wave is always negative in lead II as in case of AV junctional premature beat. It may precede, superimposed on, or follow the QRS complex that is positive and having a normal configuration as of sinus complex. If bundle branch block is also associated , QRS may assume wide and bizarre configuration. AV junctional premature complexes occurring at the rate of 60 /minute are termed as AV junctional tachycardia. If AV junctional rate is more than 60 bpm, it is termed as enhanced AV junctional rhythm. The rhythm is usually regular. AV junctional tachycardia may occur in bursts (paroxysmal) or may be continuous (Fig.176). Many times it becomes difficult to distinguish atrial tachycardia from that of AV junctional tachycardia as inverted P (negative P') waves are superimposed on the 'QRS' or 'T' complex. P'R interval is usually constant. Because of similar mechanism, atrial tachycardia and AV junctional tachycardia are termed as supraventricular tachycardia.

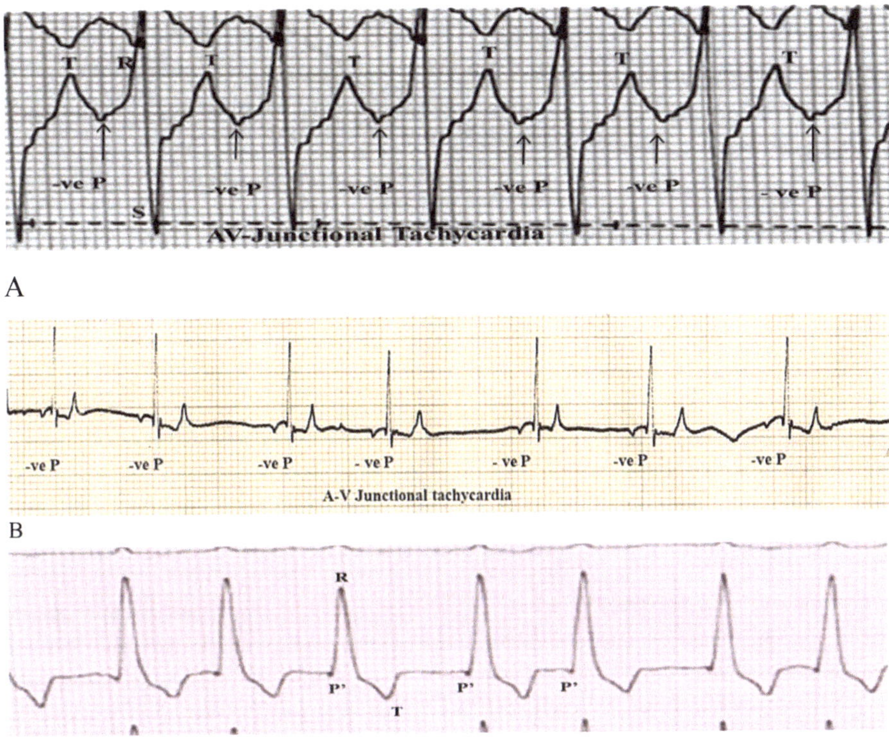

C

Fig. 176: Electrocardiograms A and B (Lead II, sensitivity 1, speed 25 mm/second) of dogs are showing atrioventicular (AV) junctional tachycardia at a rate of 120 bpm **(A)** and 90 bpm **(B)**. Note all 'P' wave are negative in both electrocardiograms. Since the rate of AV junctional beats is more than 60 and less than 100 in electrocardiogram B it is termed as enhanced AV junction rhythm. Electrocardiogram at C (sensitivity 0.5, speed 50 mm/s) is showing AV junctional rhythm. The SA node is defunct and AV junction is pacing the heart.

Ventricular Premature Beat or Contraction (VPC)

The seat of origin of ventricular premature contractions (Fig.177) is from ectopic focus in the ventricles. The impulse does not travel through specialized conduction pathway but it travels through muscles in both ventricles causing a delay in transmission leading to wide and bizarre QRS complex of large amplitude with a 'T' wave directed opposite the 'QRS' complex (Fig. 177,178) i.e. 'T' wave is negative of predominantly positive VPC and vice versa. VPCs origin can also be determined. If major deflection of 'QRS' of the VPC in lead

II is negative , the origin of ectopic beat is in left ventricle and when major deflection of QRS of VPC in lead II is positive the origin of ectopic beat is in the right ventricle. VPCs are common arrhythmias in dogs. These may be associated with normal heart rate but irregular rhythm because of premature QRS complex. VPCs are without 'P' wave. The configuration of 'P' wave of sinus complex is normal. The normal 'P' wave may precede, be within, or may be seen after VPC. VPCs are called as per their number as single (one VPC- Fig.177 B, C), pair (two VPCs in succession) or run (three VPCs in succession – Fig. 178). VPCs of similar conformation are of unifocal origin (Fig. 178) and of varying conformation are of multiform origin. Occurrence of VPCs as one sinus complex: one VPC (1:1), or two sinus complex: one VPC (2:1) / one sinus complex: two VPCs (1:2) are termed as ventricular bigeminy or trigeminy respectively.

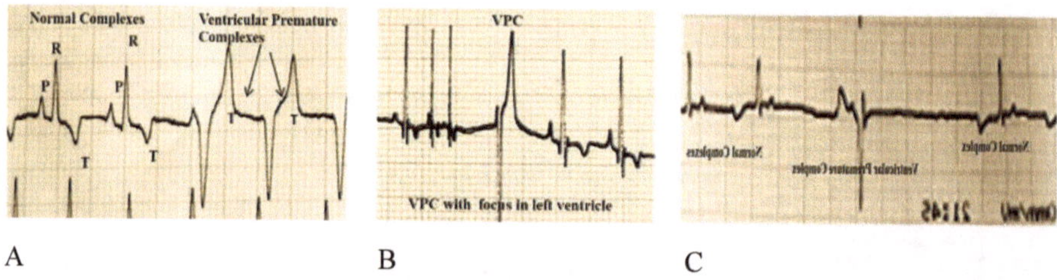

Fig. 177: Electrocardiograms (Lead II, sensitivity1, speed 25 mm/s) of dogs are showing ventricular premature contractions (VPC). QRS of these VPCs is predominantly negative therefore the origin of the ectopic beat is in the left ventricle. The QRs of the VPC is wide and bizaare and T wave is large and positive (directed opposite the predominant QRS). The 'QRS' of the sinus complexes is positive with negative 'T' wave.

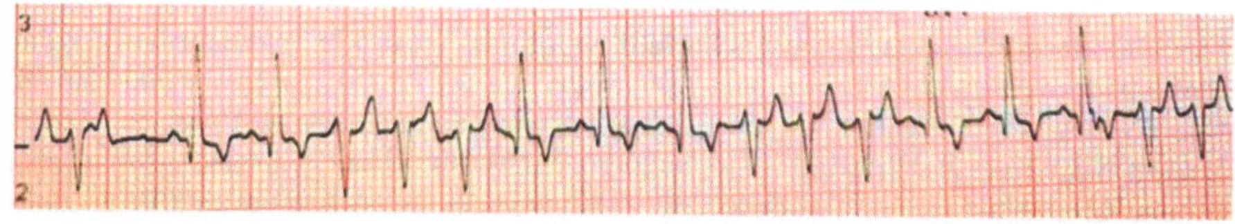

Fig. 178: Electrocardiogram (Lead II, sensitivity 1, speed 25 mm/second) of a 2.5 year old male German shepherd is showing ventricular premature complexes. Heart rate is 195 bpm. Normal rhythm is broken by VPCs. Abnormal premature beat does not have 'P' wave, its QRS is bizarre and 'T' wave is opposite of QRS. VPCs are occurring in run (three VPCs in succession) .All VPCs are of almost uniform conformation therefore their origin is unifocal.

Ventricular Tachycardia (VT)

Ectopic ventricular foci (VPCs) in continuous series is aptly termed as ventricular tachycardia (Fig.179). It may be intermittent (when three or more VPC are in row) or persistent or continuous (all complexes are VPC- Fig.

179). It is most serious tachyarrhythmia associated with underlying cardiac disease. Hypotension and congestive heart failure is common in dogs with ventricular tachycardia. Regular ventricular rhythm (VPCs) with a ventricular rate of more than 100 is usually seen in dogs with ventricular tachycardia. Heart rate is slower than the sinus tachycardia .Ventricular tachycardia with 60-100 beats per minute is termed as idio-venticular tachycardia or enhanced ventricular rhythm. When 'P' wave is seen , it is of normal configuration and is having no relationship with 'QRS', 'QRS' complex is wide and bizarre similar to VPCs. Ventricular fusion and capture complexes (Fig.180) can also be seen in electrocardiogram showing ventricular tachycardia.

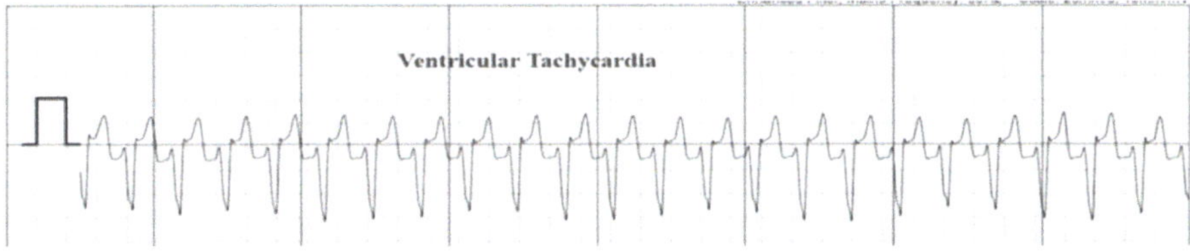

Fig. 179: Electrocardiogram (Lead II, sensitivity 1, speed 25 mm/second) of an adult dog is showing persistent or continuous ventricular tachycardia at a rate of 180 bpm. QRS complexes are wide and bizarre. All complexes are of uniform configuration reflecting their unifocal origin. There is no normal complex in the strip. Ventricular tachycardia is of left ventricular origin as QRS complexes are negative. It is most serious type of arrhythmia.

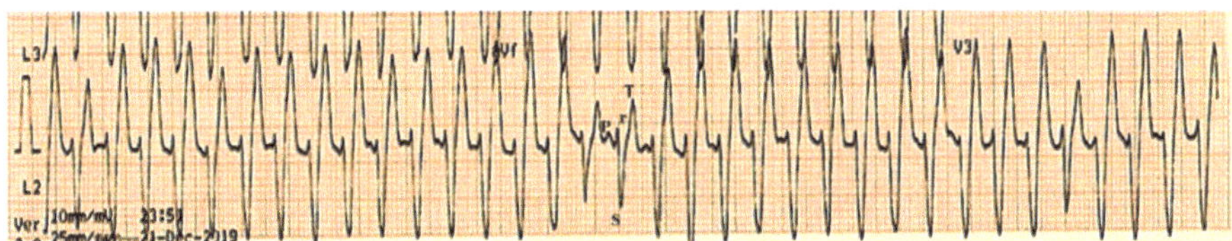

Fig. 180: Electrocardiogram (Lead II, sensitivity 1, speed 25 mm/second) of an adult dog is showing multiform ventricular tachycardia (varying configuration of VPCs) at a rate of 200 bpm. QRS complexes are wide and bizarre. A complex in the middle of the strip (marked P, rS, T) is a capture complex indicating that a normal sinus impulse has arrived at AV junction, capturing the ventricles for one complex. Ventricular tachycardia in the electrocardiogram is also of left ventricular origin because of negative complexes.

Ventricular Fibrillations/ Flutters

Ventricular flutters/fibrillations are very serious arrhythmias generally considered as terminal event leading to cardiac arrest. Well defined 'P', 'QRS' and 'T' waves are replaced by weak and uncoordinated / coarse ventricular oscillations (Fig.181). Fine base line undulations are referred as fibrillations (Fig.181A) while coarse undulations are referred as flutters (Fig.181B). Similar electrocardiographic pattern is seen in cats also (Fig.182). As seen in the following figures electrocardiogram is irregular and chaotic. Heart rate in ventricular fibrillations/flutter is very fast, irregular and uncoordinated. This type of arrhythmia is associated with shock, anoxia, severe electrolyte and acid-base imbalance, severe myocardial damage, hyperthermia, electric shock, drug reactions etc.

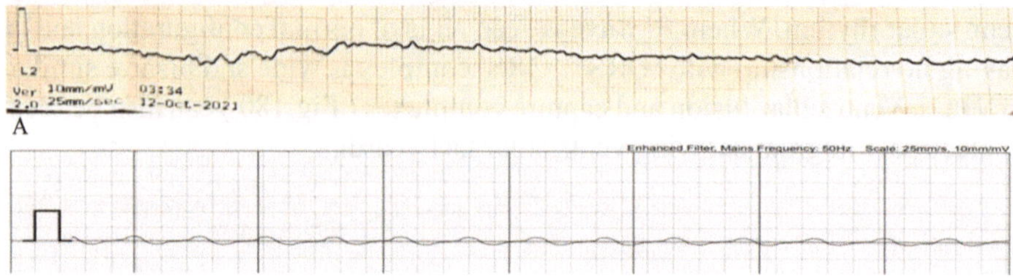

B

Fig. 181: Electrocardiograms (Lead II, sensitivity 1, speed 25 mm/second) of dogs are showing series of fine baseline undulations **(A)** and coarse baseline undulations **(B)** and absence of specific complexes ('P' and 'QRS') suggesting ventricular fibrillations **(A)** and ventricular flutter **(B)**.

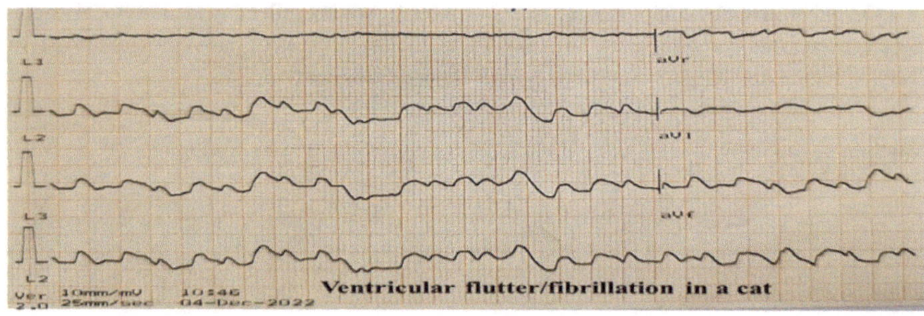

Fig. 182: Electrocardiogram (lead I ,II, III, aVR ,aVL AVF; sensitivity 1, speed 25 mm/s) of a cat with feline infectious peritonitis is showing coarse oscillations in all leads suggestive of ventricular flutter/fibrillation. Heart rate is rapid and irregular. P wave, QRS, and T wave are not recognizable

Escape Beat /Complex and Escape Rhythm

Escape beat or rhythm occurs when SA node pacemaker (of highest automaticity) slows down or ceases to function and its function is taken over by the intrinsic pacemaker of lower region of the heart (i.e. AV-junction or ventricles) to rescue the heart rhythm after a pause in the sinus rhythm (Fig. 183). In simple term the escape rhythm or beat has no 'P' wave and there is a pause after sinus beat . A single complex generated from subsidiary pacemaker of lower region (AV-node or ventricle) after a pause is termed as escape complex (Fig.183 and 184). When pacemaker of lower region (subsidiary pacemaker- AV junction or ventricles) temporarily takes over the role of pace maker of highest automaticity (SA node pacemaker) it is termed as escape rhythm (three or more escape complexes). These escape complexes are of either AV junctional or ventricular origin. When the rhythm is governed by ventricular escape impulse, it is known as idioventricular rhythm. Ventricular escape rhythm is characterized by slow heart rate, long pause before an escape beat, no 'P' wave, QRs may be wide. If it is associated with complete heart block or severe 2nd degree block, 'P' waves may be seen. Because of isolated ventricular escape complex, the rhythm becomes irregular.

When the rhythm is governed by AV-junctional escape impulse, it is known as junctional escape rhythm (Fig. 185 and 186). It is characterized by slow heart rate, long pause before an escape beat, negative P wave and normal 'QRS' configuration. The inherent rate of the AV junction is less than 60 /min.

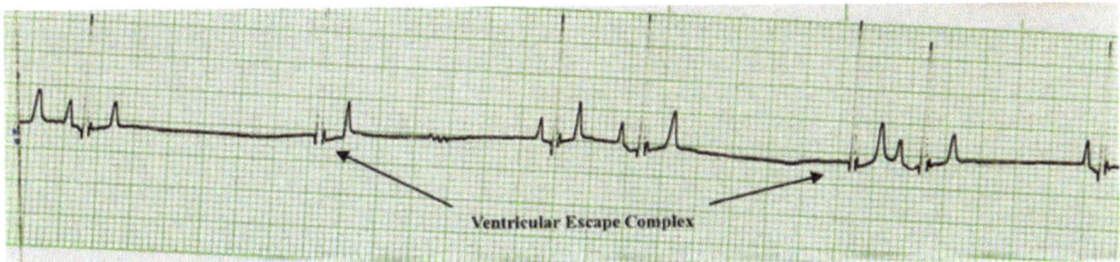

Fig. 183: Electrocardiogram (Lead II, speed 25 mm/s, sensitivity 1) of a dog is showing ventricular escape complex (2nd and 5th complexes marked with arrows). These complexes have originated from pacemaker in ventricles and are characterized by absence of 'P' wave and have appeared after a pause in the sinus rhythm (R-R interval between 1st and 2nd complex is 1.48 s; and between 4th and 5th complex is 1.2 s ; R-R interval between sinus complexes 3 and 4 is 0.48 s).

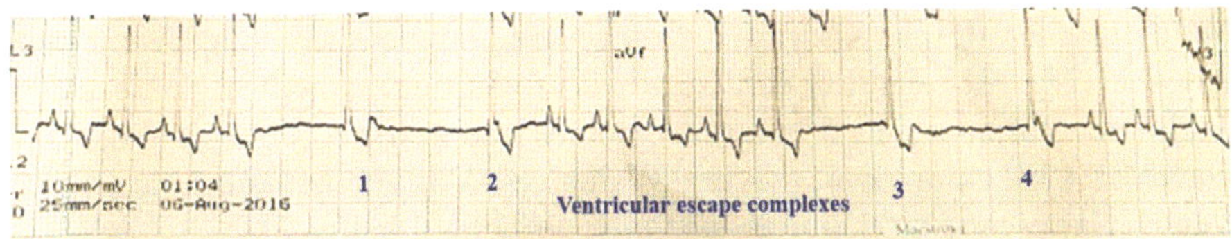

Fig. 184: Electrocardiogram (Lead II, sensitivity 1, speed 25 mm/s) of a dog is showing ventricular escape complexes (1,2,3,4) originated from ventricular pacemaker as these complexes do not have 'P' wave (no SA node pacemaker activity) and appear after a short pause. Two ventricular escape complexes are in succession. The 1st ventricular escape complex is appearing after four sinus complexes and a short pause and is followed by 2nd ventricular escape complex. The 2nd ventricular complex is followed by 5 sinus complexes. After 5 sinus complexes two ventricular escape complexes (3rd and 4th) have appeared again.

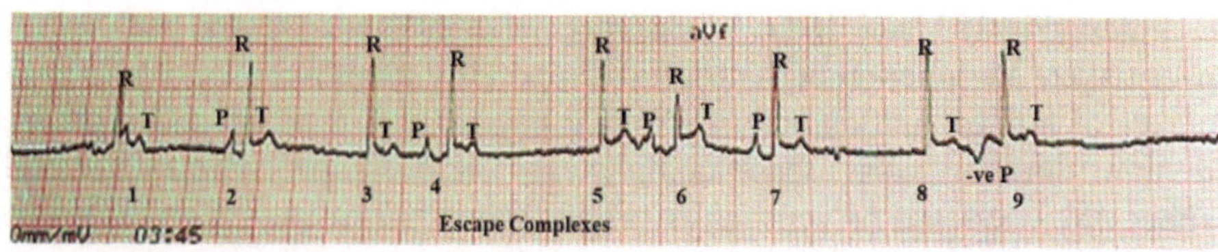

Fig. 185: Electrocardiogram (Lead II, sensitivity 1, speed 25 mm/s) of a dog is showing escape complexes (1,3,5,8 and 9). Complexes 2,4,6 and 7 are sinus complex from SA node pacemaker having P,QRS and T complexes.While complexes 1,3,5 and 8 are ventricular escape complexes originated from ventricular pacemaker. These complexes do not have 'P' wave (SA node pacemaker did not initiate the impulse) and appeared after a long pause than normal. The complex no.9 has originated from junctional pacemaker as P' wave is negative and therefore is as a junctional escape complex. The complexes in this electrocardiogram are from SA node pacemaker (sinus complex), AV junctional pace maker (9) and also from ventricular pacemaker origin (1,3,5 and 8).

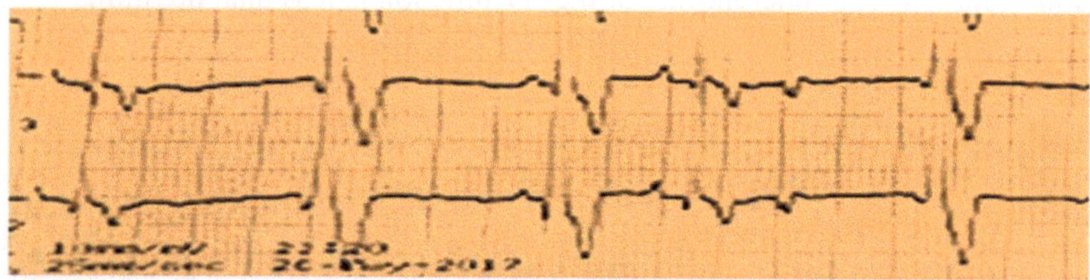

Fig. 186: Electrocardiogram (Lead II, speed 25 mm/s, sensitivity 1) of a dog is showing junctional escape complex (2nd and 5th complex).These complexes have originated from junctional pacemaker as P wave is negative in these two complexes.

Ventricular Asystole

Ventricular asystole is characterized by the absence of ventricular complexes i.e. no 'QRS' (Fig.187). P waves are of normal configuration (Fig. 187) when ventricular asystole is associated with severe complete AV block. Ventricular asystole (Fig.188) signifies cardiac arrest. If ventricular rhythm is not restored within few minutes (say 3 or 4 min), it may lead to irreversible brain damage. Severe SA block or arrest, severe 3rd degree AV-block without junctional or ventricular escape rhythm may lead to ventricular asystole.

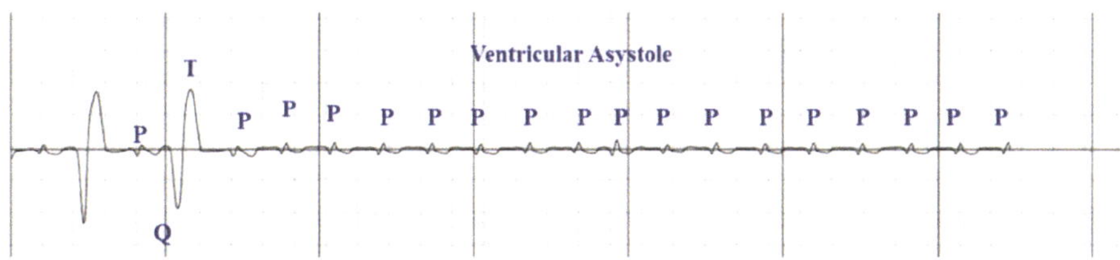

Fig. 187: Electrocardiogram (Lead II, sensitivity 1, speed 25 mm/second) of an adult dog is showing ventricular asystole with severe complete AV Block. Ventricular activity is seen only in two complexes in the beginning of the strip. Thereafter all P waves are blocked showing no ventricular activity.

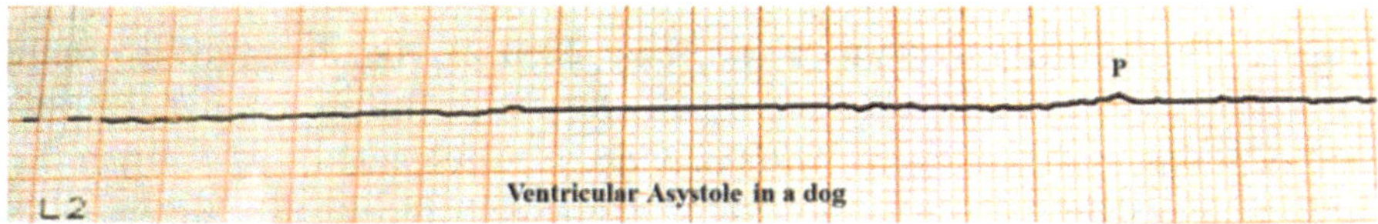

Fig. 188: Electrocardiogram (Lead II, sensitivity 1, speed 25 mm/second) is showing ventricular asystole in a dog with severe AV block. A small P wave (atrial activity) is seen at one place; there is no ventricular activity.

A-V Conduction Disturbances

Atrio-ventricular (AV) conduction time is the time period between onset of atrial depolarization and the onset of ventricular depolarization. P-R interval in electrocardiogram represents AV conduction time i.e. the total time taken by the depolarization wave in travelling from SA node to AV node plus time taken in travelling through head region of AV node plus travel time from the AV node to the initial portions of the apex of the intraventricular septum.

(AV conduction time = Time taken by depolarization wave in travelling from SA node to AV node + time taken in travelling through head region of AV node + time taken in travelling from head region to initial portion of the apex of the intraventricular septum).

Normally P-R interval in the electrocardiogram of the healthy dogs varies from 0.07 to 0.13 second with smaller duration in toy and large duration in giant breeds. Any deviation from normal values of P-R interval leads to conduction disturbances. Various types of alterations either alone or in combination occur in the electrocardiogram of the dogs affected with conduction disturbances due to delayed or blocked electrical transmission at some point in conduction system. The delay in transmission of electrical current may be located in AV node, or block in bundle of His, or block at the level of bundle branches. The conduction disturbances are classified as Heart Blocks / Atrio-ventricular (AV) blocks , Bundle branch blocks ,and Wolf-Parkinson-White Syndrome (W-P-W syndrome). Though, intracardiac electrocardiogram reliably locate the site of an AV- block, surface electrocardiogram can also be employed to ascertain the diagnosis.

When supraventricular impulse passing through the AV junction and bundle of His is either delayed or interrupted, it is termed as AV block. AV blocks are of three degrees i.e. 1st, 2nd and 3rd degree AV blocks or Heart blocks.

Bundle branch blocks are further grouped as right bundle branch block (RBBB) and left bundle branch block (LBBB).

1st degree A-V block

On surface electrocardiogram , 1st degree A-V block is manifested by usually normal heart rate with sinus rhythm, all complexes having normal 'P' wave and 'QRS' complexes, every 'QRS' having 'P' wave, and consistent but P-R interval of > 0.13 s (Fig.189). In cats 1st degree A-V block is characterized by P-R interval of >0.09 s (Fig. 190). Prolongation of P-R interval can be due to delays at any level in the conduction system. Generally 'QRS' complex is narrow or of normal duration. 1st degree block generally does not carry much clinical significance as it may be seen in clinically healthy dogs also. AV blocks may also occur in aging dogs because of degenerative changes in AV conduction system. 1st degree AV blocks are quite common in geriatric Cocker Spaniels and Dachshunds. P-R interval is inversely related to heart rate i.e. it is shorter with increased heart rate. It is positively related to age i.e. it lengthens with age. 1st degree AV blocks may be seen in severe digitalis intoxication, hyperkalemia, hypokalemia and in dogs given propranolol, quinidine or procainamide. 1st degree heart block does not need any therapeutic intervention.

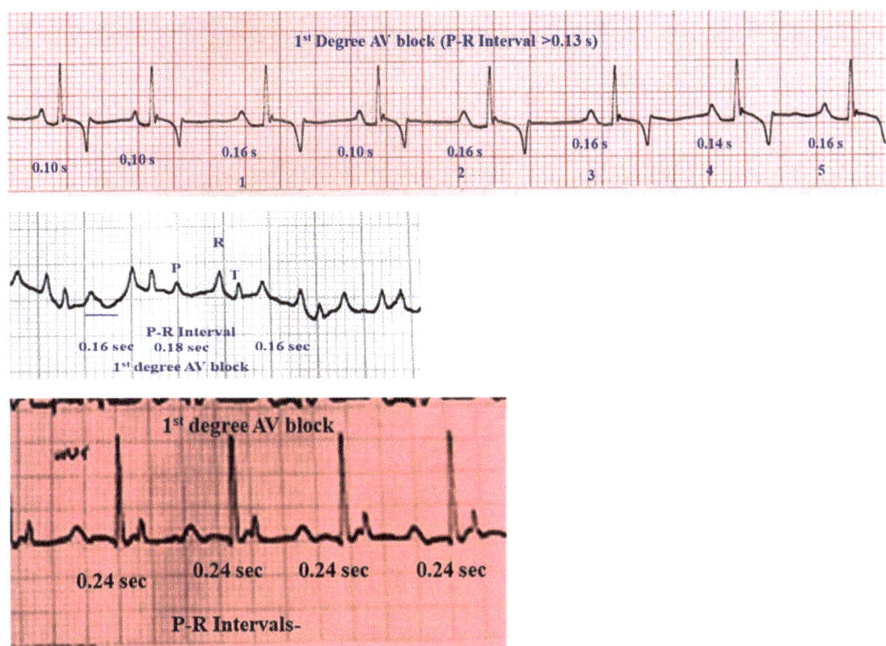

Fig. 189: Surface electrocardiograms of dogs (Lead II, sensitivity 1, speed 25 mm/second) are showing 1st degree AV Block as P-R interval is > 0.13 sec. 'QRS' complexes in all the three electrocardiograms are either narrow or normal.

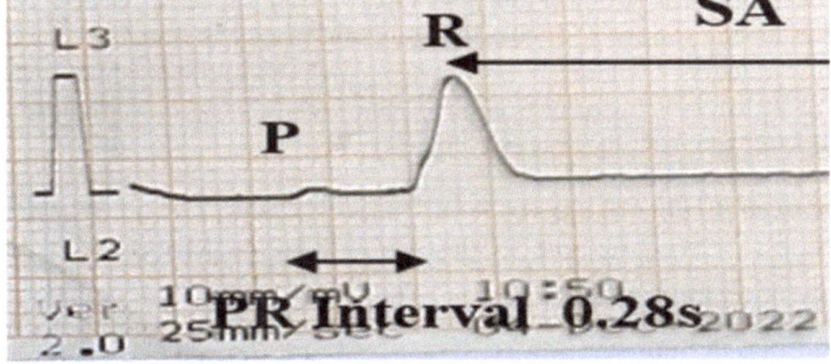

Fig. 190: Surface electrocardiogram of a cat (Lead II, sensitivity 1, speed 25 mm/second) is showing 1st degree AV Block owing to a long P-R interval of 0.28 s (> 0.09 s).

2nd degree A-V block

2nd degree A-V block or 2nd degree heart block is electrocardiographically characterized by normal or slow heart rate, rhythm broken by absence of one or several 'QRS complexes i.e. P wave (s) without 'QRS' complex (Fig. 191), normal ECG complexes with P and QRS of normal configuration. There is intermittent failure or interference in AV conduction system.

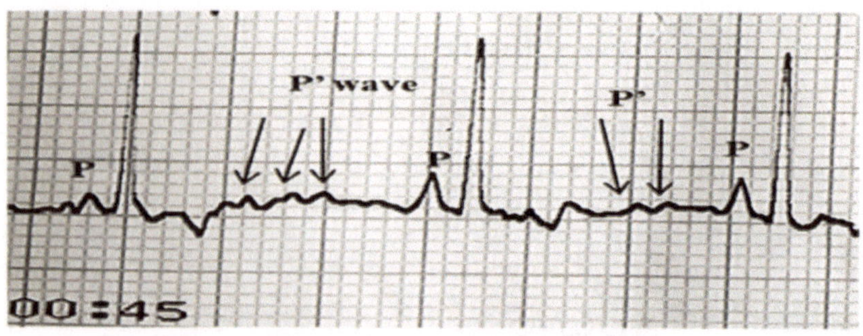

A

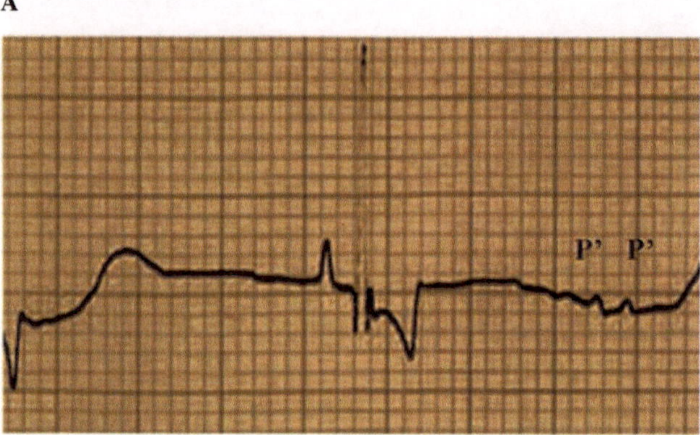

B

Fig. 191: Surface electrocardiograms (A and B) of dogs (speed 25 mm/s, sensitivity 1) are showing normal complexes having P wave with QRS complex of normal configuration. There are P' waves in both electrocardiograms. These P' waves are non-conducted and are without QRS complex. Configuration of P' waves is different from the P wave. These electrocardiographic changes are suggestive of 2nd degree A-V block or heart block.

2nd degree A-V block or heart block has been further categorized as 2nd degree A-V block Mobitz type I or type A, and 2nd degree A-V block Mobitz type II or type B.

Mobitz type I (Wenckebach phenomenon) or Type A 2nd degree A-V block is electrocardiographically characterized by progressive prolongation of P-R interval until a P wave is blocked (Fig.192). In many cases this pattern is not followed. Only longest PR interval is seen with the last conducted P wave. The block occurs in the A-V node and QRS complex is generally narrow or normal. Atrial rate is higher than the ventricular rate as there are more numbers of P waves. The rhythm is regularly irregular. Configuration of P and QRS is normal.

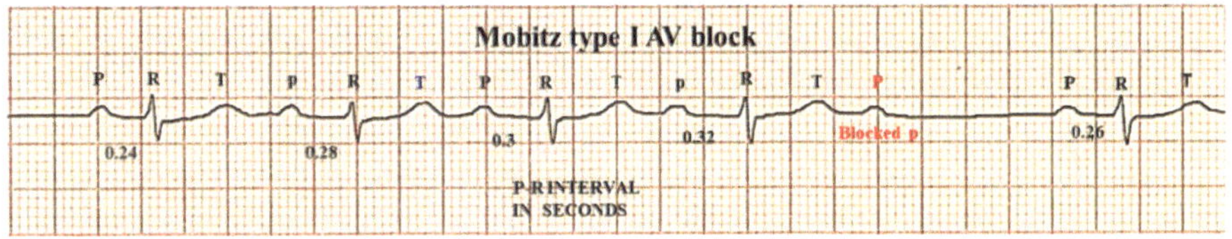

Fig. 192: Electrocardiogram (Lead II, sensitivity 1, speed 25 mm/second) of a dog is showing 2nd degree A.V Block (Mobitz type I or Type A). P (marked with red colour) is without QRS complex. P-R interval is varying and is progressively prolonged (from 0.24 to 0.32 s) before the blocked P (marked with red colour).

Mobitz type II or Type B 2nd degree A-V block in dogs (Fig.193) and in cats (Fig.194) is electrocardiographically characterized by uniform P-R interval preceding the blocked impulse and fixed relationship between atrium and ventricle depolarization. In this type of A-V block , QRS is not narrow (wide as compared to that in Mobitz type I A-V block). Atrial rate is higher than the ventricular rate. Rhythm is broken by the absence of QRS complex (one or more). P wave is of normal configuration. Abnormal QRS suggests that the defect in conduction of current is in the Bundle of His or proximal bundle branches. In this type of AV block there is fixed relationship between atria and ventricles of 2:1 (Fig.193), 3:1, 4:1 (P waves: QRS complex). PR interval is generally constant and may be normal or slightly longer. It may be normal in some young dogs and may be associated with sinus arrhythmia or may be associated with supraventricular tachycardia; microscopic fibrosis; hereditary stenosis of bundle of His in pugs; or toxicity of digitalis, low doses IV atropine, xylazine, quinidine; or electrolyte imbalances.

Usually no treatment is required in dogs with Mobitz type I (A) AV block. Dogs with Mobitz type II (B) AV block requires treatment because of wide QRS as they have the tendency to develop 3rd degree AV block. The treatment with atropine, glycopyrrolate, isoproterenol or pacemaker may be instituted as per the merit of the case.

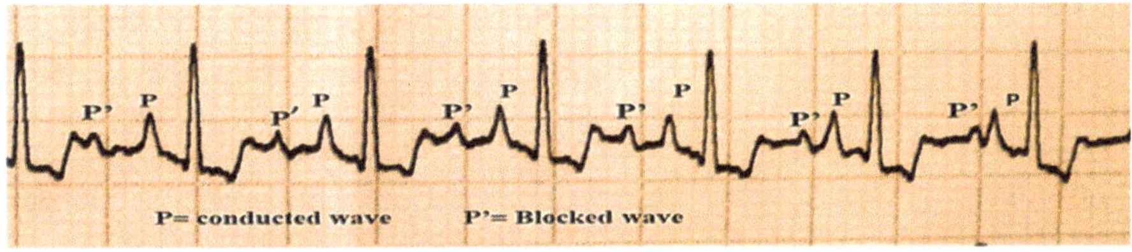

Fig. 193: Electrocardiogram (Lead II, sensitivity 1, speed 25 mm/second) of a dog is showing 2nd degree A.V Block (Mobitz type II or Type B). P' without QRS complex and PR interval preceding the blocked impulse is uniform (0.10 s). There is a fixed relationship between atrium and ventricle of 2:1 (2 P: 1 QRS).

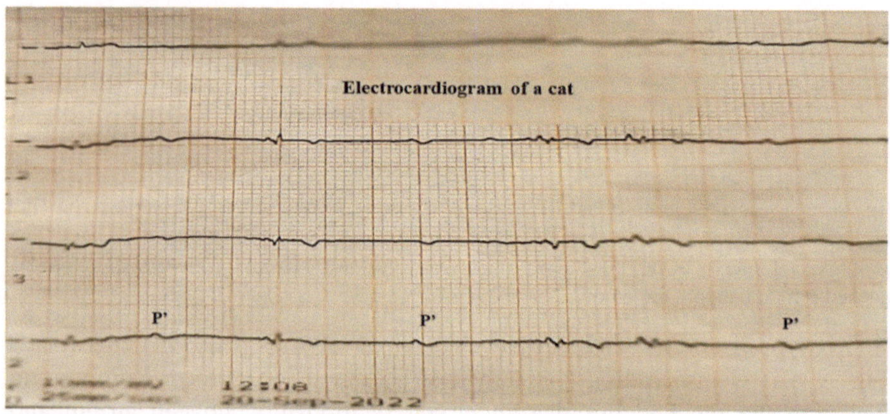

Fig. 194: Electrocardiogram (Lead I, II, III, aVR, aVL, aVF; sensitivity 1, speed 25 mm/second) of a cat is showing 2nd degree AV Block (Mobitz type II or Type B). The P' waves are without QRS complex and PR interval preceding the blocked impulse are almost uniform. The 'QRS' complex is almost normal. The 'P' wave of sinus complex is normal. Ventricular rate is slower than atrial rate.

3rd degree A-V block or Complete Heart Block

3rd degree A-V block or complete heart block (Fig.195 and 196) is electrocardiographically characterized by slow ventricular rate (< 60 bpm if junction escape rhythm or <40 if ventricular escape rhythm) , regular rhythm, more P waves than QRS complexes (ventricular rate is slower than atrial rate), varying P-R interval, no consistent relationship between atrial and ventricular beats, P waves of normal configuration , normal/bizarre QRS , no conduction between atria and ventricles, and constant P-P and R-R intervals. QRS becomes wide and bizarre when rescuing pacemaker is located in ventricle or in lower AV junction with bundle branch block. There is no AV conduction in 3rd degree AV block and pacemakers below the area of the block control ventricles i.e. atria and ventricles are activated by different pacemakers leading to no relationship between P waves and QRS complexes. Clinically 3rd degree AV block is associated with syncope or sometimes with congestive heart failure. Complete heart block has been associated with isolated congenital AV block, aortic stenosis, ventricular septal defect (VSD), digitalis toxicity, infiltrative cardiomyopathy, hypertrophic cardiomyopathy, amyloidosis, neoplasia, idiopathic fibrosis (old Cocker Spaniels), hyperkalemia, myocardial infarction and bacterial endocarditis.

Though treatment with atropine, isoproterenol and corticosteroids can be attempted, it is usually futile. In symptomatic dogs artificial pacing is required. A permanent cardiac pacemaker is the only solution for long term relief. Drugs for ventricular arrhythmias are not advised unless pacemaker is in place.

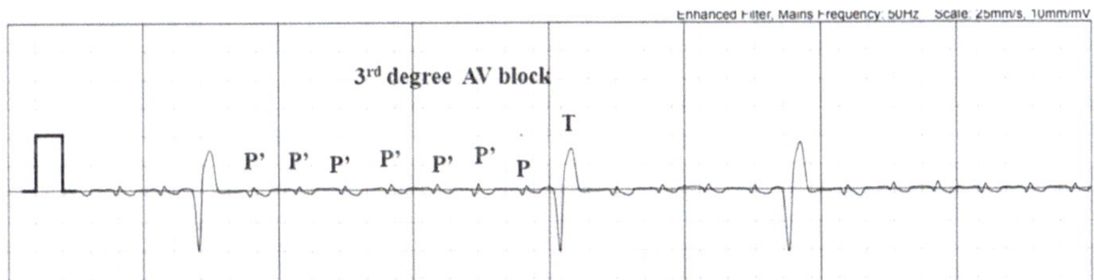

Fig. 195: Electrocardiogram (Lead II, sensitivity 1, speed 25 mm/second) of a dog is showing 3rd degree AV block. The ventricular rate is slow (30 beats per minute). There are number of P waves that are blocked with a slow ventricular rate.

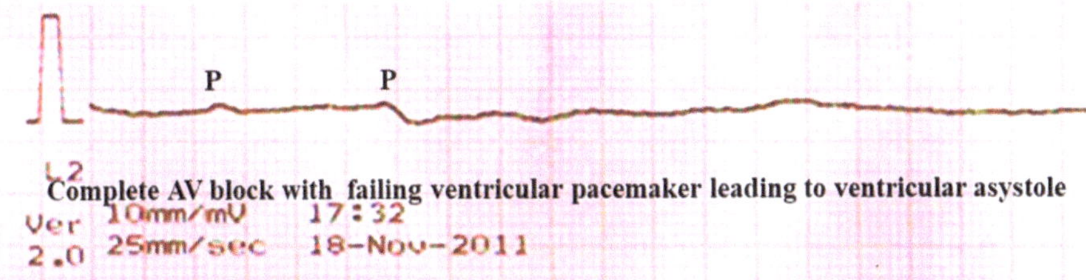

Fig. 196: Electrocardiogram (Lead II, sensitivity 1, speed 25 mm/second) of a dog is showing complete heart block with failing ventricular pacemaker leading to ventricular asystole. Both P waves are blocked and there is no ventricular activity.

Bundle Branch Block

Bundle of His divides in to left and right bundle branches. Left bundle branch is further divided into anterior and posterior fascicles interconnected with septal fascicle. Block may occur in left anterior or posterior fascicles or right bundle branch (Fig.197). Bundle branch block or intraventricular conduction defect is characterized by delay or block in any conduction pathways below the Bundle of His. Right bundle branch, left bundle branch, anterior and posterior fascicle of the left bundle branch are the major components of intraventricular conduction system (Fig.197). Delay or block occurring in any one, two or three pathways at a time may lead to delayed depolarization of ventricles causing changes in 'QRS' configuration. 'QRS' is generally broadened due to delay in depolarization.

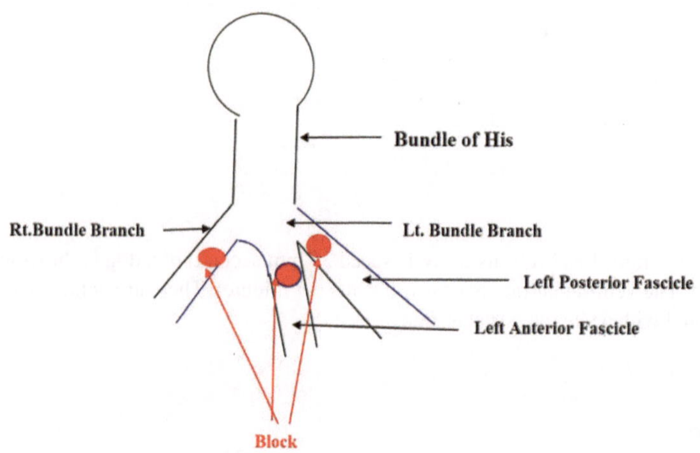

Fig. 197: Diagram is showing location of bundle branch and fascicular blocks.

Left Bundle Branch Block (LBBB)

Left bundle branch block in dogs (Fig.198) is electrocardiographically characterized by normal mean electrical axis (MEA) on frontal plane ; wide (0.07 second -Fig.199 and 200) and sloppy 'QRS'; wide and positive 'QRS' complex in leads I, II, III , aVF (Fig.199) , CV_6LL and CV_6LU; a small 'Q' wave in lead II (Fig.200), III and aVF (incomplete LBBB); a small 'Q' wave in lead I and left precordial leads (CV_6LL and CV_6LU); and inverted 'QRS' in lead aVR, aVL and CV5RL. These electrocardiographic features along with radiographic absence of left ventricular enlargement are indicative of left bundle branch block. If these features are associated with 1st or 2nd degree AV block (Fig. 201), involvement of right bundle branch is also speculated (Fig. 201). When broad QRS complexes are seen intermittently and fulfill the other criteria, they are termed as intermittent left bundle branch block (Fig.199 B).

Left bundle branch block is not very common in cats. It is electrocardiographically characterized by broad QRS (> 0.06 s) ; positive QRS in lead I,II,III and avF; and inverted QRS in aVR and aVL (Fig. 202). When 1st or 2nd degree AV blocks (Fig.202) are associated with broad QRS, right bundle branch block is also speculated.

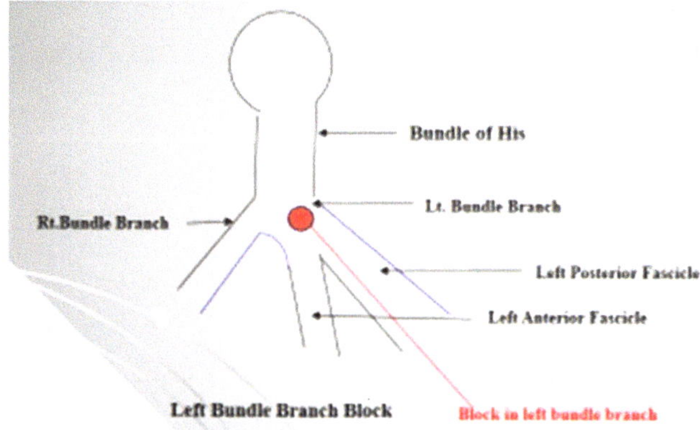

Fig. 198: Diagram is showing left bundle branch block

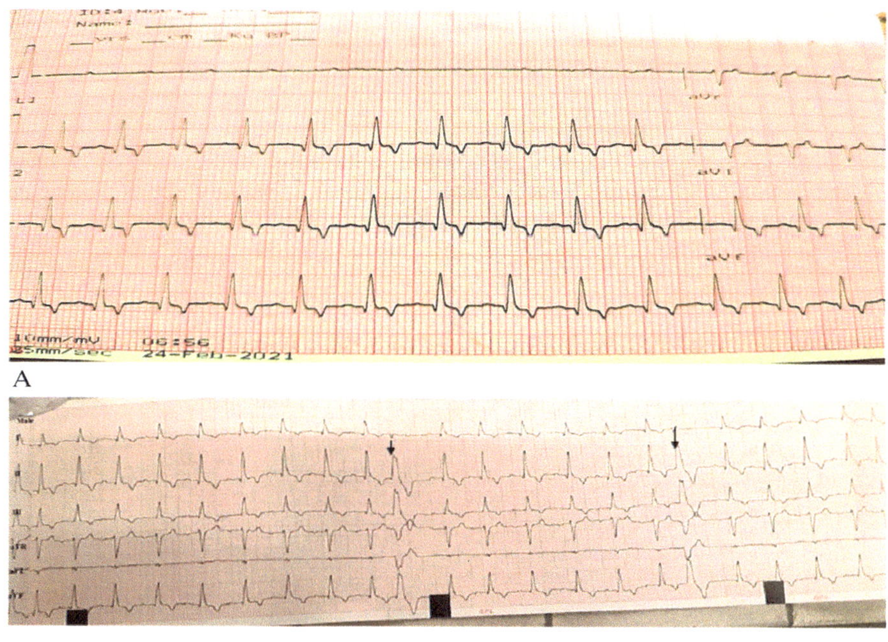

A

B

Fig. 199: A. Electrocardiogram (Lead I, II,III, aVR, aVL and aVF, sensitivity 1.0, speed 25 mm/second) of a dog is showing wide (> 0.07 second) and positive 'QRS' in Lead I,II,III and aVF; inverted broad 'QRS' in aVR and aVL and normal amplitude of QRS (R 0.8 mV) suggesting left bundle branch block. **B.** Electrocardiogram (Lead I, II,III, aVR, aVL and aVF, sensitivity 1.0, speed 50 mm/second) of a Pug with dilated cardiomyopathy is showing wider (0.08 second) QRS in the 10th and 17th complexes in Lead II (marked by black arrow), III and aVF; these broad QRS are inverted in aVR and aVL ; amplitude of QRS is normal suggesting intermittent left bundle branch block.

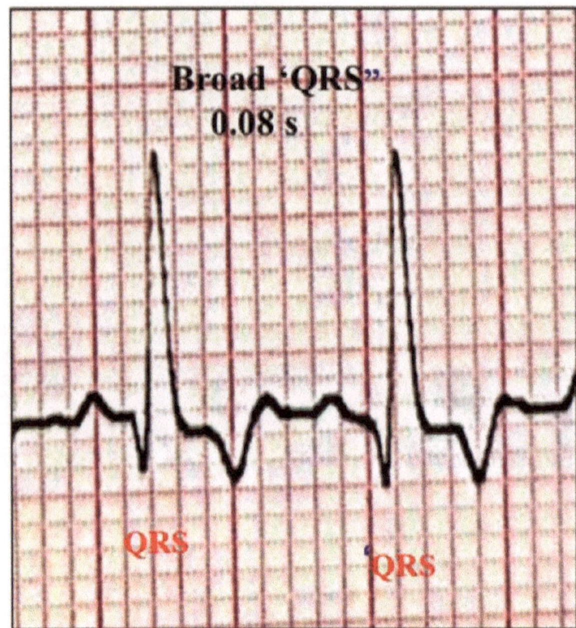

Fig. 200: Electrocardiogram of a dog (Lead II, sensitivity 1.0, speed 25 mm/second) is showing wide and positive (0.08 second) 'QRS' in lead II with normal amplitude of the 'R' wave (1.9 mV) and small 'Q' (0.2 mV) in lead II suggesting Incomplete left bundle branch block.

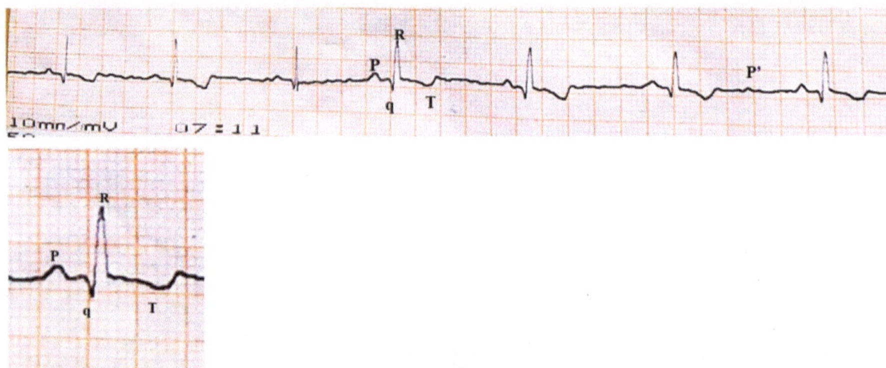

Fig. 201: Electrocardiogram of a dog (lead II, sensitivity 1, speed 25 mm/s) is showing incomplete left bundle branch block and intermittent right bundle branch block. In first three complexes the 'QRS' is narrow (< 0.03 mV) while in 4th, 5th, 6th, and 7th complexes the 'QR' is wide (0.08 mV) with a small 'q' wave. The blocked P' wave (2nd degree AV block) suggests a probable intermittent right bundle branch block also. The ECG is suggestive of incomplete left bundle branch block with intermittent right bundle branch block.

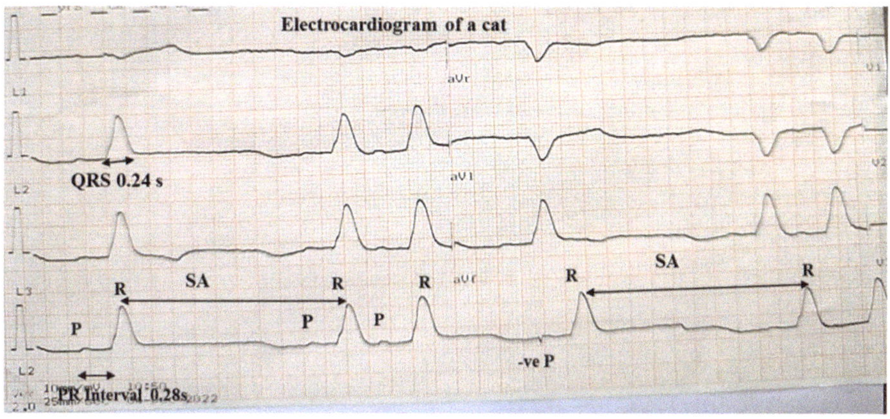

Fig. 202: Electrocardiogram of a cat (lead I, II, III, aVR, aVL and aVF; sensitivity 1, speed 25 mm/s) is showing wide (0.24 s) and positive 'QRS' in lead I, II, III and aVF; inverted QRS in lead aVR and aVL; long pauses of 2.08 s (> twice of normal R-R interval of 0.68 s); negative P wave (4th from the left) ; and long P-R interval (0.28 s > 0.09 s). This electrocardiogram is suggestive of left bundle branch block (due to wide QRS) along with involvement of right bundle branch block also (due to long P-R interval – 1st degree AV block), sinus arrest (due to long pauses (R-R interval), and AV junctional premature complex (-ve P wave 4th from the left).

Fascicular Block

Anterior and posterior fascicles are the division of left bundle branch. Block may occur in left anterior or left posterior fascicles. Block in the fascicles slightly prolongs ventricular depolarization.

Left anterior fascicular block (Fig.203) is electrocardiographically characterized by QRS of normal duration ; left deviated mean electrical axis (MEA) on frontal plane ; small q and tall R in lead I and aVL; and deep S in leads II,III and aVF . Left anterior fascicular block has been seen in cases of ventricular pre-excitation, hyperkalemia, left ventricular hypertrophy, and changed position of the heart within thorax.

In cats, left anterior fascicular block is electrocardiographically characterized by QRS of normal duration, tall R wave in lead I and aVF, deep S in lead II,III and aVF, isoelectric aVR, and left axis deviation (Fig.204). A small q wave in lead I and aVL has also be seen in humans.

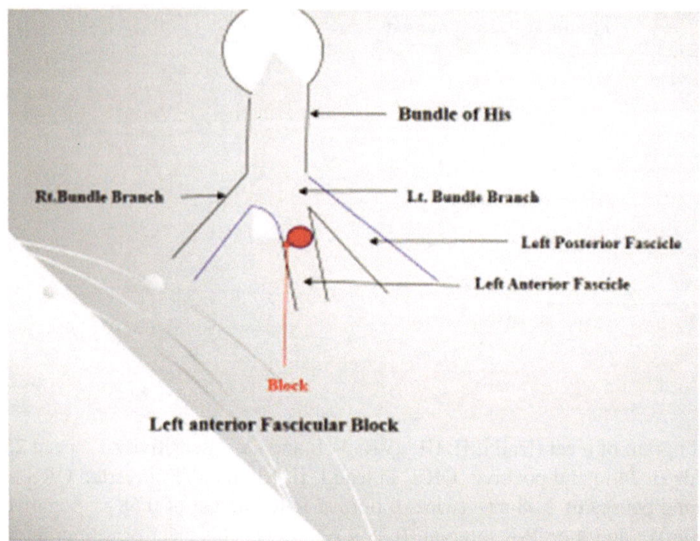

Fig. 203: Diagram is showing left anterior fascicular block.

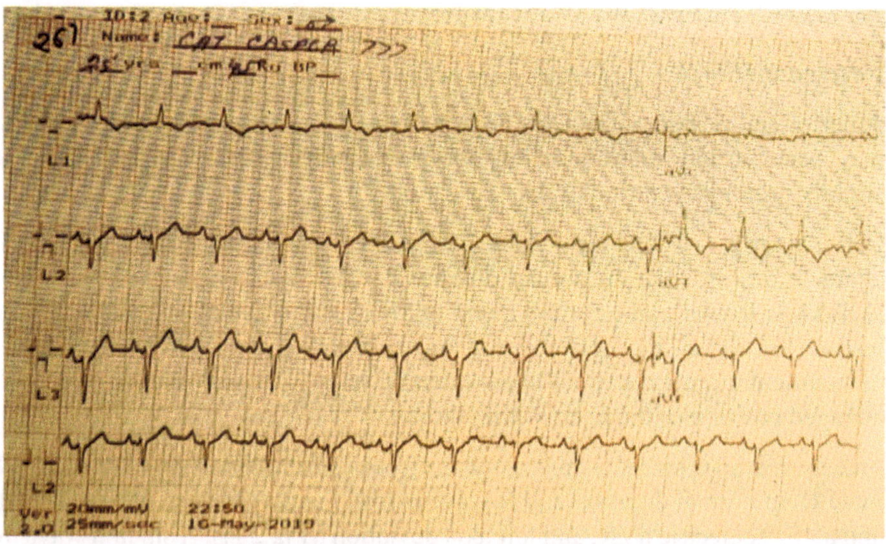

Fig. 204: Electrocardiogram (Lead I, II,III, aVL, and aVF ,sensitivity 2.0, speed 25 mm/second) of a cat is showing tall R wave in lead I and aVL; normal QRS (0.03-0.04 s) ; deep S in lead II,III and aVF exceeding r wave, isoelectric aVR and left axis deviation (-65^0) suggesting left anterior fascicular block. There is no small q waves in lead I. It may be seen sometimes.

Left posterior fascicular block in dogs is characterized by normal thoracic radiograph, right axis deviation, rs pattern of QRS in leads I, aVF; qR pattern with large R in leads II,III and aVF. Not much information is available about left posterior fascicular block in dogs.

Right Bundle Branch Block (RBBB)

Right bundle branch block (Fig. 205) is electrocardiographically (Fig. 206,207, 208) characterized by right axis deviation on frontal plane (MEA >104^0), positive QRS in aVR, aVL and CV5RL, wide QRS (>0.07 second) showing 'RSR' or 'rsR' pattern , wide 'S' (in lead I,II,III, aVF, CV6LL, CV6LU), 'S' wave or W pattern in lead V10. 'QRS' of normal duration having any 2 to 4 other criteria such as right axis deviation, positive QRS (lead aVR, aVL , CV5RL), wide 'S' (lead I,II,III, aVF, CV6LL, CV6LU), or 'S' wave or 'W' pattern in lead V10 is indicative of incomplete right bundle branch block (RBBB). Radiographic absence of right ventricular enlargement in dogs with these electrocardiographic features can differentiate between right bundle branch block and right ventricular enlargement. The presence of 1st or 2nd degree AV block in the electrocardiograms with the features of right bundle branch block may indicate involvement of left bundle branch also.

Right bundle branch block in cats is electrocardiographically characterized by broad QRS; right axis deviation (Fig. 209); positive QRS in aVR (Fig.209) and CV5RL; wide QRS (M shaped, rsR or RSR pattern) in CV5RL; large S wave in lead I,II,III, aVF (Fig.209), CV6LL, and CV6LU. If 1st and 2nd degree AV block is also seen in the electrocardiogram with changes mentioned earlier, left bundle branch block is also associated. QRS of normal duration with right axis deviation, positive QRS in aVR and large S in lead I, II, III, aVF is suggestive of incomplete right bundle branch block in cats (Fig.209).

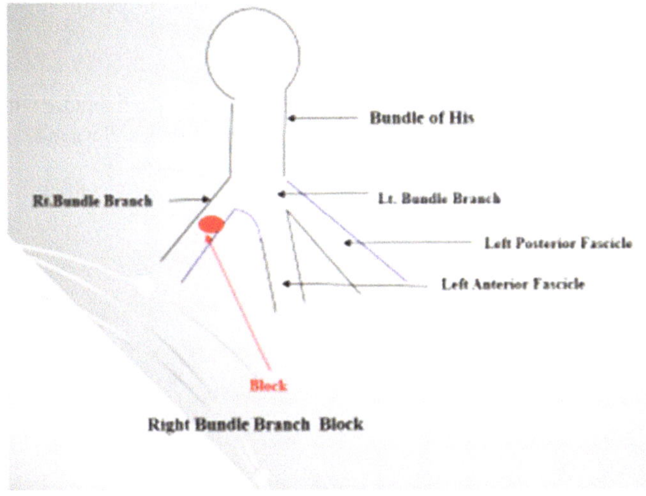

Fig. 205: Diagram is showing right bundle branch block

Right bundle branch block has been observed in healthy dogs also. It is also associated with congenital heart disease, chronic valvular fibrosis, cardiac tumour, trauma, cardiac needle puncture, cardiac surgery, or chronic *Trypanosoma cruzi* infection.

Generally therapy is instituted for the primary heart disease. Right bundle branch block usually does not cause much clinical problem. When right bundle branch block is associated with complete heart block, treatment becomes essential.

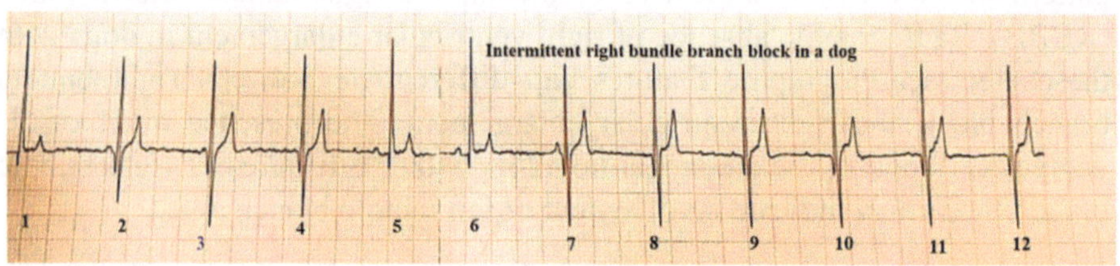

Fig. 206: Electrocardiogram (Lead II, sensitivity 1.0, speed 25 mm/second) of a geriatric Labrador dog is showing intermittent right bundle branch block. Complexes 1, 5, 6 are normal while complexes 2,3,4,7,8,9,10,11 and 12 are showing right bundle branch pattern. Wide (0.07 second) 'QRS' with deep 'S' wave (0.9 mV to 1.2 mV in complexes 2 to 4 and 7 to 12) interrupted with normal QRS (1,5,6) are suggesting intermittent right bundle branch block.

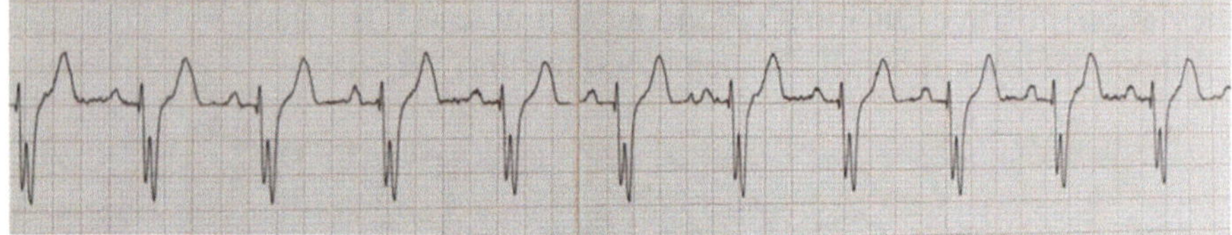

Fig. 207: Electrocardiogram (Lead II, sensitivity 1.0, speed 50 mm/second) of a Labrador with congestive heart failure is showing right bundle branch block. The QRS is 0.08 s. S wave is deep (1.5 mV).

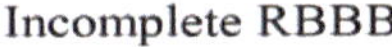

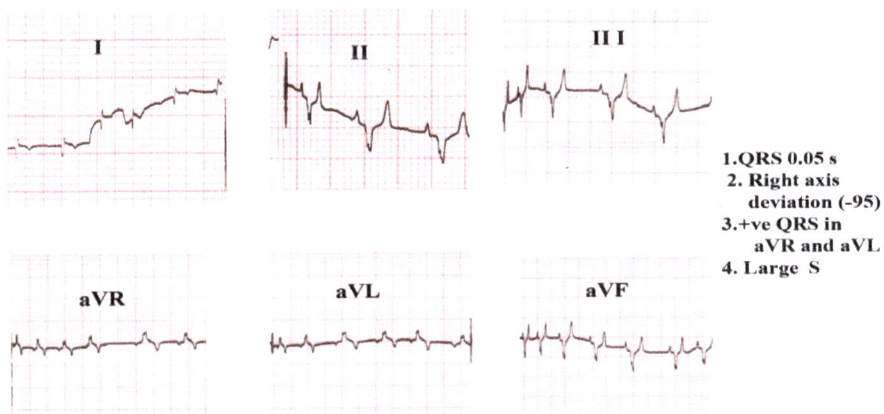

Fig. 208: Electrocardiogram (Lead I, II, III, aVL and aVF, sensitivity 1, speed 25 mm/s) of a dog is showing QRS of 0.05 s, right axis deviation (-95^0), positive QRS complex in aVR and aVL leads and deep S in lead I,II,III and aVF suggesting incomplete right bundle branch block.

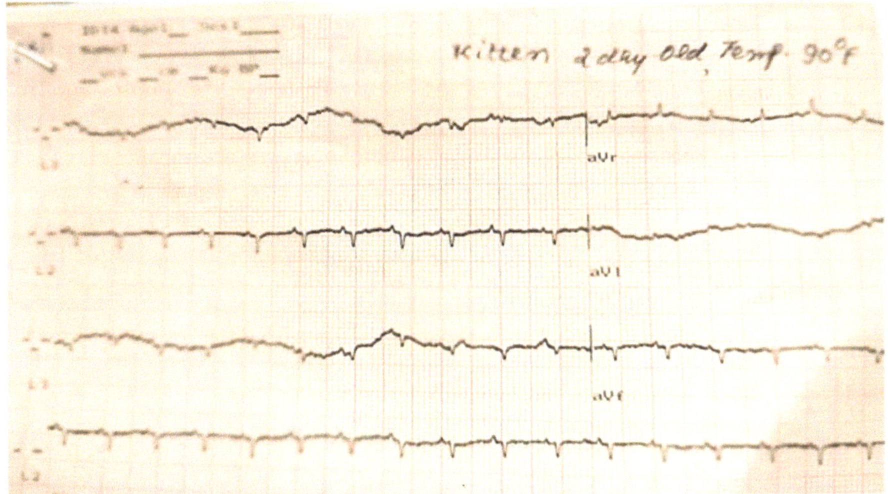

Fig. 209: Electrocardiogram (Lead I,II,III, aVR, aVLand aVF sensitivity 1, speed 25 mm/s) of a two day old kitten with hypothermia (rectal temperature 90^{0}F) is showing QRS of 0.04 s, right axis deviation (-120^0), positive QRS complex in aVR and large S in lead I, II, III, avF suggesting incomplete right bundle branch block.

Right Bundle Branch and Left Anterior Fascicular Block

Right bundle branch with left anterior fascicular block (Fig.210) is electrocardiographically characterized by marked left axis deviation

(< + 40°) on frontal plane, broad 'QRS' (>0.07 s), rsR or RSR pattern of QRS in CV_5RL, wide and deep 'S'(lead I,II,III, aVF and CV6LU), tall 'R' and small 'q' (in lead I and aVL).

Electrocardiographic features of right bundle branch block and anterior fascicular block in cats are wide QRS, marked left axis deviation (> -60°), long and broad S wave in leads I,II,III,aVF and CV_6LU, and wide QRS in CV_5RL.

Right bundle branch and left anterior fascicular block has been associated with hypertrophic cardiomyopathy, causes of hyperkalemia and left ventricular hypertrophy, myocardial infarction and post-surgical repair of cardiac defects.

Right bundle branch and left anterior fascicular block, in itself, does not warrant any treatment as hemodynamic abnormalities are not severe. Generally treatment is directed at the primary underlying etiology. The right bundle branch and left anterior fascicular block may lead to symptomatic severe 2nd or 3rd degree AV block requiring insertion of pacemaker.

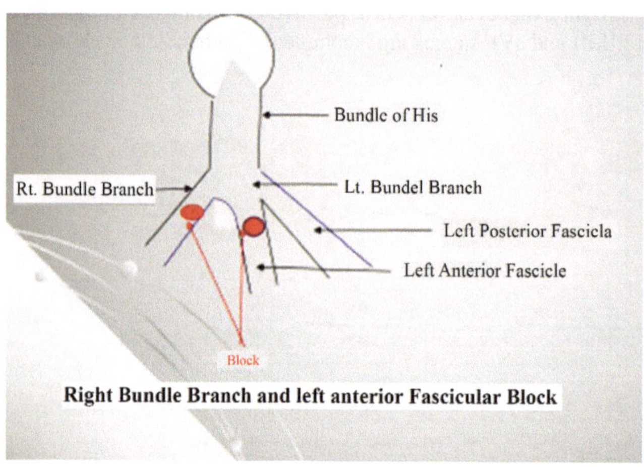

Fig. 210: Diagram is showing right bundle branch and left anterior fascicular block.

Further Readings

Boswood, A.M.A. (2007). ECG Interpretation. Proceedings, WSAVA world congress.

Côté, E.(2010) . Electrocardiography and Cardiac Arrhythmias. pp. 1159–1187. In: Textbook of Veterinary Internal Medicine, 7th ed. (Ettinger, S. J. and Feldman, E. eds.) WB Saunders, Philadelphia

Tilley, L. P. (1992). Analysis of canine P-QRS-S deflections. In: Essentials of Canine and Feline Electrocardiography. 3rd ed., Lea and Febiger, Philadelphia. pp 59-99.

11

Therapeutics of Arrhythmias and Conduction Disturbances

Though the treatment for arrhythmias has been recommended for even a single premature beat, in the current scenario the treatment is indicated when there are more than 17 VPCs per minute. In certain situations the side effects or proarrhythmic effects of drugs can lead to morbidity or mortality. As a result, new guidelines are proposed when evaluating the need for treatment of arrhythmias. Keeping the adverse effects of antiarrhythmic agents in mind, one should be selective about which arrhythmias are to be treated. The goal of antiarrhythmic therapy includes the treatment of an existing arrhythmia or prophylaxis for anticipated arrhythmias. The use of antiarrhythmic agents for prophylaxis should be considered carefully, as only a few antiarrhythmic agents have been approved for the use in veterinary medicine and these agents may have considerable risk associated with their use. The successful prophylactic use of beta-blocking antiarrhythmic agents in human medicine has stimulated interest in the prevention of arrhythmias in veterinary patients with conditions that are also associated with sudden death, such as dilated cardiomyopathy. Sudden cardiac death can occur from ventricular fibrillation, ventricular asystole, or electrical-mechanical dissociation. The antiarrhythmic drugs can reduce the frequency of dangerous arrhythmias alleviating the related clinical signs and thus reduce the risk of death. However, these drugs can have antiarrhythmic effects without anti-fibrillatory effects and vice versa. Most antiarrhythmic drugs exert its effects on normal myocardium to some extent and may have intrinsic arrhythmogenic properties termed as proarrhythmic properties. In general, the antiarrhythmic drugs are used to manage life threatening arrhythmias to minimise the risk of sudden cardiac arrest. In other words, treatment of arrhythmias is aimed to alleviate clinical signs such as, syncope and weakness that precipitate heart failure; and to prolong survival period.

Till date, the Vaughan-Williams classification system is the most commonly used that attempts to group antiarrhythmic drugs based on their major ion channel or receptor effect. Besides treating arrhythmias alone, its underlying cause should also be identified for sustainable outcome. For example, atrial standstill as a result of hyperkalaemia in a dog associated with cystic calculi or obstruction, is best addressed by correcting the underlying etiology rather than attempting antiarrhythmic therapy towards hyperkalemia.

As most of the antiarrhythmic drugs work at the level of the relevant ion channels, a basic knowledge on the electrophysiology associated with the generation of the cardiac action potential is essential. The pacemaker cells of the sinoatrial node are responsible for the generation of the normal sinus rhythm. The sinus node depolarizes, followed by the atrial depolarization wave, atrioventricular nodal conduction, bundle branch conduction, and ventricular depolarization. The shape of the action potential differs between the cardiac myocytes and pacemaker cells, reflecting the prominent role that differences in ion channels play in the function of cardiac tissues. The pharmacological action of most of the antiarrhythmic drugs are complex and also differ with species, age, tissue-drug concentration, acid-base and electrolyte balance, presence or absence of myocardial damage, and indirect hemodynamic or autonomic actions. In order to overcome certain limitations of the existing Vaughan-Williams system, electrophysiologists attempted to develop the Sicilian Gambit in 1991. The Vaughan Williams system divides the antiarrhythmic drugs into four classes on the basis of their major electrophysiological effects on the myocardium. Because antiarrhythmic drugs are associated with electrophysiological effects on the myocardium, these antiarrhythmic drugs share the paradoxical side effect of being proarrhythmic. Electrolyte abnormalities will potentiate this arrhythmogenic effect, underscoring the value of correcting any underlying or concurrent electrolyte abnormalities whenever possible.

Classification of Antiarrhythmic Drugs

The classification of antiarrhythmic drugs is typically based on their predominant electrophysiologic effect on myocardial cells. Further, this classification scheme does not always aid in selection of a specific antiarrhythmic for a specific condition.

- Class I: Na channel blockers
- Class II: β-blocker
- Class III: K channel blockers
- Class IV: Ca channel blockers

Class I Antiarrhythmic

These agents are commonly known as "membrane-stabilizing agents" that work by selectively blocking a proportion of the fast sodium channels in cardiomyocytes, leading to depression of phase 0 of the action potential that finally result in a reduction in conduction velocity. The relative potency of their sodium channel effects, whether blockade of the activated or inactivated channel occurs, and their effects on other channels and receptors determine their subclassification. Based on their concurrent effects on repolarization, these agents are further sub-classified into three subclasses (a, b, and c).

• Class Ia Agents

These agents have a powerful, fast sodium channel–blocking effect along with moderate blockade of the rapid component of the delayed rectifier potassium current, resulting in prolongation of action potential thus resulting in proarrhythmic effects in certain cases. Quinidine, procainamide, and disopyramide are the drugs in this group.

Quinidine is basically an antimalarial drug , absorbed rapidly after oral administration, has membrane-stabilizing properties relevant to class I agents and also has indirect, antivagal (atropine-like) effect in the atria. It is indicated in atrial fibrillation, supraventricular and ventricular arrhythmias. It has the potential to convert atrial fibrillation to sinus rhythm. The atropine-like effects of quinidine may result in increased impulse conduction through the AV node to the ventricles and paradoxical acceleration in ventricular response in animals with atrial fibrillation. In general, quinidine use should be avoided in dogs with severe myocardial failure or in dogs that have, or have had, heart failure. Quinidine should not be used in cats. The quinidine is administrated @5.0–10.0 mg/kg, IV, qid, or 6.0–20.0 mg/kg, PO, TID or QID in dogs.

The effects of procainamide are similar to those of quinidine. However, its effects on the autonomic nervous system are significantly weaker (less antivagal effect). Procainamide depresses conduction velocity and prolongs the effective refractory period in a wide variety of tissues, including the atrial and ventricular myocardium, accessory atrioventricular (AV) pathways, and retrograde fast AV nodal pathways. Procainamide can thus be effective in a wide variety of arrhythmias, either as a single agent or combined with other agents. It can be administered parenterally for acute termination of severe ventricular or supraventricular tachyarrhythmias. It must be administered slowly intravenously (over 5 to 10 minutes) to prevent hypotension. Agents that prolong AV nodal conduction time are given first for initial treatment of atrial tachyarrhythmia, because procainamide can enhance AV nodal conduction, thus worsening the ventricular response rate. Procainamide is more effective than lidocaine for acutely terminating these rhythms in human patients. It is rapidly and almost completely absorbed after oral administration and biotransformed extensively by the liver to inactive metabolites in dogs. It is administered @ 6.0 to 8.0 mg/kg IV over 5 to 10 minutes or 6.0 to 20 mg/kg IM in dogs. A constant rate infusion (CRI) of 20 to 40 µg/kg/min can be used once a therapeutic response is obtained with bolus administration. Its adverse effects are hypotension and AV block (IV administration only), proarrhythmia and altered coat colour (long term administration), and GI disturbances (with the oral formulations). Gastrointestinal side effects such as anorexia, nausea, and vomiting are seen most commonly in dogs.

- **Class I b Agents**

Lidocaine, mexiletine, and tocainide are the common agents under class I b antiarrhythmic drugs. Among these the lidocaine is most commonly used. Lidocaine is well absorbed from the GI tract, but is extensively metabolized and subject to a high first-pass effect, resulting in poor bioavailability. It is used predominantly for treatment of acute ventricular arrhythmias. It has no efficacy against supraventricular arrhythmias and minimal effects on the autonomic nervous system. It is an ideal drug for treatment of acute ventricular arrhythmia because it has a rapid onset of action and short half-life (~1 hr in a dog) and is effective and safe. It exerts its antiarrhythmic action by blocking inactive sodium channels for a short duration of time. It is the drug of choice for ventricular tachyarrhythmias. It has the benefit of minimal hemodynamic, sinoatrial, and AV nodal effects at standard dosages. Liver disorders such as hepatitis or cirrhosis that effects hepatic blood flow, prolong its half-life as it is predominantly metabolized in the liver. Heart failure, hypotension, and severe hepatic disease can therefore result in decreased lidocaine metabolism and predispose the patient to lidocaine toxicity. Lidocaine is available only as a parenteral formulation for IV administration. Care should be taken to avoid the administration of lidocaine through the same catheter or line as other medications. The standard dose in dogs is to administer @ 2 mg/kg, IV boluses over 1 min to effect (slowing the ventricular arrhythmia or conversion to sinus rhythm) or to a cumulative dose of 8 mg/kg over 30 min. Due to its short half-life, it may be repeated as boluses or a CRI (25–75 mcg/kg/min) to maintain rhythm control. There are generally few side effects associated with orally administered lidocaine, but rapid IV administration can cause hypotension and seizures. There is some evidence to suggest that the use of combinations of Class 1a and 1b antiarrhythmics (procainamide, quinidine, tocainide, and mexiletine) may increase longevity, as reported in a retrospective study of Doberman Pinchers with severe ventricular arrhythmias.

Mexiletine is an oral analogue of lidocaine used to treat ventricular arrhythmias in dogs and it is highly protein bound and eliminated by renal excretion. It is rarely used as monotherapy for ventricular arrhythmias. It is most often an adjunctive treatment in severe, chronic ventricular arrhythmias not well controlled by sotalol alone or in dogs that do not tolerate sotalol. It should be administered at its lowest effective dose with food to limit toxicity. Its indications and common side effects are similar to those of lidocaine. It has been used in dogs in which ventricular tachyarrhythmias are acutely responsive to lidocaine and can be combined with class I a, II, or III agents. It is administered at a standard dose of 4 to 6 mg/kg PO TID. Anorexia, vomiting, tremors, and hepatic toxicity are some of the common side effects.

Tocainide, another lidocaine congener to treat ventricular arrhythmias, is rarely used in dogs because of the high incidence of serious side effects (CNS and GI disturbances, hypotension, renal failure and corneal dystrophy) . It can be used in dogs that do not tolerate sotalol and also as an add-on therapy for severe chronic ventricular arrhythmias. The drug is used @ 15.0 – 20.0 mg/kg, PO, TID in dogs.

• Class I c Agents

Flecainide, encainide and propafenone are some of the class I c antiarrhythmic drugs available but has only been used in dogs under experimental conditions. Flecainide exhibits a prolonged blockage of fast Na+ channels and it is particularly efficacious in prolonging the atrial action potential at fast heart rates, unlike the class Ia agents, making it useful for the therapy of atrial fibrillation and supraventricular tachycardia in humans.

Class II Antiarrhythmic

Class II antiarrhythmic drugs are β-adrenergic receptor blocking agents useful particularly in the blockade of arrhythmias enhanced by catecholamines. These β-Blockers can be either nonselective (block both β_1 and β_2 receptors) or selective (block predominantly β_1 receptors). As these agents decrease the down-regulation of β receptors in CHF, they can also be beneficial in allowing activation of receptors during times of stress and exercise. Further, all the β-blockers are dose-dependent and can act as negative inotropes and chronotropes. As a class these agents started as nonselective beta blockers such as, propranolol and subsequently in order to limit the adverse effects associated with β_2-receptor blockade, selective β_1-receptor blockers (atenolol) were identified. Currently available third-generation β-blockers (carvedilol) were developed that are more complete adrenergic blockers blocking β_1, β_2 and α_1-receptor.

Propranolol is a non-selective beta receptor blocking agent that should be avoided or cautiously used in dogs with asthma (as it cause bronchospasm). The drug is used at the dose of is 0.2–1 mg/kg, PO, TID

Atenolol is most commonly used selective beta blocker in dogs as it selectively blocks β_1 receptors. The drug can safely be given in dogs with respiratory diseases as it doesn't affect bronchospasm. The drug is used at the dose of 0.2–1 mg/kg, PO, BID in dogs, particularly in a gradual up titration. Similarly, the drug can be discontinued by titrating down gradually. The most potent side effects are usually dose related and more likely if underlying systolic function is present. Adverse effects include myocardial depression, bradycardia (sinus and AV block), and hypotension.

Carvedilol is a recent generation β-blocker with complete adrenergic blocking spectrum. In addition to β_1, β_2, it also blocks α_1 receptors along with certain ancillary antioxidant properties. Though it is commonly used in the treatment of human heart failure, a meagre reports are available for its potential survival benefits in canine DCM with and without CHF. If β-blockers are used for this indication, the general thumb rule is to never initiate in the face of active heart failure (pulmonary edema), start low (initial dose), go slow (and titrate up), and aim high (target dose tolerated). The initial dosage in dogs is 0.15–0.25 mg/kg, PO, BID, titrated up by increasing the dose ~25% every 2 week while monitoring for clinical signs suggestive of decompensation. The target dosage is 1 mg/kg, PO, every 2 hr (if tolerated). Higher doses may be indicated in dogs concurrently receiving pimobendan and in dogs with cardiovascular disease (vs those with DCM).

Class III Antiarrhythmic

These drugs act on blocking the potassium channel and thus prolong the cardiac action potential and its refractory period. Sotalol and amiodarone are the classic drugs under this category.

Sotalol, a nonselective β-blocking agent, is most commonly used in long-term management of ventricular arrhythmias. It can be used as a sole drug or combined with mexiletine if rhythm control is suboptimal with sotalol alone. Apart from this combination, the drug is also used in combination with other cardiac drugs viz., ACE inhibitors, furosemide, spironolactone, and pimobendan. Only precaution while using this drug is that the sotalol should not be combined with other β-blockers like atenolol or other negative inotropes (diltiazem) and with another class III agent (amiodarone). This drug can be used at the dose rate of 1.0 –2.5 mg/kg, PO, BID . Its possible adverse effects include negative inotropy, bradyarrhythmia (sinus and AV block), and proarrhythmia.

Amiodarone prolongs the refractory period of atrial and ventricular myocardium and the AV junction. Apart from this electrophysiological affect, this drug has a combination of properties viz., sodium channel–blocking properties (class I effects), β- and α-receptor blockade (class II effects) and calcium channel blockade (class IV effects). Amiodarone is used to treat refractory conditions associated with life-threatening ventricular arrhythmias and atrial fibrillation. Similar to sotalol, amiodarone is also often used in combination with other drugs like ACE inhibitors, furosemide, spironolactone, and pimobendan. As it has β-blocking effects it should not be combined with other β-blockers or other negative inotropes and with another class III agent (sotalol). Its adverse effects include gastro-intestinal signs, blood dyscrasias and proarrhythmia. The hepatic dysfunction is another common adverse effect encountered clinically and are typically reversible after cessation of the therapy. The oral dosage of amiodarone in dogs is 8.0–10.0 mg/kg, PO, OD/BID for 7–10 days, and then decrease dose to 4.0–6.0 mg/kg/day for long-term treatment. It can also be used parenterally in dogs @ 2–5 mg/kg, IV, infused over 30–60 min.

Class IV Antiarrhythmic

The commonly used antiarrhythmic agents in this class are diltiazem and amlodipine, having a predominant electrophysiologic effect on blockade of the slow calcium channels in cardiac cells and vascular smooth muscle. The relative affinity of a drug in this class for cardiac versus vascular tissue determines its predominant effect. Amlodipine is most active in vascular smooth muscle where it causes vasodilation and is thus considered to be a vasodilator. While the diltiazem is most active in cardiac cells.

Diltiazem is most commonly used class IV antiarrhythmic agent in veterinary medicine, which slows AV conduction and sinus rate. It blocks entry of calcium into cardiomyocytes during the action potential, leading to a dose-dependent reduction in calcium release from the sarcoplasmic reticulum, limiting the availability of calcium to the contractile apparatus, and resulting in negative inotropy and positive lusitropy. It also blocks calcium channels in the specialized conduction tissue in the heart, on which automaticity of intrinsic pacemaker cells and AV conduction depend for normal function.

Blockade of calcium channels can slow heart rate and AV conduction. Diltiazem is therefore typically indicated for treatment of atrial fibrillation and other supraventricular arrhythmias in dogs. Diltiazem has no effect on ventricular arrhythmias. Its dosage in dogs is 0.05–0.2 mg/kg IV over 5 min, which can be repeated to a cumulative dose of 0.3 mg/kg, after which the dog should be reassessed or an oral formulation initiated. In dogs, the dosage of the standard oral formulation is 0.5–2 mg/kg, PO, TID, and of the sustained-release formulation 1.0–4.0 mg/kg, PO, BID. Blood pressure, heart rate and rhythm should be monitored during IV therapy. Possible adverse effects include systemic hypotension, negative inotropy and bradycardia (sinus or AV block), and exacerbation of CHF. Diltiazem is often used in combination with other drugs commonly used to treat heart disease and heart failure, including ACE inhibitors, furosemide, spironolactone, and pimobendan. Because diltiazem is a negative inotrope and chronotrope, it should not be administered concurrently with a β-blocker.

Amlodipine acts as a selective calcium-channel blocker in vascular smooth muscle, with minimal effects on cardiac calcium transport and hence it is recommended for hypertension in dogs. Its common side effects include swelling, tiredness, abdominal pain, and nausea. Serious side effects may include hypotension. Amlodipine works partly by increasing the size of arteries. Amlodipine has an inhibitory effect on calcium influx in smooth muscle cells to inhibit contraction leading to significant reduction in total vascular resistance without decreasing cardiac output. Treatment with amlodipine lasting for a month enhances cardiac output significantly . Unlike verapamil which has efficacy in moderation of emotional arousal and reduces cardiac load without lowering cardiac output demands, amlodipine increases the cardiac output response concomitantly with increased functional cardiac load. Amlodipine is also used to treat congestive heart failure due to mitral valve regurgitation in dogs. By decreasing resistance to forward flow in the systemic circulation it results in a decrease in regurgitant flow into the left atrium. Similarly, it can be used on dogs and cats with left-to-right shunting lesions such as ventricular septal defect to reduce the shunt. In dogs, the primary side effect is gingival hyperplasia.

Treatment of Arrhythmias as per their Nature

Guidelines for the treatment of arrhythmias as per their nature is given below in table no.3.

Table 3: Guidelines for the Treatment of Arrhythmias as per their Nature

Arrhythmia	Drugs used for treatment	Remarks
Sinus Tachycardia	Generally treatment is not needed	1. Underlying etiology is to be ascertained. 2. Sinus tachycardia due to excitement may be treated with tranquilizers. 3. Sinus tachycatdia due to CHF may be treated with digoxin.
Sinus Bradycardia	Atropine or glycopyrrolate intravenously. Followed by Isoproterenol CRI (cases unresponsive to atropine)	Only when sinus bradycardia is associated with clinical signs
Sinus Arrhythmia	Generally no treatment is given	Keep under observation
Wandering pace maker	No treatment is required	
Atrial Premature complexes (APCs)	Digoxin is the drug of choice.	Few APCs do not require any treatment. Underlying etiology should be addressed
Atrial Tachycardia	Digoxin is the drug of choice Calcium channel blockers (Diltiazem) are also effective	Carotid or ocular pressure should be tried first. In emergency thump on the chest may be tried
Atrial Flutter	Digoxin is the drug of choice. Quinidine is another drug Verapamil is quite effective	Carotid or ocular pressure may be tried. In emergency thump on the chest may be tried
Atrial Fibrillation	Digoxin followed by Verapamil or propranolol to reduce ventricular rate if required. Quinidine is used for conversion to sinus thythm	
A-V Junctional Premature Complexes	Same as for APCs	If due to digitalis toxicity, discontinue it.
A-V Junctional Tachycardia	Phenytoin may be used to restore sinus rhythm. Atropine may be tried to increase activity of SA pace maker to overcome junctional focus.	If due to digitalis toxicity, discontinue it. Check serum Potassium level. In case K+ is low give Potassium intravenously. Carotid sinus or ocular pressure may be helpful in cases not associated with digitalis toxicity.
Escape Rhythms	Generally no treatment is needed.	Being a secondary phenomenon, underlying etiology should be ascertained.

Arrhythmia	Drugs used for treatment	Remarks
Ventricular Premature Complexes	Treatment is needed if VPCs are more than 16 per minute or VPCs are in run or multiform or there is R on T phenomena. Lidocaine is the drug of first choice. If heart failure is there then digoxin may be tried to eliminate VPCs. Other drugs recommended for treatment of VPCs are procainamide, quinidine, propranolol, diazepam, phenytoin.	Ascertain underlying etiology. Supportive drugs to overcome acid-base imbalance or to correct electrolyte abnormalities.
Ventricular Tachycardia(VT)	Same as Ventricular premature complexes	Treatment should be started immediately as soon as diagnosis of VT is made. In lidocaine unresponsive cases with haemodynamic crisis electrical cardioversion starting with low watt-seconds should be considered.
Ventricular Fibrillation	Cardiac resuscitation procedure should be followed. Debrillator may be used. Intracardiac epinephrine or calcium chloride can convert fine fibrillations into coarse fibrillations. Lidocaine and sodium bicarbonate is another option if fibrillations are still persisting. A mixture of 1.0 mEq potassium / kg BW and acetylcholine/kg BW intra cardiac has also been reported effective.	Treatment should be started immediately as it is a serious arrhythmia.
Ventricular Asystole	Cardiac resuscitation procedure should be followed. Intracardiac epinephrine and sodium bicarbonate. Calcium chloride can be considered intracardiac or intravenously. When it is associated with severe bradycardia or AV block, atropine should be considered. Dopamine may also be tried when there is electro-mechanical dissociation.	Treatment should be started immediately as it is a serious end stage condition.

Arrhythmia	Drugs used for treatment	Remarks
Sinoatrial Arrest (SA- arrest) or Sinoatrial Block (SA-block)	No therapy is needed for asymptomatic SA arrest or block. Severe cases may be treated with atropine, glycopyrrolate or isoproterenol. More severe cases may require pace maker implantation.	
Persisent Atrial Standstill	Pace maker implantation is needed. Complications of heart failure are to be treated accordingly.	
1st Degree AV block	No treatment is needed	Constant observation is needed for progression when bundle branch block is associated.
2nd degree AV block Mobitz type I	Generally treatment is not needed. Cases with 2nd degree AV block Mobitz type 1 required to be treated with atropine, glycopyrrolate ,isoproterenol or artificial pace maker.	If digitalis is being administered, stop it. When associated with broad QRS treatment is necessary.
3rd degree AV block	Atropine, isoproterenol and corticosteroids are of little value. Epinephrine or isoproterenol can be used till pace maker is implanted.	Artificial pace maker is needed.

Table 4: Anti-arrhythmic Drugs As per their Class– A Ready Reckoner

Class I Drugs: Sodium Channel Blockers				
Class I A				
S.No.	Drugs	Indications	Dose	Contraindications
1	Quinidine	• Supra ventricular arrhythmias • Acute atrial fibrillation	Dogs: 6-20 mg/kg, PO, 3-4 times daily Cats: 4-8 mg/kg, IM, 3 times daily Horses: 20mg/kg, PO, every 2 hrs. by stomach tube until arrhythmia is abolished. : 1mg/kg, IV, every 5-10 minutes.	Contra indicated in patients with complete AV block, intraventricular conduction defect, aberrant ectopic impulses, myasthenia gravis, hepatic impairment
Class I B				
1	Lidocaine	• Ventricular arrhythmias	Dogs: 1-2 mg/kg, IV bolus, followed by 30-50 µg/kg/min, IV CRI Cats: 0.25-0.75 mg/kg,slow IV, followed by 10-40 µg/kg/min, IV CRI Large animals: 0.25-0.5 mg/kg, IV.	Contraindicated in patients with known hypersensitivity to the amide class local anaesthetics. It should not be used in atrial flutter. Contraindicated during 3rd degree AV blocking owing to its ability to suppress Purkinje cell automaticity. Ineffective in the presence of hypokalaemia.
2	Mexiletine	• Ventricular tachyarrhythmias, especially frequent ventricular premature beats	Dogs: 4-8 mg/kg, PO, 3 times daily: 4-8 mg/kg, IV,followed by 5-10 µg/kg/min, IV infusion.	Contraindicated during bradycardia, AV conduction defects, hypotension ,hepatic failure or severe myocardial failure. Not recommended for cats
3	Tocainide	• Long term control of ventricular arrhythmias	Dogs: 15-20 mg/kg, PO, 3 times daily	Contraindicated during bradycardia, AV conduction defects
4	Phenytoin	• Ventricular arrhythmias	Dogs: 10 mg/kg, IV, 3 times daily, usually in increments of 2-4 mg/kg : 30 mg/kg, PO, 3 times daily. Cats: 2-3mg/kg, PO, once daily	Its use is controversial in cats

5	Aprindine	• Pre mature ventricular beats and ventricular tachycardia	Dogs: 0.1 mg/kg, IV infusion for 5 min, repeated at 10 min intervals till arrhythmia is controlled. This is followed by 3 mg/kg, PO, 3 times daily.	------
Class I C				
1	Flecainide	• Atrial fibrillation in horses	Dogs: 5-10 mg/kg, PO, 3 times daily Horses: 1-2mg/kg, iv	Contraindicated during severe heart failure and pre existing atrio ventricular or bundle branch abnormalities
Class II				
1	Propranolol	• Supra ventricular tachycardia • Atrial fibrillations • Atrial and ventricular depolarizations	Dogs: 0.1 mg/kg, PO, 3 times daily. Dose may be increased to a maximum of 1 mg/kg, 3 times daily over 3 -5 days, if required : 0.02-0.06 mg/kg slow IV over 2-3 minutes Cats: 2.5 mg(total), PO, 3 times daily. Dose may be increased to 10mg (total), 3 times daily over 3 -5 days, if required Horses: 175 mg(total), PO, 3 times daily on days 1 and 2, followed by 275 mg (total) 3 times daily on day 3 and 4. Then 350mg (total), 3 times daily on days 5 and 6. : 0.1-0.3 mg/kg, slow IV, 2 times daily.	Contraindicated in patients with heart failure, sinus bradycardia, shock, severe hypotension and bronchospastic lung disease. It should be used cautiously in diabetic patients.
2	Atenolol	• Supra ventricular tachyarrhythmias • Systemic hypertension • Hypertrophic cardiomyopathy	Dogs: 6.5-25 mg(total), PO, 2 times daily Cats :6.5-12.5 mg (total), PO, once daily : 0.01mg/kg,slow IV, over 5 minutes.	---------

3	Esmolol	• Immediate therapy of tachycardia	Dogs and cats: 0.5-1 mg/kg, slow IV as loading dose followed by 0.05-0.2 mg/kg/ min IV infusion.	------
4	Sotalol	• Ventricular tachycardia • Wolff-parkinson-white syndrome • Atrial flutter	Dogs: 0.5 – 3 mg/kg, q12h PO	-------
Class III				
1	Amiodarone	• Supra ventricular and ventricular arrhythmias	Dogs: 10-15mg/kg, PO, 2 times daily for 1 week, then 5-7.5 mg/kg, 2 times daily for 2 weeks, followed by maintenance dose of 7.5 mg/kg, once daily Cats: 10-20mg/kg, IV	Contraindicated in thyrotoxicosis, severe SA node dysfunction with severe sinus bradycardia, 2nd or 3rd degree heart block and hypertension
2	Dronedarone	• Atrial fibrillation and atrial plutter	Dogs: 10-20 mg/kg, PO, twice daily	----
3	Bretylium	• ventricular arrhythmias	Dogs: 5-20 mg/kg, IV Pigs: 0.02 mg/kg/min, IV infusion.	----
CLASS IV Calcium Channel Blocker				
Diphenylalkylamine Derivatives				
1	Verapamil	• Supra ventricular tachyarrhythmias • Sustained and paroxysmal tachycardia • Excessive ventricular hypertrophy • Atrial flutter and fibrillation	Dogs: 1-5 mg/kg, PO, 3 times daily : 0.05-0.2 mg/kg, slow IV, administered over a period from 2 to 5 minutes followed by IV infusion of 2-10 µg/kg/minute. Cats :1-3 mg/kg, PO, 3 times daily.	Contraindicated in sick sinus syndrome, cardio genic shock, severe CHF,AV block , myocardial failure, bradycardia and cardiac glycosides toxicity.
2	Gallopamil	• Cardiac arrhythmias	Dogs: 0.5 – 1.0 mg/kg, PO	-----

Benzothiazepine Derivatives				
1	Diltiazem	• Atrial fibrillation • Supra ventricular tachycardia • Hypertrophic cardiomyopathy • Systemic hypertension	Dogs: 0.5-1.25 mg/kg, PO, 3 to 4 times daily. : 0.25 mg/kg, IV, over 2 minutes. Dose may be repeated if required. Cats: 0.5-2.5 mg/kg, PO, 2 to 3 times daily. : 0.15-0.25 mg/kg, IV over 2 minutes, and then 1-8 µg/kg/minute	Contraindicated in sick sinus syndrome, atrio ventricular node conduction disturbances, bradycardia, impaired left ventricle function, COPD.
2	Clentiazem	• Atrial fibrillation • Supra ventricular tachycardia • Hypertrophic cardiomyopathy • Systemic hypertension	Dogs: 8–10 mg/kg, PO, once to twice daily for 7–10 days, and then decreased to 4–6 mg/kg/day for long term treatment	----

Table 5: Drugs Commonly Used in the Treatment of Arrhythmias and Conduction Disturbances- At a Glance

Name of the drug	Presentation	Indications	Doses D: Dogs C ; Cats	Remarks
Amiodarone	Tab: 200 mg Inj: 50 mg/ml	Indicated for severe refractory atrial and ventricular arrhythmias.	D: Loading dose of 10 mg/kg PO q 12hr for 1 week, thereafter 5 mg/kg PO q 12 – 24 hr. C: None	Class III anti arrhythmic with some class I II & IV effects. Use as last resort for recurrent unstable ventricular tachycardia, Takes weeks to achieve therapeutic levels. Side effects include anorexia, liver, thyroid and pulmonary dysfunction.
Atenelol	Tab: 25, 50, 100mg Oral suspension: 25 mg/ml Inj: 0.5 mg/ml	Atrial and ventricular arrhythmias, Hypertropic cardiomyopathy (outflow obstruction) Systemic hypertension, Aortic stenosis, Cardiac manifestations of Hyperthyroidsm.	D: 0.25 – 2 mg/kg PO q 12 – 24 hrs C: 6.25 – 12.5 mg/kg PO q 12 – 24 hrs.	Beta I selective beta blocker. Less bronchoconstriction and vasoconstriction than non-selective betablockers. Taper dose while discontinuing the therapy. Avoid in CHF. Can be Cautiously used once congestion is controlled.
Atropine Sulphate	Inj: 0.05, 0.1, 0.3, 0.4, 0.5, 0.8, 1 mg/ml	Sinus bradycardia, AV block, Sick sinus syndrome, Cardiac arrest.	D: 0.01 – 0.04 mg/kg IV, IM, IO. 0.02 – 0.04 mg/kg SC q 6 – 8 hrs (IT: Double dose) C: same	Anticholinergic. May transiently worsen bradyarrhythmia. Preoperatively, use with caution and only with bradycardia in cardiac cases.

Name of the drug	Presentation	Indications	Doses D: Dogs C ; Cats	Remarks
Digoxin	Tab: 0.0625, 0.125, 0.1875, 0.25 mg Elixir: 0.05 mg/mL	Supraventricular arrhythmias (Especially atrial fibrillation). myocardial failure	D: Maintenance dose: 0.003-0.005 mg/kg PO q12h. Max. dose for Dobermans 0.25 mg q12h Oral loading dose: Twice the maintenance dose for the first 24-48 hours C: 0.01 mg/kg PO q48h	Digitalis glycoside. Toxicity potentiated by hypokalaemia, hypercalcemia, hypothyroidism, hyponatremia, hypoxia . Dose on lean body weight. Reduce dose 10%-15% with elixirs. Therapeutic range. 0.5-1 ng/mL; 8 hours after a dose.
Esmolol	Inj: 10 mg/mL	Short term management of supraventricular tachyarrhythmias, ventricular tachycardia, and systemic hypertension	D.C: 50-100 µg/kg IV bolus every 5 min (up to 500 µg/kg max) 25-200 µg/kg/min CRI	Ultra-short-acting **β□- selective beta adrenergic blocker**
Glycopyrrolate	Inj: 0.2 mg/ml	Sinus bradycardia, AV block, sick sinus syndrome	D: 0.005-0.01 mg/kg IV, IM 0.01-0.02 mg/kg SC C: Same	Anticholinergic. Longer duration of action. Preoperatively, use with: caution and only with bradycardia in cardiac cases
Hyoscyamine	Tab: 0.125 mg	Rate control in sick sinus syndrome and AV block	D: 0.003- 0.006 mg/kg PO q8h	Anticholinergic
Isoproterenol	Inj: 1:5000 (0.2 mg/mL)	Short-term management of severe bradycardia unresponsive to atropine (sinus bradycardia, AV block, sick sinus syndrome)	D: 0.04-0.09 µg/kg/min IV (titrate up to effect) 10 µg/kg/min IM, SC q6h C: Same	Sympathomimetic agent. Used as an emergency treatment until artificial pacing is accomplished.

Name of the drug	Presentation	Indications	Doses D: Dogs C ; Cats	Remarks
Lidocaine	Inj: 5, 10, 15, 20, mg/ml. (without epinephrine)	Ventricular arrhythmias	D: 2 mg/kg slowly IV or 10 (double the dose IT) in 2 mg/kg boluses followed by IV drip at 30-80 (occasionally up to 100) ug/kg/min CRI C: 0.25-0.75 mg/kg IV over 5 min	Class I antiarrhythmic . Use with caution in cats as may cause seizures. Drug of choice for initial control of ventricular tachycardia . Effects increased by high potassium and decreased by low potassium
Metoprolol	Tab: 25, 50, 100 mg Inj: 1 mg/mL	Atrial and ventricular arrhythmias, hypertrophic cardiomyopathy, systemic hypertension, myocardial failure	D: 0.25-1.0 mg/kg PO q8h C: Same	1 selective beta blocker Less bronchoconstriction, and interference with insulin therapy than with nonselective beta blockers. Taper dose when stopping. Dose slowly titrated over weeks with myocardial failure.
Procainamide	Cap: 250, 375, 500 mg Tab: 250, 375, 500 mg Tab: CR, SR: 250, 500, 750. 1000 mg Inj 100, 500 mg/mL Some oral formulations may be unavailable.	Ventricular and supraventricular arrhythmias. WPW	D: 10-30 mg/kg IM, PO q6h 2 mg/kg IV Over 3-5 min up to total dose of 15 mg/kg 25-50 µg/kg/min CRI C: 2-5 mg/kg PO q6-8h	Class 1 antiarrhythmic agent. Beware hypotension with IV administration . Effects increased by high potassium and decreased by low potassium . Monitor ECG: 25% prolongation of QRS is sign of toxicity. May be difficult to obtain. Use with caution in cats. Reduce dose with severe renal and liver disease.
Propantheline bromide	Tab: 7.5, 15 mg	Rate control in sick sinus syndrome and AV block	D. C: 0.25-0.5 mg/kg PO q8-12h	Anticholinergic

Name of the drug	Presentation	Indications	Doses D: Dogs C ; Cats	Remarks
Propranolol	Tab: 10, 20, 40, 60, 80 mg Cap: 60, 80, 120, 160 mg Inj: 1 mg/mL Solution: 4.mg/mL	Atrial and ventricular arrhythmias, Hypertrophic cardiomyopathy Systemic hypertension, Thyrotoxicosis	D: 0.2-1.0 mg/kg PO q8h 0.02-0.06 mg/kg IV over 5-10 minutes C: <4.5 kg: 2.5-5 mg PO q8-12h	Nonselective ß blocker. Start with low dose and titrate to effect. Taper dose when discontinue therapy. Beware of possible bronchoconstriction.
Quinidine gluconate	Tab SR: 324 mg Inj: 80 mg/mL	Ventricular and supraventricular arrhythmias, WPW. conversion of atrial fibrillation	D: 6-20 mg/kg PO, IM q6h 6-20 mg/kg PO q8h with sustained release products 5-10 mg/kg IV (very slowly) C: None Note: Dose calculated for quinidine base equivalent.	Rarely used, replaced by mexiletine and sotalol for managing ventricular arrhythmias. Class 1 antiarrhythmic . Reduce dose in CHF, hepatic disease, and hypoalbuminemia Quinidine base in each quinidine salt; quinidine gluconate: 324 mg tab = 200 mg quinidine; quinidine sulphate: 300 mg tab = 250 mg quinidine
Quinidine sulfate	Tab SR: 300 mg			
Sotalol	Tab: 80, 120, 160 mg	Atrial and ventricular arrhythmias	D: 1-2 mg/kg PO q12h (medium- size dogs start 40 mg per dog, then increase to 80 mg. if needed.) C: 2 mg/ kg PO q12h	Antiarrhythmic agent with class II (beta blocking) and class III effects . Monitor closely with CHF due to negative inotropic properties.
Verapamil	Tab: 40, 80, 120 mg Inj: 2.5 mg/mL	Supraventricular arrhythmias	D: 0.05 mg/kg slow IV (1-2 min) boluses given at 10-30 minute intervals (to effect) to a maximum cumulative dose of 0.2 mg/kg C: 0.05 mg/kg slow IV, may repeat twice as described for dog	Calcium channel blocker. Diltiazem is a safer alternative in heart failure. Potent vasodilator and negative inotrope.

Further Readings

Varshney, J.P. (2020). Electrocardiography in Veterinary Medicine. Springer Nature, Singapore, Pte, Ltd.

Varshney, J.P. (2023). Heart Failure in Animals: Current Concepts. New India Publishing Agency (NIPA), New Delhi.

12

Electrocardiograms for Self-Exercise

This chapter on electrocardiograms for self-exercise is designed to provide opportunities to the readers to assess their understanding of reading and interpreting electrocardiograms and to increase their confidence. Each electrocardiogram has its detail and a question to answer. On the reverse side of each electrocardiographic tracing, detailed reading and interpretation is provided to match your assessment and to improve your interpretation skill. It is to be remembered that each electrocardiogram should be evaluated in conjunction with complete data base (history, clinical manifestations, laboratory investigations, radiological observations, and echocardiographic observations). The study of a long strip (lead II) is valuable for accurate analysis of cardiac rhythm and rate. It is to be remembered that a normal electrocardiogram does not always rule out cardiac disease and therefore, interpreting an electrocardiogram in isolation may be erroneous or misleading.

ECG 1

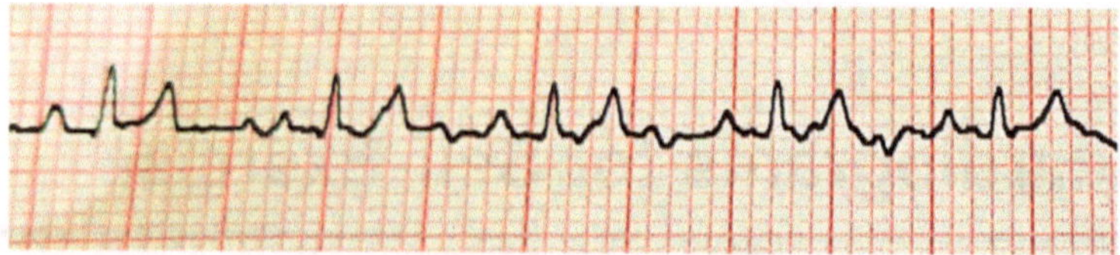

Question. It is an electrocardiogram of an adult dog recorded at the speed of 25 mm/s and sensitivity of 1 in lead II. Is it a normal or abnormal electrocardiogram? What is your interpretation?

ECG 2

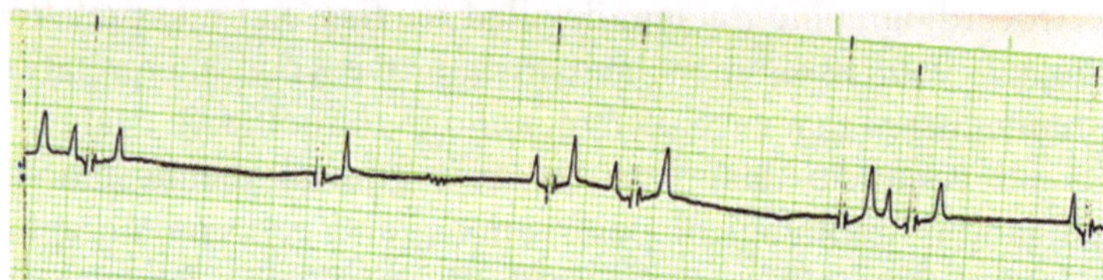

Question. It is an electrocardiogram of an adult male German shepherd recorded at the speed of 25 mm/s and sensitivity of 1 in lead II. What is your interpretation?

ECG 1

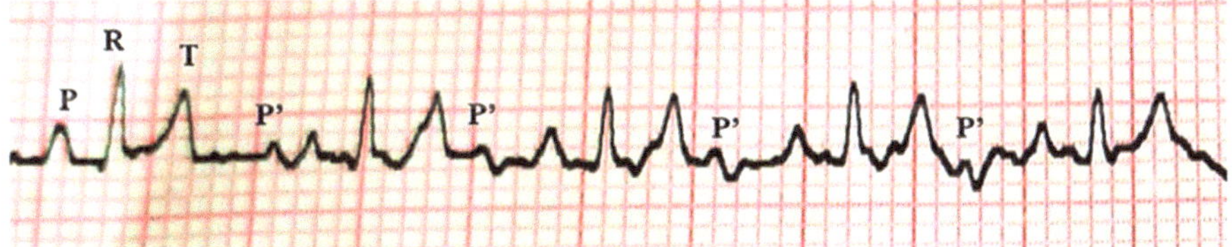

Answer. It is not a normal electrocardiogram**.** Rhythm is not normal. There are regular P' wave that are not followed by 'QRS' and 'T' complexes i.e. P' waves are blocked and the current is not conducted to ventricles. When P is conducted it is followed by QRS and T complexes . All the complexes of conducted P wave are of normal configuration . Ventricular rate is 150 bpm while atrial rate is 270 bpm. There is a fixed relationship between atria and ventricles of 2:1 (2P : 1 QRS). P-R interval in this case is almost constant (0.1 s – 0.12 s). Since QRS of the conducted P wave is normal, P' wave is blocked and rhythm is regularly irregular, it is 2nd degree AV block of Mobitz type II with normal bundle branch conduction.

ECG 2

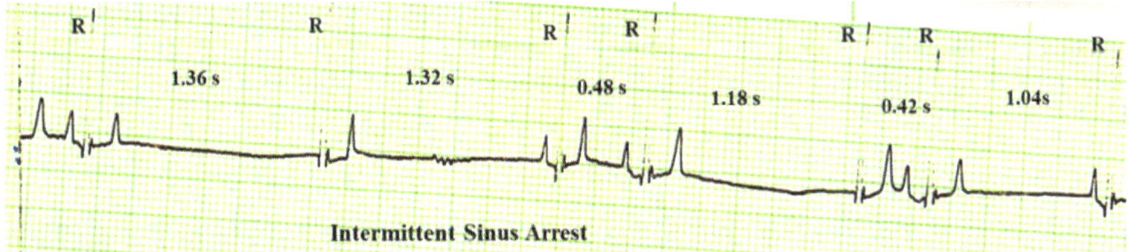

Answer. Electrocardiogram (lead II, sensitivity 1, speed 25 mm/s) of an adult German shepherd is suggestive of intermittent Sinus Arrest. The pauses between complexes 1and 2; 2 and 3; 4 and 5; 6 and 7 (1.04 to 1.36 s) are greater than twice of the normal R-R interval (0.42 s).

ECG 3

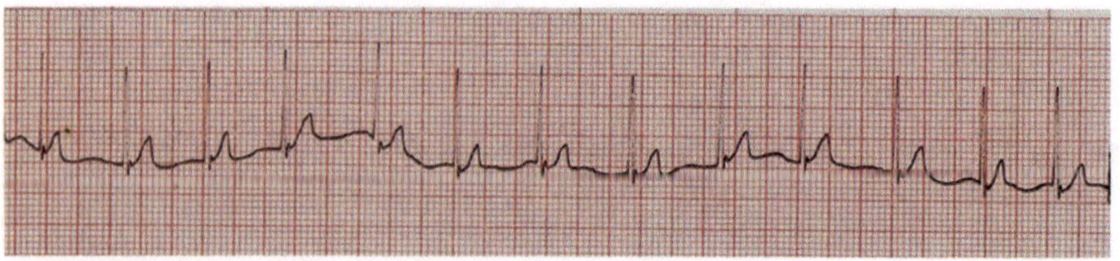

Question. It is an electrocardiogram of an aged male Pomeranian dog taken at the speed of 25 mm/s and sensitivity of 1 in lead II. What is your interpretation?

ECG 4

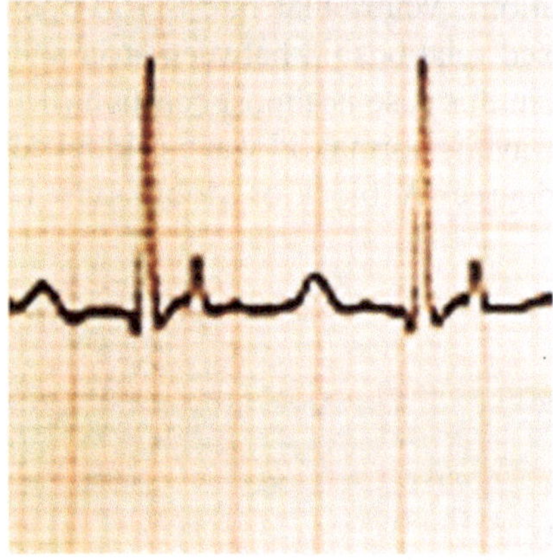

Question. It is an electrocardiogram of a dog taken at the speed of 25 mm/s and sensitivity of 1 in lead II . What is your interpretation?

ECG 3

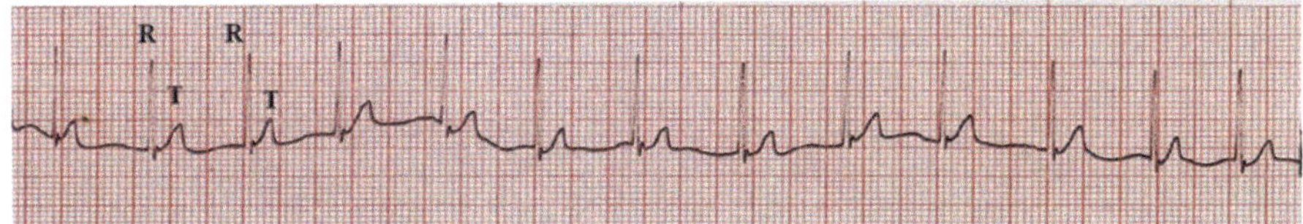

Answer. Electrocardiogram (lead II, sensitivity 1, speed 25 mm/s) of an aged male Pomeranian dog is showing only QRS and T complexes. P wave (atrial depolarization) is absent. R wave is of 1.5 mV. QRS is narrow (0.03-0.04 s). T wave is of 0.4 to 0.5 mV and 0.08 s. Absence of P wave is suggestive of atrial standstill

ECG 4

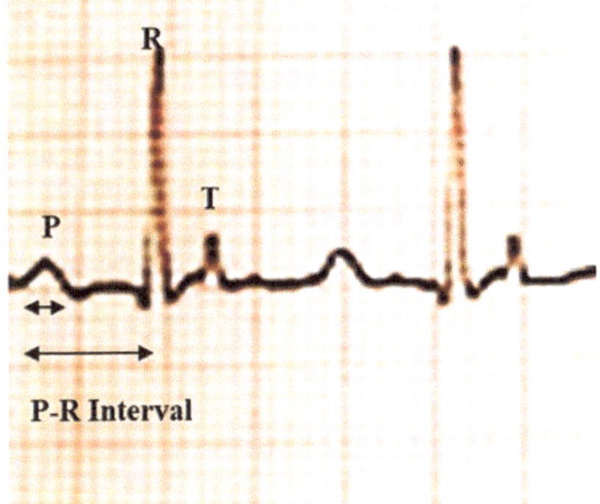

Answer. Electrocardiogram (lead II, speed 25 mm/s, sensitivity 1) of a dog is showing broad P wave (0.08 s) and prolonged P-R interval (0.24 s). Broad P wave is suggestive of left atrial enlargement (P mitrale). Prolonged P-R interval is suggestive of 1st degree AV block. The QRS complex is normal. This ECG shows P mitrale with 1st degree AV block.

ECG 5

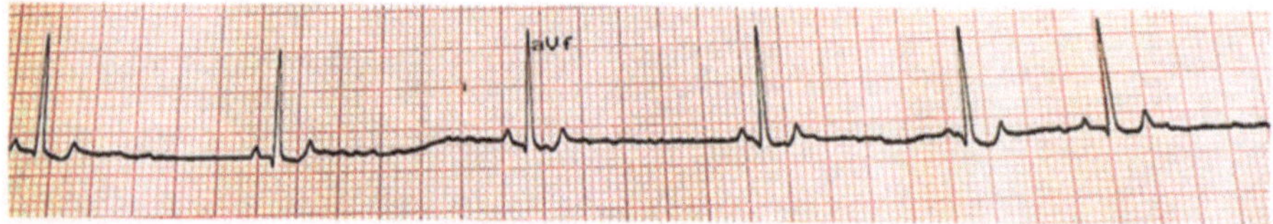

Question. It is an electrocardiogram of an adult Labrador dog taken at the speed of 25 mm/s and sensitivity of 1 in lead II. What is your interpretation?

ECG 6

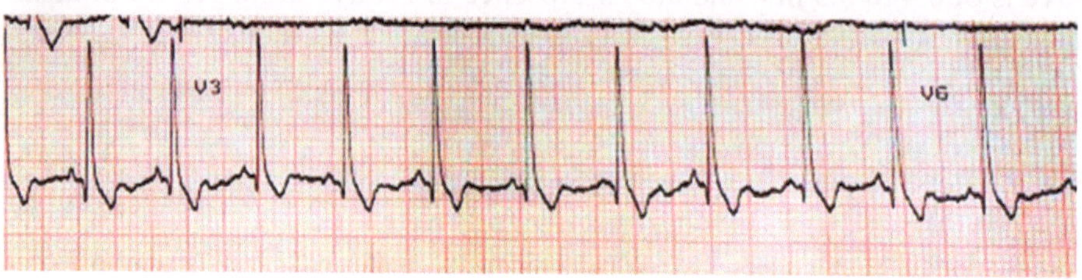

Question. It is an electrocardiogram of an adult non-descript dog taken at the speed of 25 mm/s and sensitivity of 1 in lead II. What is your interpretation?

ECG 5

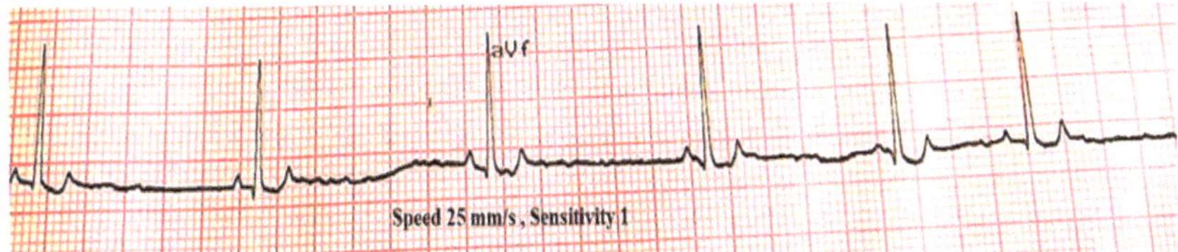

Answer. Electrocardiogram (lead II , speed 25 mm/s, sensitivity 1) of a Labrador is showing normal P (0.1 mV, 0.04 s),QRS (small q of 0.05 to 0.1mV, R of 1.4 mV, QRS of 0.04 s duration), T (+ ve T of 0.2 mV and 0.06 s duration) complexes; P-R interval (0.1s), S-T segment (isoelectric, 0.08 s duration); variable R-R interval (0.7 to 1.22 s) ; normal Q-T interval (0.18 s); and slow heart rate (60 bpm) suggesting Brady arrhythmia.

ECG 6

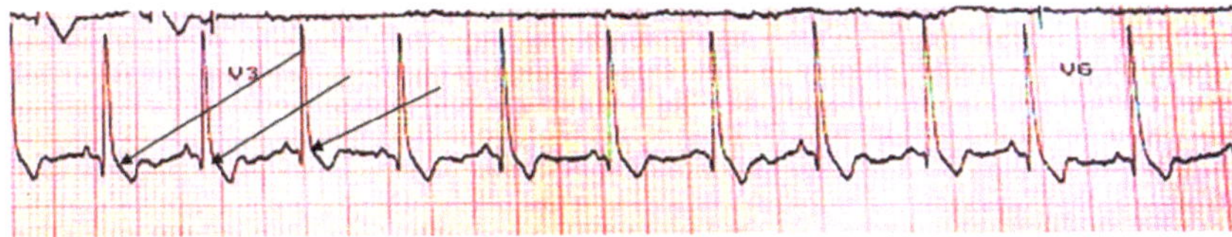

Answer. Electrocardiogram (lead II, speed 25 mm/s, sensitivity 1) of a non-descript dog is showing a displaced S-T segment or S-T coving or S-T slurring (arrows). It is seen in left ventricular enlargement or left bundle branch block provided other criteria are also met with.

ECG 7

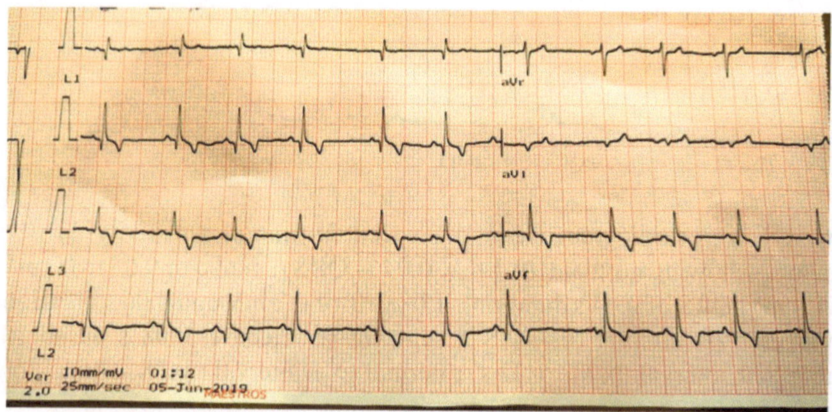

Question. It is an electrocardiogram (speed 25 mm/s and sensitivity 1 in standard bipolar limb leads and augmented unipolar limb leads) of a male 13 year old Labrador . Read the electrocardiogram and also find mean electrical axis (MEA) on the frontal plane. Is there any deviation of the heart?

ECG 8

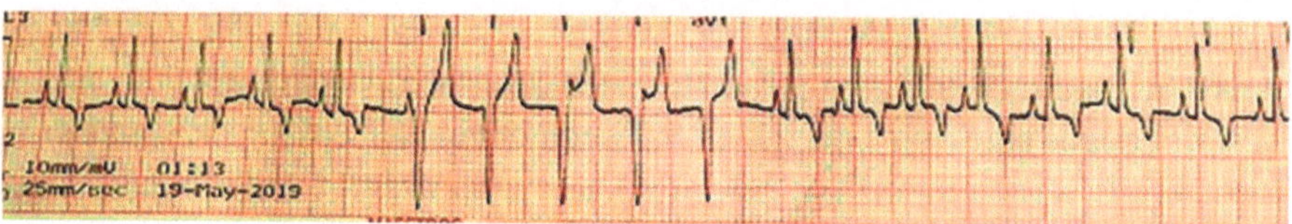

Question. It is an electrocardiogram (Lead II, speed 25 mm/s, sensitivity 1) of a 7 year old German shepherd, bitten by a snake. What is your opinion about the abnormality in this electrocardiogram?

ECG 7

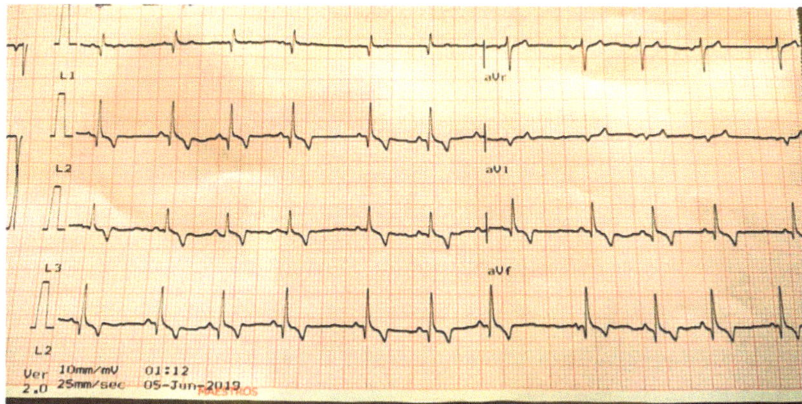

Answer. Electrocardiogram (Bipolar and augmented leads, speed 25 mm/s, sensitivity 1) of a male 13 year old Labrador is showing almost sinus rhythm with a heart rate of 100 bpm. The electrocardiographic complexes P (0.1 mV, 0.04 s), q(0.2 mV), R (0.7 mV), QRS (0.04 s), T (0.3 mV, 0.08s); segments (P-R segment 0.04 s, S-T segment 0.08 s, T-P segment 0.24-0.52 s); and intervals (P-R interval 0.08-0.1 s, Q-T interval 0.2 s, R-R interval 0.52-0.82 s) are within normal range. Mean electrical axis on frontal plane is +90 ^{0}. (isoelectric lead is I i.e. 0 ^{0} and perpendicular line to this lead is at +90^0). Therefore mean electrical axis of the heart on frontal plane is within normal range and there is no deviation of the heart.

ECG 8

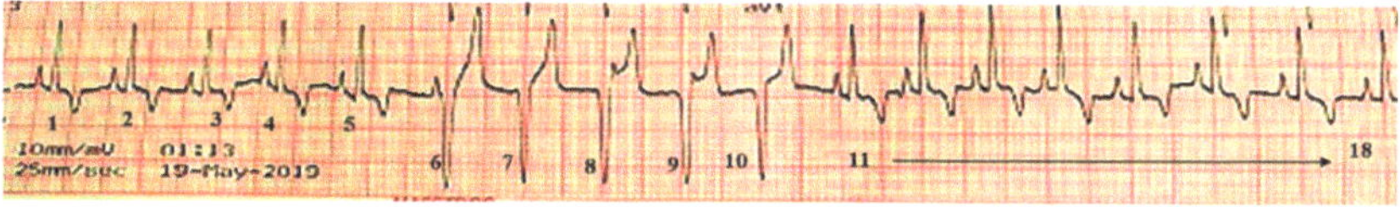

Answer. Electrocardiogram (lead II, sensitivity1, speed 25 mm/s) of a seven year old German Shepherd, bitten by a snake , is showing normal (1 to 5 and 11 to 18) and abnormal complexes (6 to 10). The normal rhythm has been broken by abnormal complexes. The abnormal complexes (6 to 10) do not have a 'P' wave, their QRS complexes are premature, bizarre and of large amplitude, and the T wave is opposite to the dominant QRS. These are premature complexes and are termed as ventricular premature complexes (VPCs). As VPCs are in a row of 5 (> three) and intermittent, it is appropriately termed as intermittent ventricular tachycardia. The deflection of major QRS is negative in lead II, the ectopic focus lies in the left ventricle. The rate of VPCs is 150 /minute, it can be termed as idioventricular tachycardia or enhanced ventricular rhythm.

ECG 9

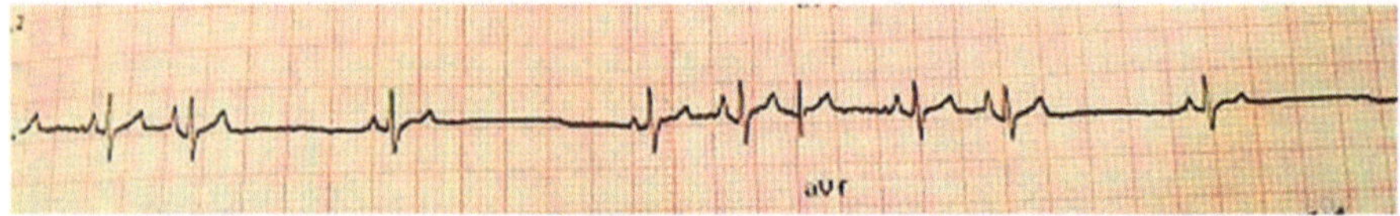

Question. It is an electrocardiogram of a dog taken at the speed of 25 mm/s and sensitivity of 1 in Lead II. What is your interpretation?

ECG 10

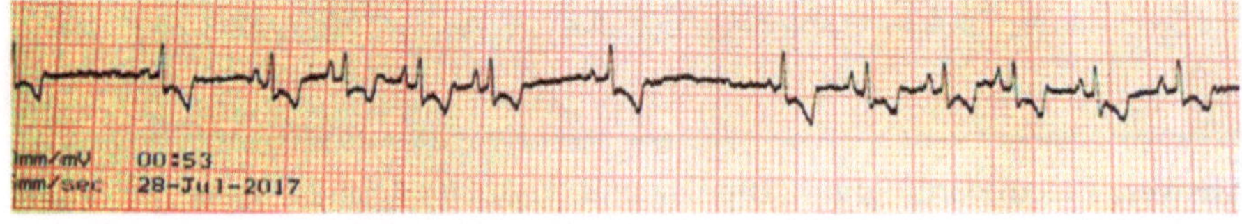

Question. It is an electrocardiogram of a dog taken at the speed of 25 mm/s and sensitivity of 1 in Lead II. What is your interpretation?

ECG 9

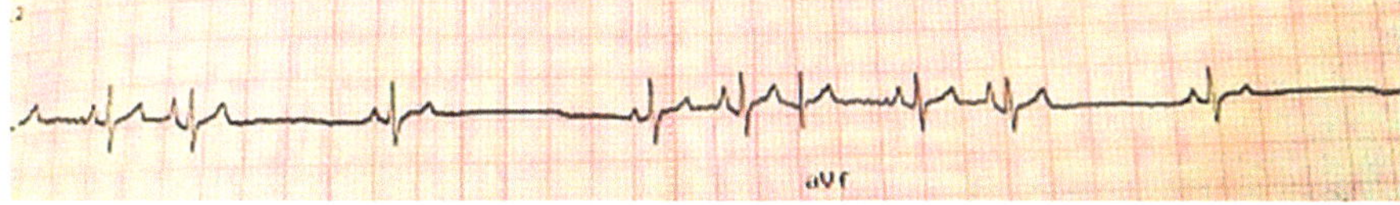

Answer. Electrocardiogram (lead II, sensitivity1, speed 25 mm/s) of a dog is showing sinus arrest at four places, wandering pacemaker (P wave amplitude is varying), and low voltage complexes (R amplitude < 0.5 mV). The pauses (R-R interval varying from 0.88 to 1.2 s) are greater than the twice of normal R-R interval (0.28-0.54 s).

ECG 10

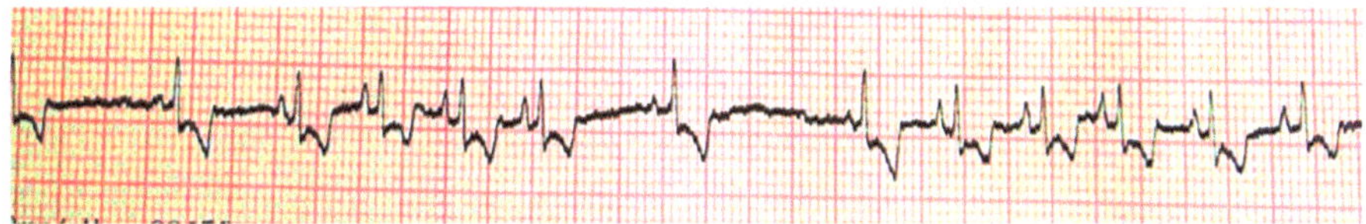

Answer. Electrocardiogram (lead II, sensitivity1, speed 25 mm/s) of a dog is showing sinus arrhythmia (HR 132 bpm, R-R interval varying from 0.36 to 0.88 second) ,sinus arrest at one place (R-R interval 0.88 s) wandering pacemaker (P wave amplitude is varying from 0.075 to 0.15 mV), low voltage complexes (R amplitude < 0.5 mV), negative T wave, and S-T segment depression (0.15 -0.2 mV).

ECG 11

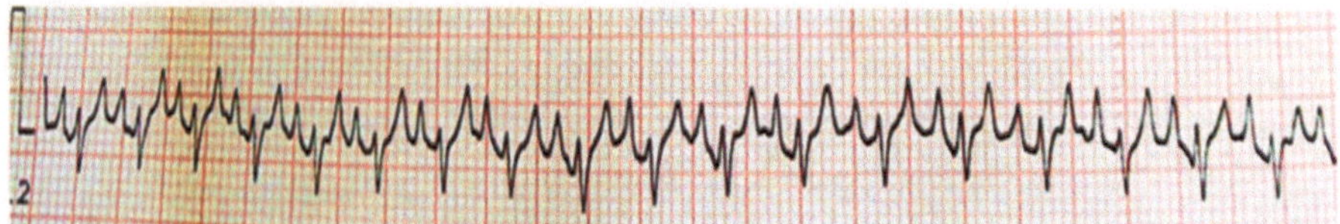

Question. It is an electrocardiogram of a dog taken at the speed of 25 mm/s and sensitivity of 1 in Lead II. What is your interpretation?

ECG 12

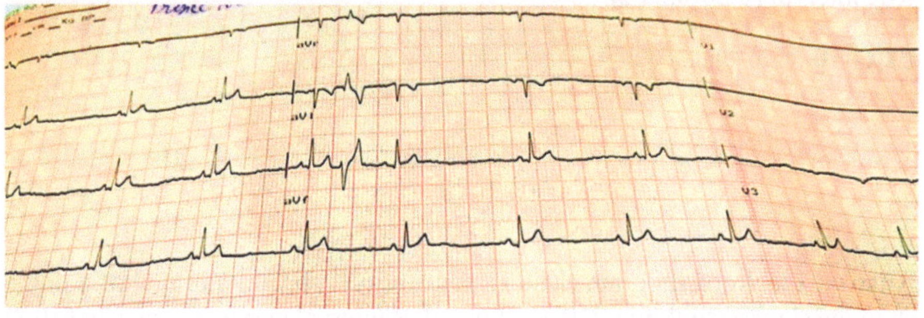

Question. It is an electrocardiogram of a dog taken at the speed of 25 mm/s and sensitivity of 1 in Lead I, II, III, aVR, aVL and aVF. What is your interpretation?

ECG 11

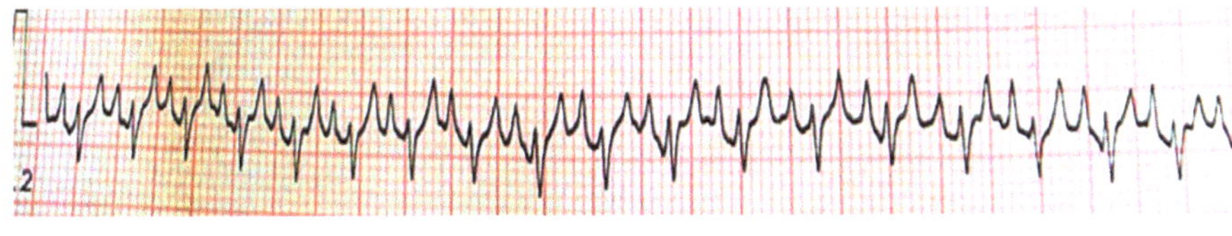

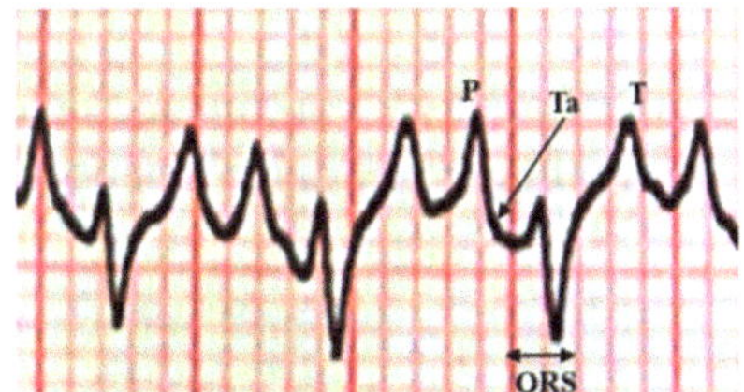

Answer. Electrocardiogram (lead II, sensitivity1, speed 25 mm/s) of a dog is showing Ta wave (a slight depression of baseline following the P wave), rS pattern of QRS, S (0.4 mV) and QRS duration of 0.08s suggesting right atrial enlargement (Ta wave) and right bundle branch block (S wave and broad QRS).

ECG12

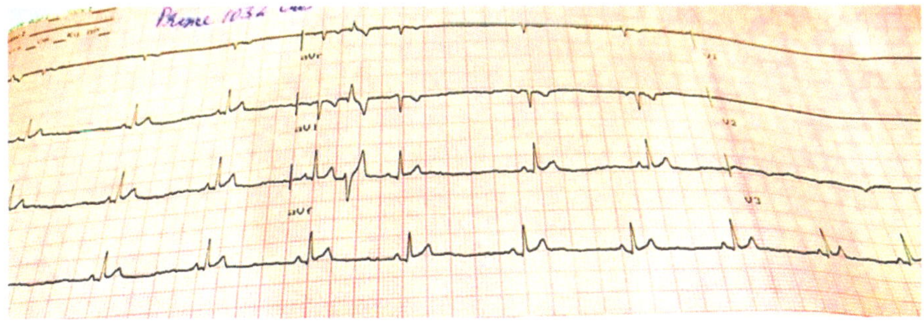

Answer. Electrocardiogram (lead I, II, III, aVR, aVL, aVF; sensitivity1, speed 25 mm/s) of a dog is showing almost sinus rhythm with a heart rate of 70 bpm. P, QRS and T complexes, P-R interval, S-T segment are within limits. There is no electrocardiographic abnormality in this electrocardiogram.

ECG 13

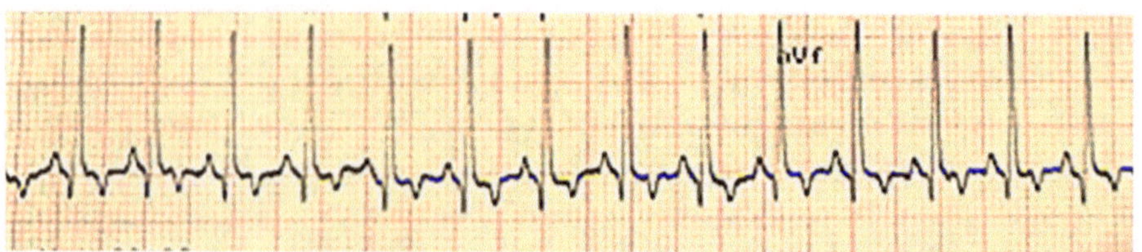

Question. It is an electrocardiogram of an adult Labrador dog taken at the speed of 25 mm/s and sensitivity of 1 in Lead II. What is your interpretation?

ECG 14

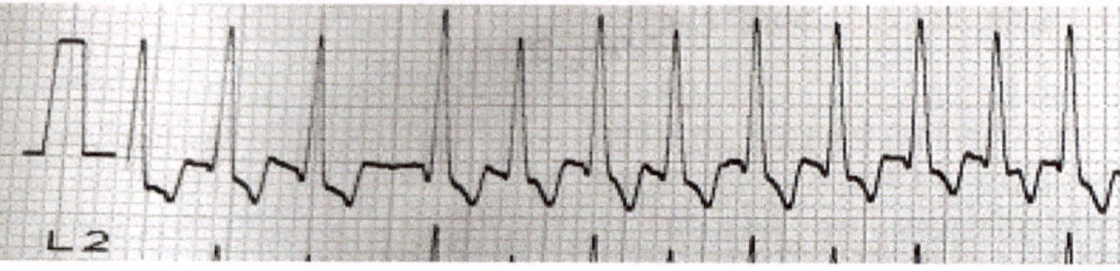

Question. It is an electrocardiogram of an adult dog taken at the speed of 25 mm/s and sensitivity of 1 in Lead II. Is it a normal electrocardiogram? If not. What is your opinion?

ECG 13

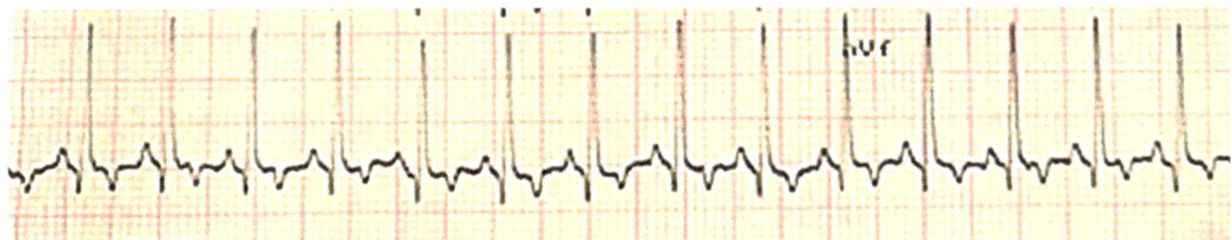

Answer. Electrocardiogram (lead II, sensitivity1, speed 25 mm/s) of a dog is showing heart rate of 180 bpm with sinus rhythm (R-R interval 0.32-0.36 s) and no other abnormality suggesting sinus tachycardia.

ECG 14

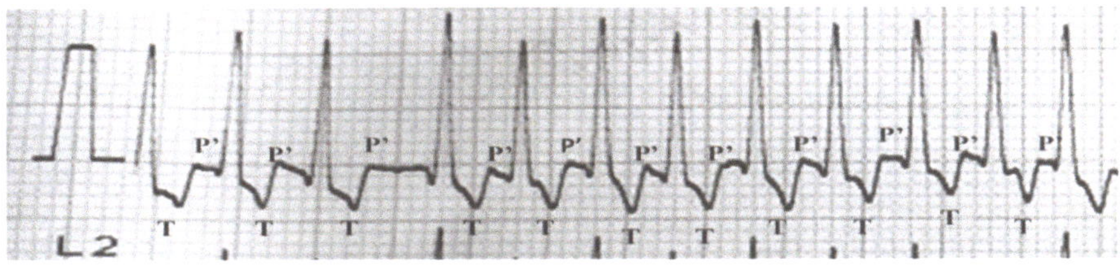

Answer. It is not a normal electrocardiogram. Electrocardiogram (lead II, sensitivity1, speed 25 mm/s) of a dog is showing premature P' wave in all complexes. The hint of P' wave is in previous T wave in each complex. The focus of premature P' wave is in atria but away from SA node. Configuration of P' wave is slightly different from the normal P wave. The rhythm appears regular. QRS complex is of normal configuration. The atrial premature complexes are more than three in series, it is called as atrial tachycardia.

ECG 15

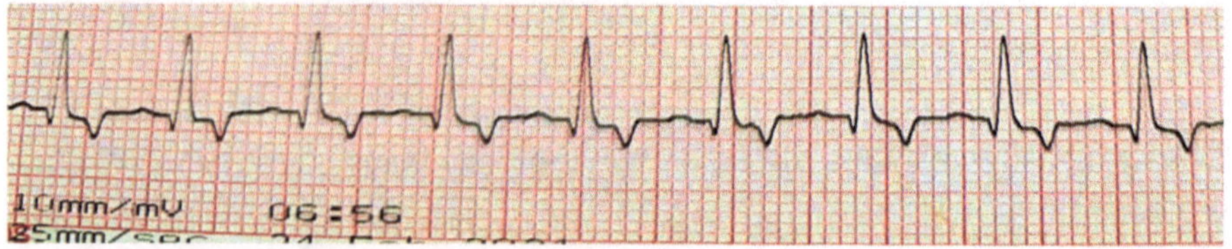

Question. It is an electrocardiogram of a dog taken at the speed of 25 mm/s and sensitivity of 1 in Lead II. What is your interpretation?

ECG 16

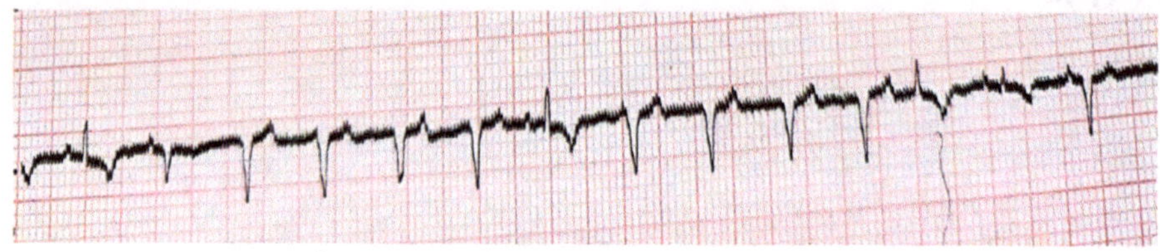

Question. It is an electrocardiogram of a dog taken at the speed of 25 mm/s and sensitivity of 1 in Lead II. What is your interpretation?

ECG15

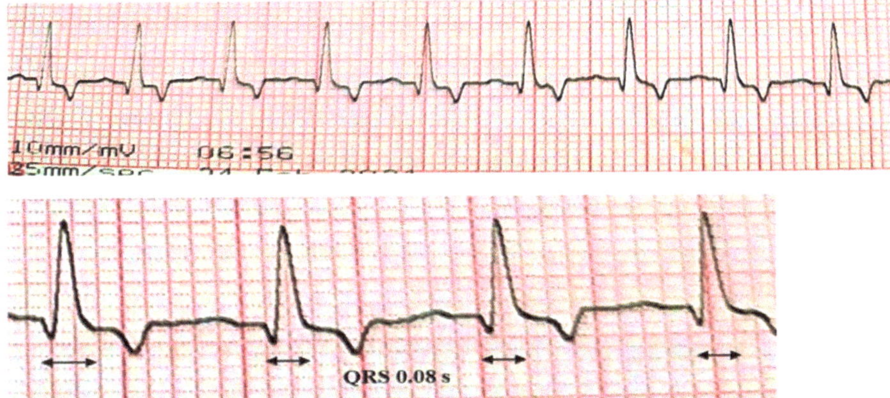

Answer. Electrocardiogram (lead II, sensitivity1, speed 25 mm/s) of a dog is showing left bundle branch block. The QRS complexes are wide (0.07s - 0.08s) but the 'R' wave amplitude is within the range (0.9 to 1.0 mV).

ECG16

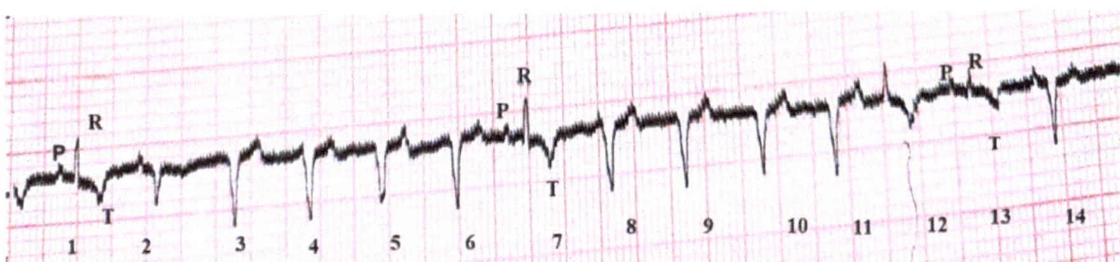

Answer. Electrocardiogram (lead II, sensitivity1, speed 25 mm/s) of a dog is showing multiform ventricular tachycardia at an average of 150 /min. The complexes1, 7,12 and 13 are normal complexes. While complexes 2 to 6, 8 to 11 and 14 are ventricular ectopic complexes (ventricular premature complex) of varying configuration. The ectopic complexes are in the row of 4 or 5. Hence it is called as ventricular tachycardia. The QRS deflection of VPC is predominantly negative, therefore the ectopic focus is in left ventricle. The 7th, 12th and 13th complexes are capture complex. Besides multiform ventricular tachycardia, the electrocardiogram also shows electrical interference (60-cycle).

ECG 17

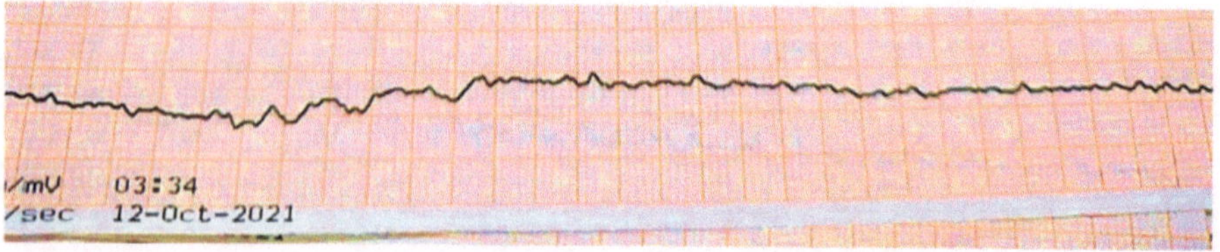

Question. It is an electrocardiogram of a dog taken at the speed of 25 mm/s and sensitivity of 1 in Lead II. What is your interpretation?

ECG 18

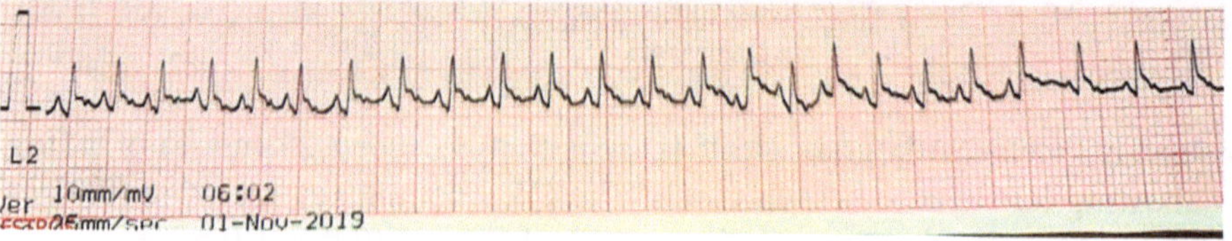

Question. It is an electrocardiogram of a dog taken at the speed of 25 mm/s and sensitivity of 1 in Lead II. What is your interpretation?.

ECG 17

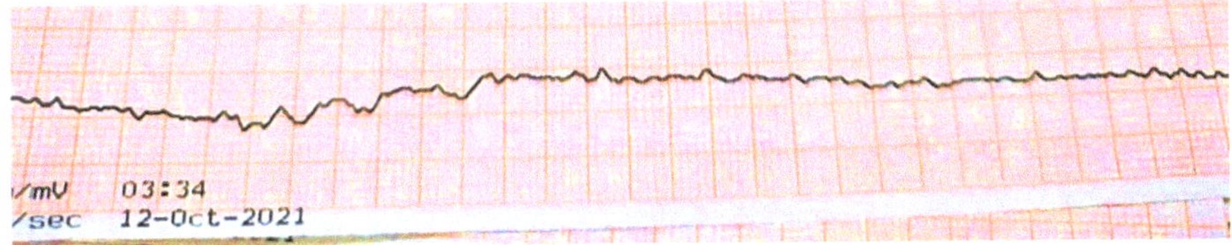

Answer. Electrocardiogram (lead II, sensitivity1, speed 25 mm/s) of a dog is showing no recognizable P, QRS and T complexes. The heart rate is fast, irregular, chaotic and bizarre. Only coarse fibrillations are seen .The fibrillations/oscillations are suggestive of ventricular fibrillations/flutters. Ventricular fibrillations/ flutters are generally a terminal event and may lead to cardiac arrest.

ECG 18

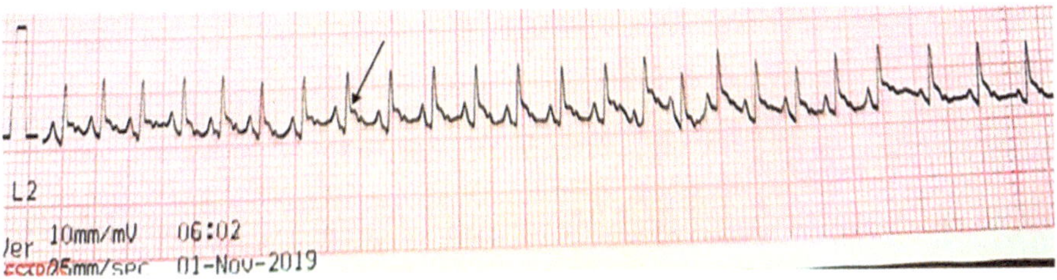

Answer. Electrocardiogram (lead II, sensitivity1, speed 25 mm/s) of a dog is showing S-T segment elevation of 0.2 mV, and sinus tachycardia (HR 220 bpm, R-R interval of 0.27 s).

ECG 19

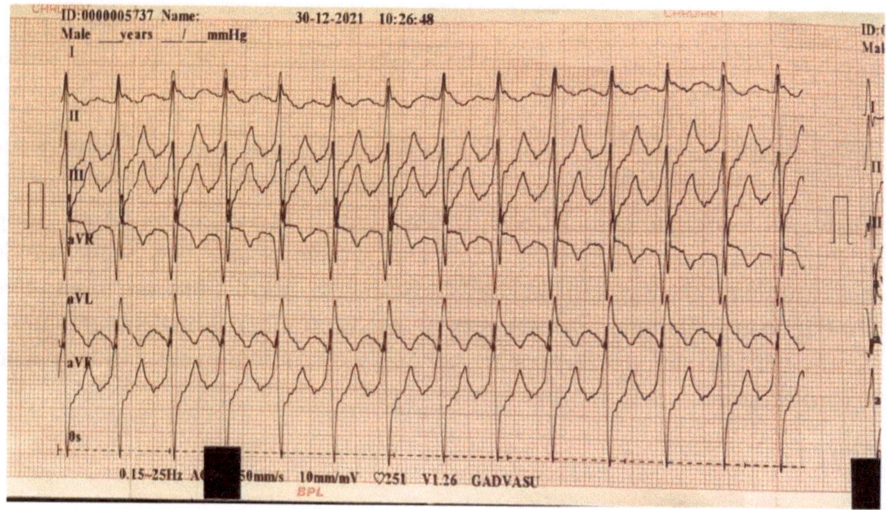

Question. It is an electrocardiogram of a young dog , with tricuspid insufficiency, taken at the speed of 50 mm/s and sensitivity of 1 in Lead I,II, III,aVR, aVF and aVL .What is your interpretation?.

ECG 20

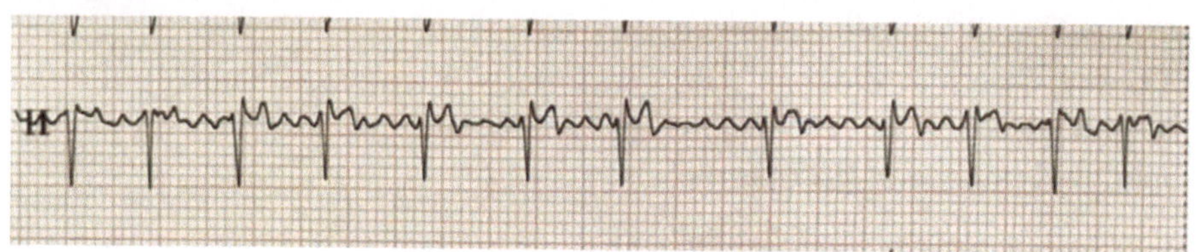

Question. It is an electrocardiogram of a dog taken at the speed of 25 mm/s and sensitivity of 0.5 in Lead II. What is the abnormality in this electrocardiogram?

ECG 19

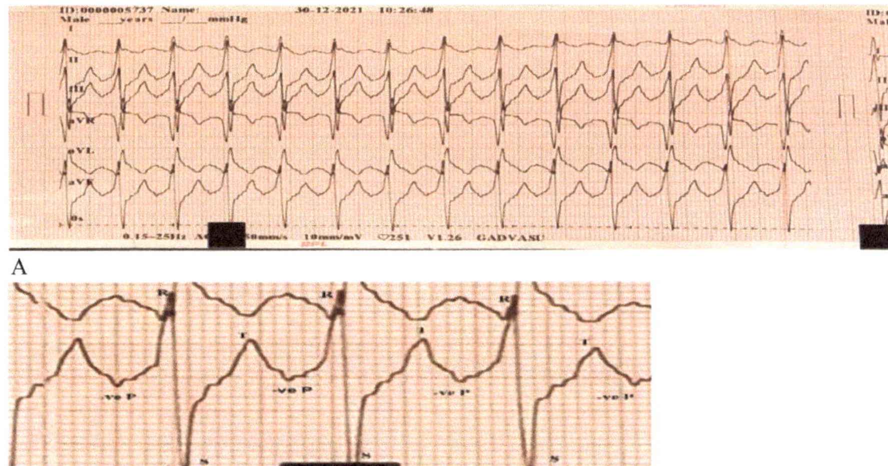

B

Answer . Electrocardiogram (lead I, II, III, aVR, aVL and aVF ;sensitivity 1 and speed 50 mm/s) of a young dog with tricuspid insufficiency (A) and magnified view of few complexes (B) is showing negative P wave (-ve) , R wave of 1.0-1.2 mV, S wave of 1.3-1.4 mV, QRS of 0.06 s and T wave of 0.5 mV and 0.06 s . S wave is deep in lead I, II, III and aVF . The electrocardiogram is suggestive of AV junctional tachycardia with right ventricular enlargement.

ECG 20

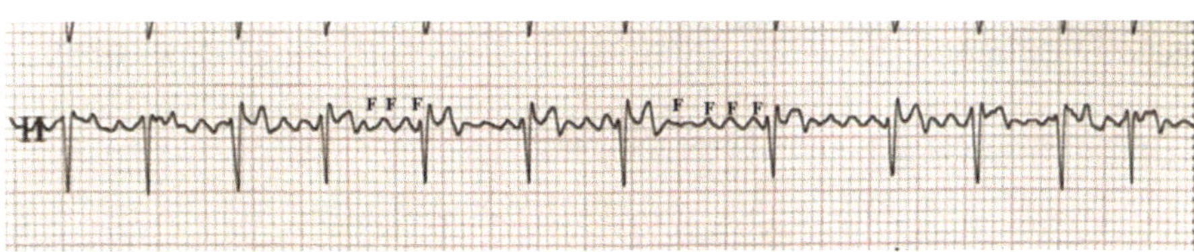

Answer. Electrocardiogram of a dog (Lead II, speed of 25 mm/s and sensitivity of 0.5) is showing atrial flutter (F waves) at the rate of 380 /min. The average ventricular rate is 160 /min..

ECG21

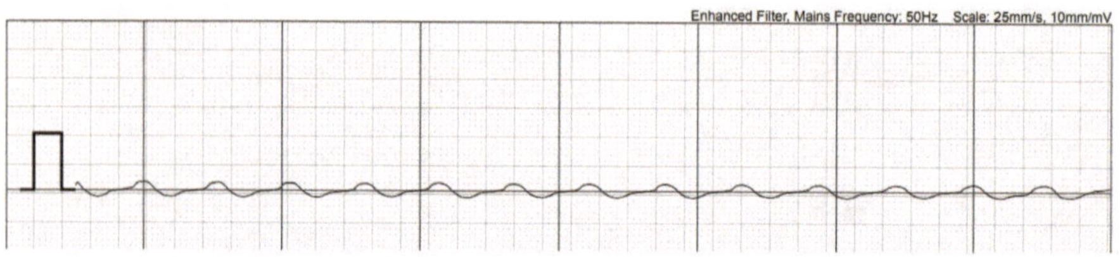

Question. It is an electrocardiogram of a dog taken at the speed of 25 mm/s and sensitivity of 1 in Lead II. What is your interpretation?

ECG 22

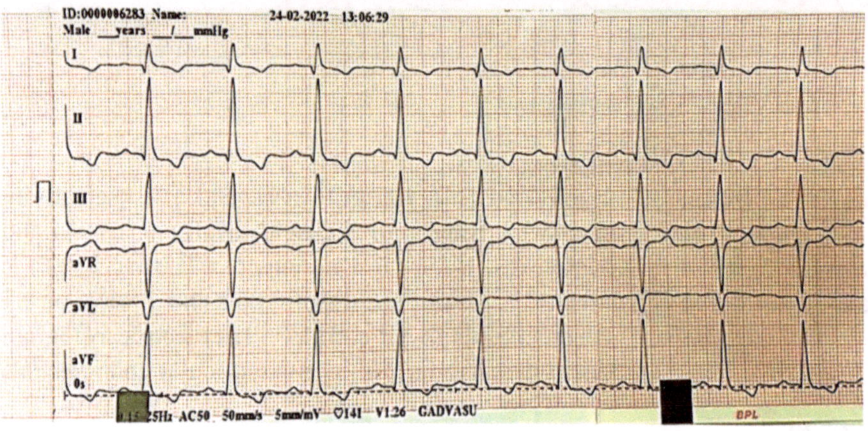

Question. It is an electrocardiogram of an adult large breed dog taken at the speed of 50 mm/s and sensitivity of 0.5 in Lead I, II. III, aVR, aVL, aVF. Calculate the wave's amplitude and duration, intervals and segments. Find out its mean electrical axis and interpret the findings.

ECG 21

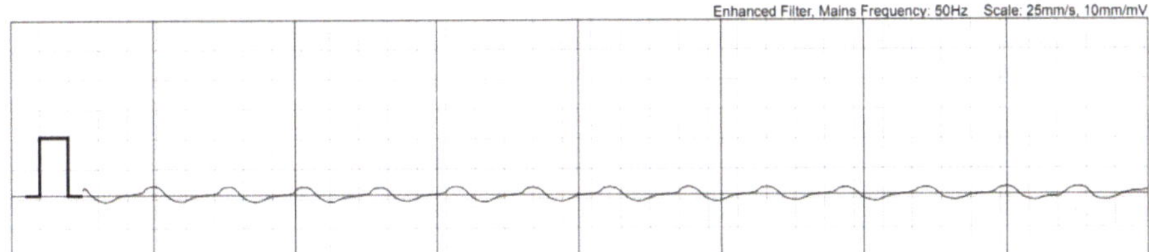

Answer. Electrocardiogram (lead II, sensitivity1, speed 25 mm/s) of a dog is showing ventricular flutter. There is no recognition of P, QRS and T complexes. There are only fine oscillations.Ventricular flutter/fibrillations are serious arrhythmias as it can lead to cardiac arrest.

ECG 22

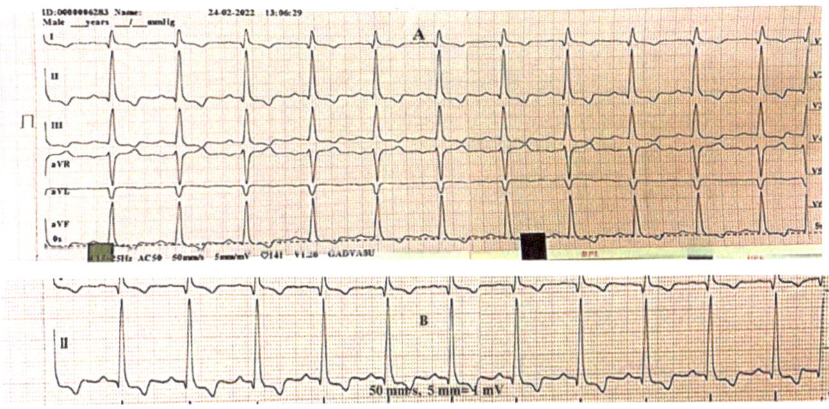

Answer. Electrocardiogram (speed 50 mm/s ,sensitivity 0.5) of an adult large breed dog in standard bipolar limb leads and augmented unipolar leads (A) and Lead II has been cropped out for calculation of amplitude, segments and intervals (B). Analysis of lead II reveals heart rate as 140 bpm, sinus rhythm (R-R interval 0.42), normal P wave (0.2 mV, 0.04 s), small q(0.2 mV), increased amplitude of R wave (3.8 mV), broad QRS (0.07-0.08 s), normal T (negative 0.4 mV, 0.06 s), normal P-R segment (0.06 s), normal P-R interval (0.1 s), isoelectric S-T segment (0.06 s), normal Q-T interval (0.2 s) and almost constant R-R interval (0.42 s). The mean electrical axis on frontal plane is + 78 $^{0.}$ Increased amplitude of R wave in lead II, III, aVF and broad QRS is suggestive of left ventricular enlargement.

ECG 23

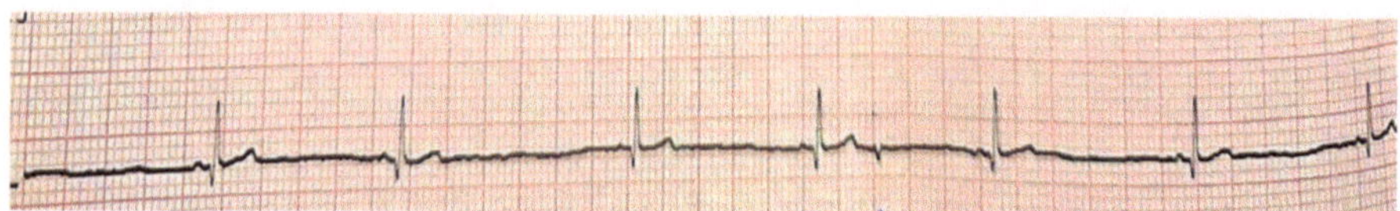

Question. It is an electrocardiogram of a dog taken at the speed of 25 mm/s and sensitivity of 1 in Lead II. Find out heart rate variability.

ECG 24

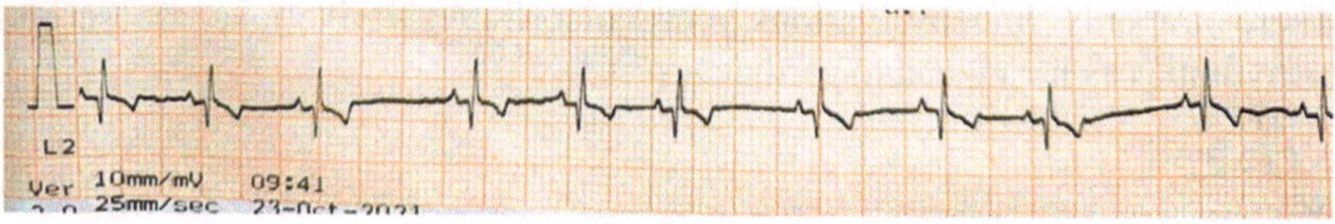

Question. It is an electrocardiogram of a dog taken at the speed of 25 mm/s and sensitivity of 1 in Lead II. Find out Q-T interval variability.

ECG 23

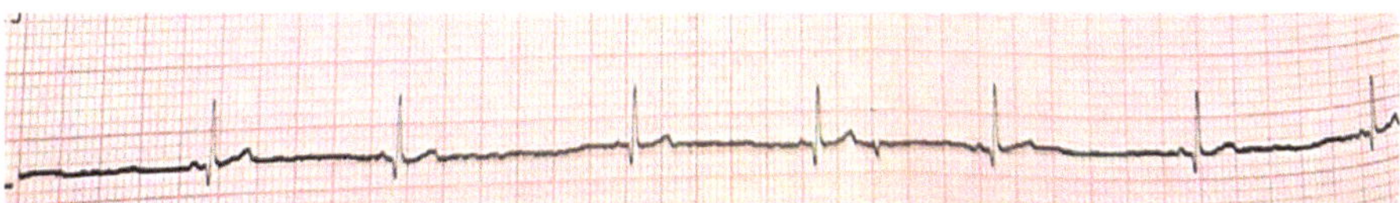

Answer. Electrocardiogram of a dog (lead II, sensitivity1, speed 25 mm/s) showing seven complexes and 6 R-R intervals. HR variability can be calculated as per the following formula (given in chapter 4).

VVTI = $L_n (SD_{R-R})^2$, Where L_n = Mean of 10 consecutive R-R interval, $(SD_{R-R})^2$ = Variance of R-R interval. VVTI = Vasovagal Tonus Index.

VVTI is the measure of calculating heart rate variability. Heart rate 60 bpm. R-R interval is varying from 1.0 to 1.28 second (1.0, 1.28, 1.04, 1.0,1.12, 1.08 seconds)with a mean of 1.086 second . In this case VVTI is 0.010 second or 10 millisecond. VVTI is a reliable indicator of heart rate variability. It means there is beat to beat difference of 10 milliseconds.

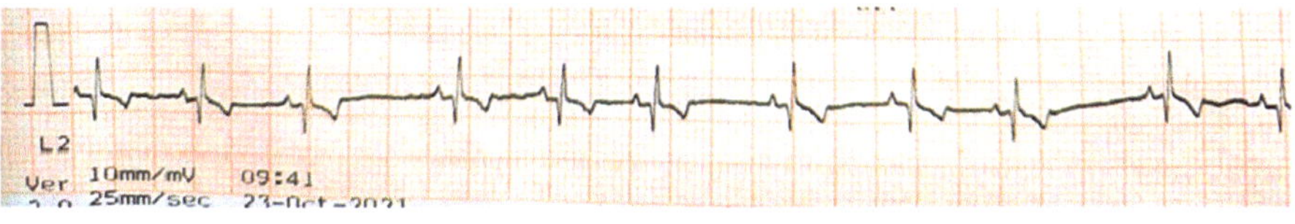

ECG24

Answer. Electrocardiogram of a dog (lead II, sensitivity1, speed 25 mm/s) showing 11 complexes. Q-T interval variability can be calculated as per the following formula (given in chapter 4).

Q-Tc = Q-T/ $\sqrt{}$R-R, Where Q-T c = Q-T interval corrected, Q-T = Mean of 10 Q-T intervals, $\sqrt{}$R-R= square root of R-R interval (mean of 10 intervals)

Heart rate 120 bpm. The mean R-R interval is 0.586 second (mean of 10 consecutive R-R interval). Mean of 10 consecutive Q-T interval is 0.208 second or 208 millisecond (Q-T interval 0.22,0.20,0.20,0.20,0.20,0.22,0.20,0.22, 0.22 and 0.20 second). Q-T –c in this case is 0.271 second or 271 millisecond.

ECG 25

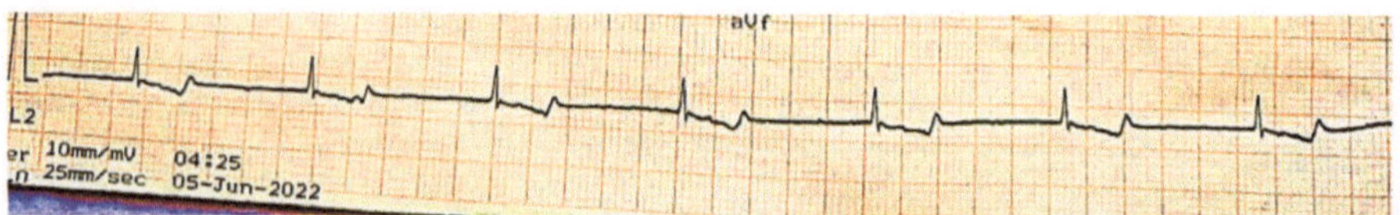

Question. It is an electrocardiogram (Lead II, speed 25 mm/s, sensitivity 1) of a seven year old female cat of 2.3 kg weight with hypothermia (92.0 ^{0}F), lethargy, depression, weak hardly palpable femoral pulse , increased capillary refill time (> 2 second) and mammary tumor. What is your interpretation?

ECG 26

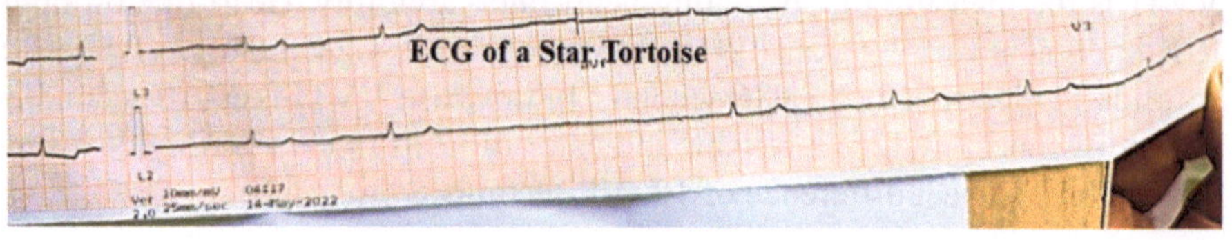

Question. It is an electrocardiogram (lead II, speed 25 mm/s, sensitivity 1) of a star tortoise (800 g) with flaccid body, and no movement. Is it a normal electrocardiogram?

ECG 25

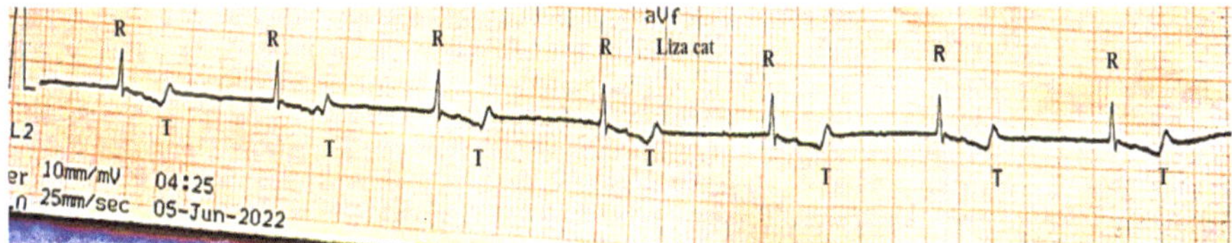

Answer. Electrocardiogram (lead II, sensitivity 1, speed 25 mm/s) of a seven year old female cat of 2.3 kg weight with hypothermia (92.0 ^{0}F), lethargy, depression, weak hardly palpable femoral pulse , increased capillary refill time (>2 second) and mammary tumor is showing regular rhythm (R-R interval 1 second), bradycardia (heart rate 60 bpm), all QRS complexes without P wave, QRS complexes of normal duration (0.03-0.04s, 0.4-0.45 mV), and 60 cycle disturbances suggestive of probable ventricular escape rhythm or idioventricular rhythm or idionodal rhythm. The pacemaker of highest automaticity (SA node pacemaker) has stopped working and its role has been taken over by a pacemaker of a lower region. It is a disorder of impulse formation of SA node pacemaker

ECG 26

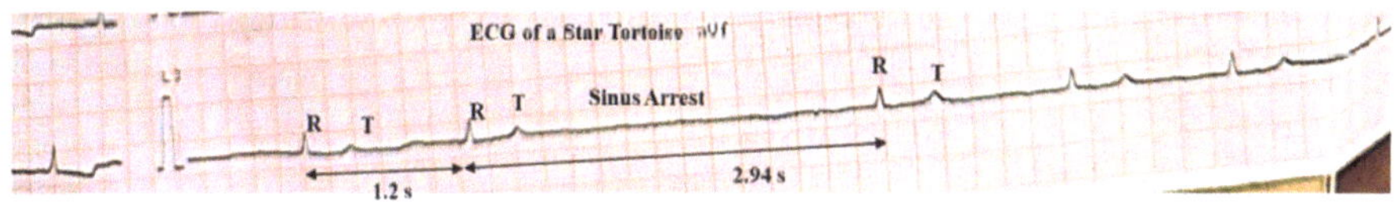

Answer. Electrocardiogram (lead II, speed 25 mm/s, sensitivity 1) of a star tortoise (800 g) with flaccid body, and no movement is showing sinus arrest. The pause (2.94 s) is greater than twice the normal R-R interval (1.2 s). P wave is imperceptible; R and T waves are of low amplitude. These are the characteristics of the tortoise electrocardiogram. The heart rate is 40 bpm. In tortoise/turtles heart continues to beat for sometimes even after death.

ECG27

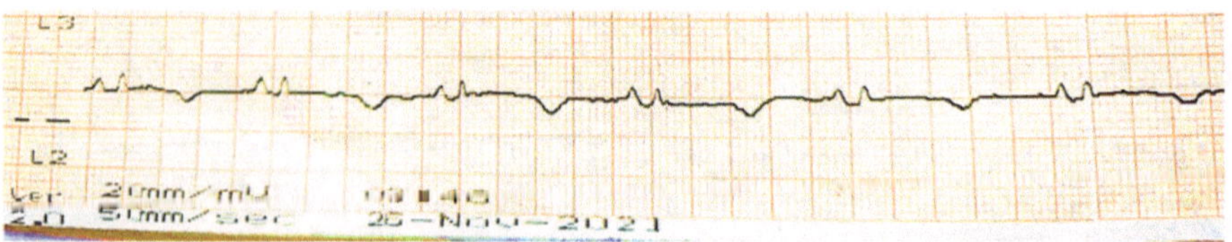

Question. It is an electrocardiogram (lead II, speed 50 mm/s, sensitivity 2) of a 15 day old kitten with unconsciousness, hypothermia (92.2°F) and imperceptible femoral pulse. Calculate the heart rate and measurements of electrocardiographic complexes, intervals and segments.

ECG 28

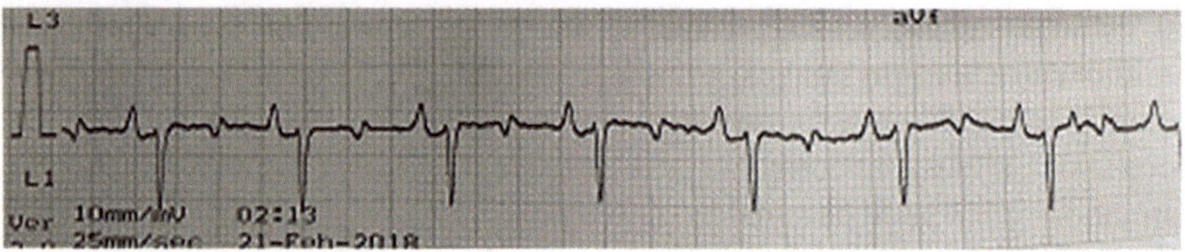

Question. It is an electrocardiogram (lead I, speed 25 mm/s, sensitivity 1) of a one month old cow calf. Calculate heart rate. Is rhythm abnormal? Comment on T wave.

ECG 27

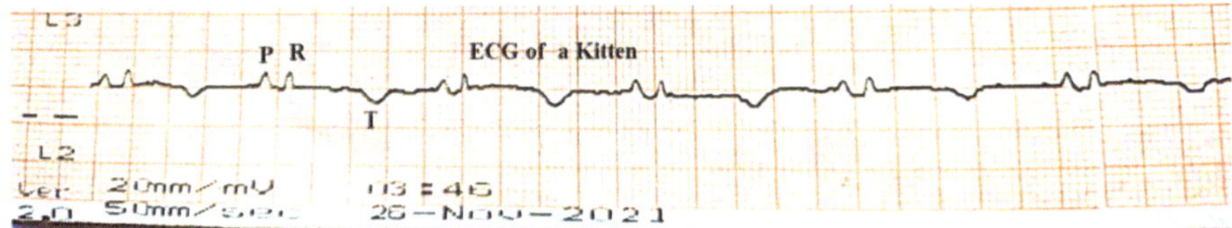

Answer. Electrocardiogram (Lead II, speed 50 mm/s, sensitivity 2) of a 15 day old kitten with unconsciousness, hypothermia (92.2°F) and imperceptible femoral pulse is showing sinus rhythm (R-R interval 0.5 s); bradycardia (HR 120 bpm); normal amplitude and duration of P wave (0.1 mV, 0.02- 0.03 s), QRS (0.1-0.125 mV,0.02 s), T wave (0.05-o.1 mV,0.06 s); normal P-R segment (0.03-0.04 s), normal P-R interval (0.08-0.09 s); S-T segment on baseline (0.14-0.18s); prolonged Q-T interval (0.24-0.28 s) due to slow heart rate. This ECG is suggestive of sinus bradycardia.

ECG 28

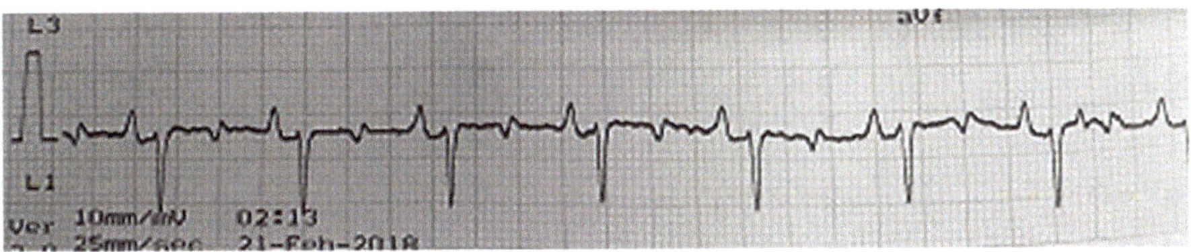

Answer. Electrocardiogram (lead I, speed 25 mm/s, sensitivity 1) of a one month old cow calf is showing sinus rhythm (R-R interval 0.6 s), QRS of rS type. Heart rate is 100 bpm. P wave is normal (0.2 mV, 0.04 s).There is very small r wave. S wave is deep (0.8 mV). T wave is biphasic.

ECG29

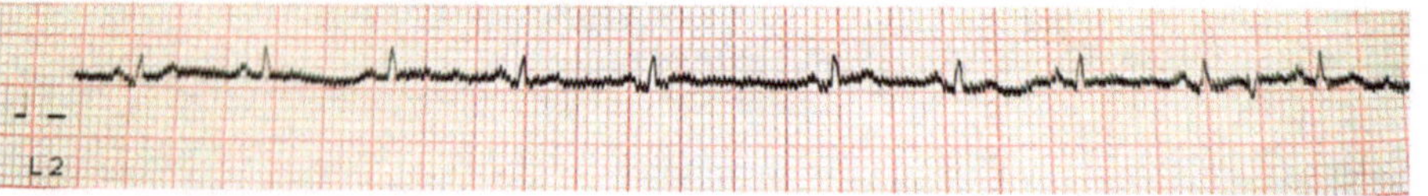

Question. It is an electrocardiogram (lead II, speed 25 mm/s, sensitivity 1) of a pug with ascites. What is the predominant abnormality in this electrocardiogram?

ECG30

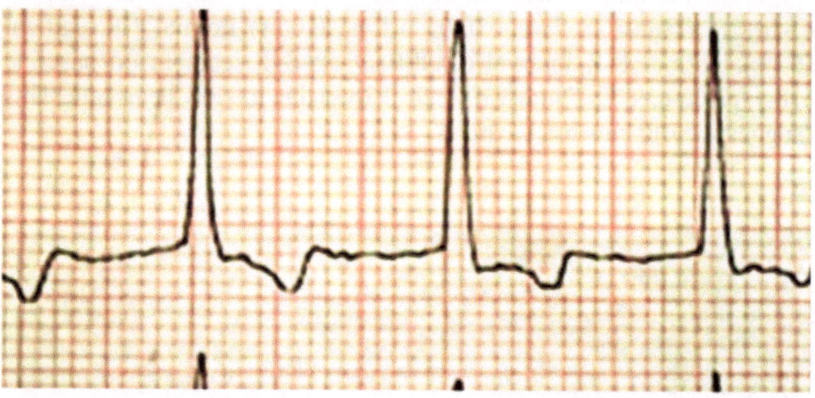

Question. It is electrocardiographic complexes of a dog (lead II, speed 25 mm/s, sensitivity 1) with the history of syncope. Are these complexes normal?

ECG 29

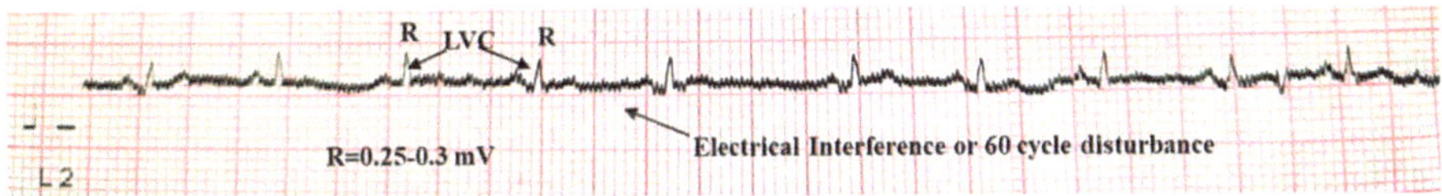

Answer. Electrocardiogram (lead II, speed 25 mm/s, sensitivity 1) of a pug with ascites is showing electrical interference commonly called as 60 cycle disturbance and low voltage complex as amplitude of R wave is < 0.5 mV.

ECG 30

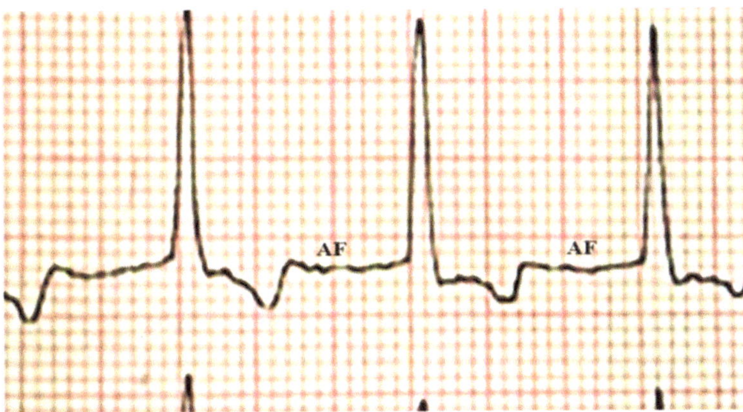

Answer. Electrocardiographic complexes of the dog with syncope (lead II, sensitivity 1, speed 25 mm/s) are not normal because there is no distinct P wave. P waves have been replaced by fine fibrillations. QRS is broad (0.08 sec) and R amplitude is within range (1.6 mV) suggesting atrial fibrillations and left bundle branch block.

ECG 31

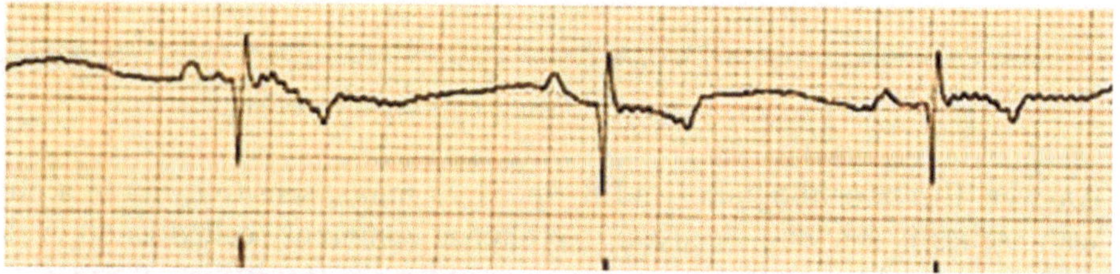

Question. It is an electrocardiogram (lead II, speed 50 mm/s, sensitivity 1) of a male dog . What is the type of QRS pattern?

ECG 32

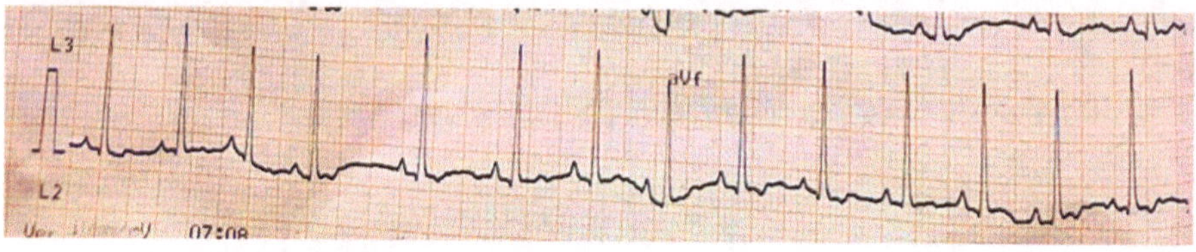

Question. It is an electrocardiogram (lead II, speed 25 mm/s, sensitivity 1) of a male Labrador dog with edema on ear pinna, hind limbs, abdomen; hepato and splenomegaly. What abnormality is seen in this electrocardiogram?

ECG 31

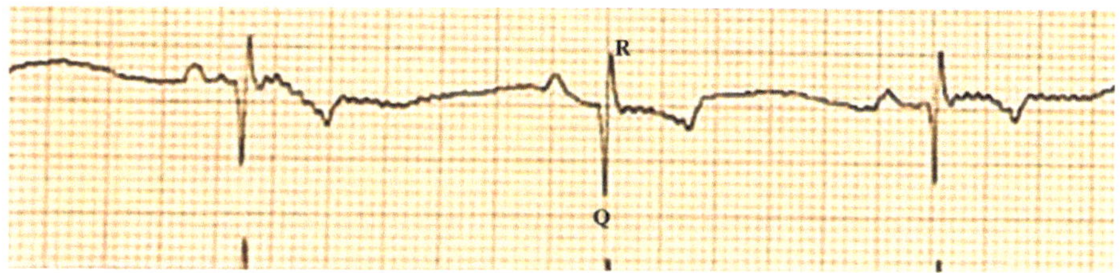

Answer. Electrocardiogram (lead II, sensitivity 1, speed 50 mm/s) of the male dog is showing QR type of QRS pattern. The Q wave is deep (0.8 mV). QRS is normal (0.04 s).It may be due to right ventricle enlargement / right bundle branch block. Differentiation of these two conditions require study of other leads as well as of chest radiograph.

ECG 32

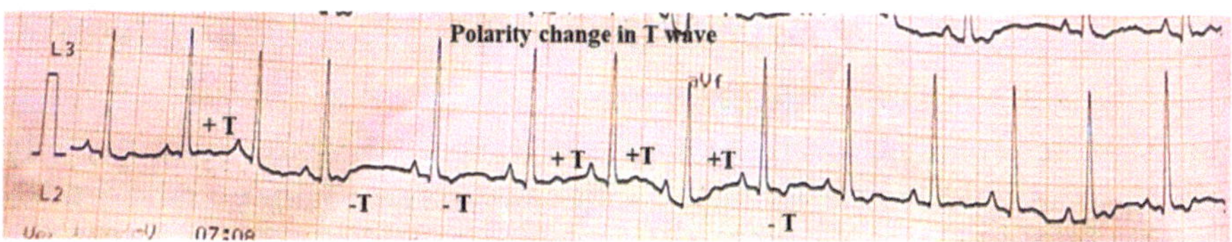

Answer. Electrocardiogram (lead II, speed 25 mm/s, sensitivity 1) of a male Labrador dog with edema on ear pinna ,hind limbs, abdomen ; hepato and splenomegaly is showing polarity change in T wave. Polarity of T wave in complex 1,2,3,6,7 and 8 is +ve; and in complex 4, 5, 9, 10, 13 and 14 is negative.

ECG 33

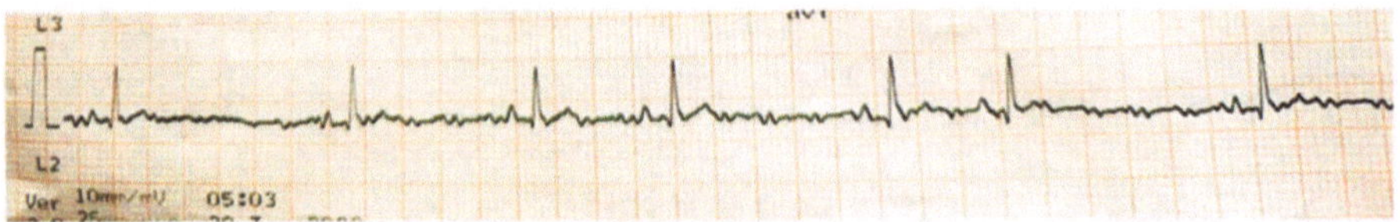

Question. It is an electrocardiogram (lead II, speed 25 mm/s, sensitivity 1) of a five year old male German Shepherd dog with edema of both hind limbs and scrotum. The dog was negative to brucellosis. What are main abnormalities in this electrocardiogram?

ECG 34

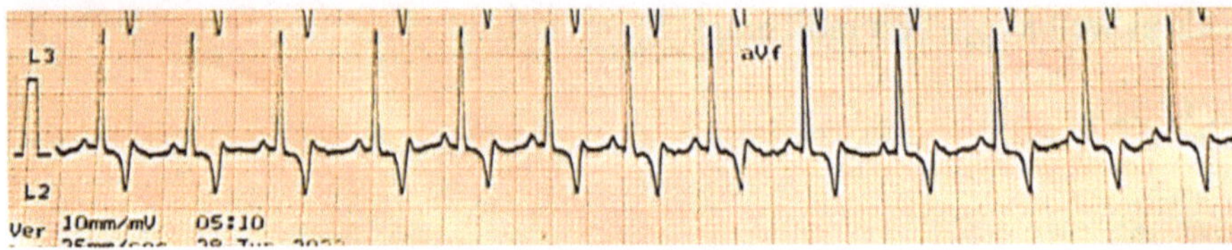

Question. It is an electrocardiogram (lead II, speed 25 mm/s, sensitivity 1) of a 62 month old female Labrador with chronic renal failure grade 5 (Hb 5.5 g/dl, total erythrocytes 2.62 x $10^{6}/mm^{3}$. HCT 17.4%, serum creatinine 10.12 mg/dl, BUN 122.7 mg/dl calcium 9.0 mg/dl, serum phosphorus 10. 0 mg/dl, sodium 146 mEq/L, potassium 5.2 mEq/L, chloride 101.7 mEq/L, urine protein ++, pus cells 60-65 /hpf, epithelial cell 10-12/hpf, sp.gr. 1.025). What is your interpretation?

ECG 33

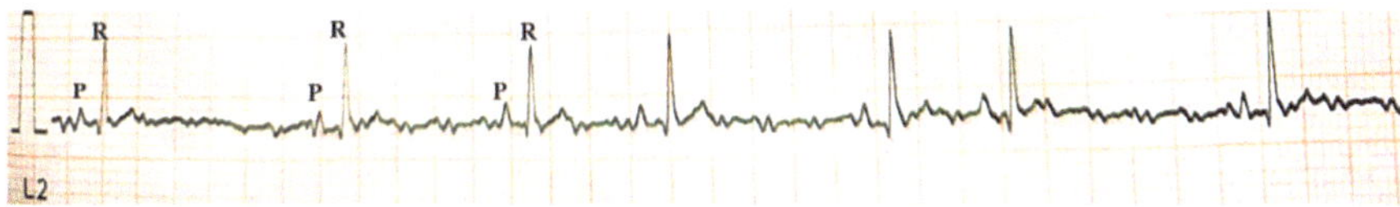

Answer. Electrocardiogram (lead II, speed 25 mm/s, sensitivity 1) of a five year old male German Shepherd dog with edema of both hind limbs and scrotum, is showing irregular rhythm (R-R interval varying from 0.56, to 1.34 s indicating sinus block/sinus arrest) ,a heart rate of 70 bpm and artifacts due to muscle tremors. At many places P wave is difficult to identify clearly while ventricular rhythm is easily identifiable. The T wave is also difficult to identify clearly. The rapid and irregular vibrations of baseline are giving an impression of atrial flutter/fibrillation.

ECG 34

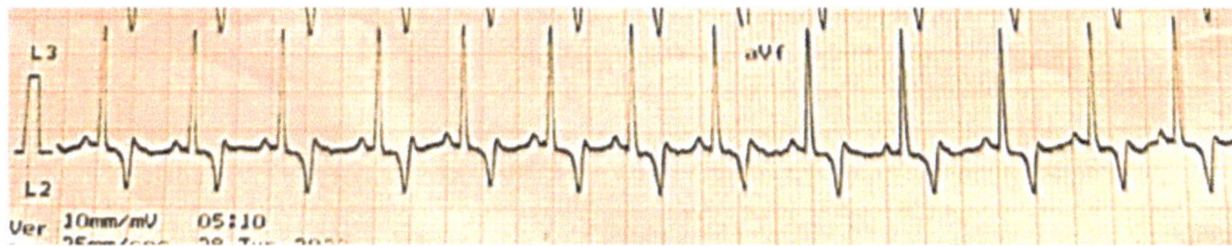

Answer. Electrocardiogram (lead II, speed 25 mm/s, sensitivity 1) of a 62 month old female Labrador with chronic renal failure grade 5 (Hb 5.5 g/dl, Total erythrocytes 2.62 x 10^6/mm^3, HCT 17.4%, serum creatinine 10.12 mg/dl, BUN 122.7 mg/dl calcium 9.0 mg/dl, serum phosphorus 10. 0 mg/dl, sodium 146 mEq/L, potassium 5.2 mEq/L, chloride 101.7 mEq/L, urine protein ++, pus cells 60-65 /hpf, epithelial cell 10-12/hpf, sp.gr. 1.025) is showing a heart rate of 120 bpm with sinus rhythm (R-R interval 0.5 s) ; normal P wave (0.1 mV, 0.04 s), P-R interval (0.08 s), QRS complex (R 1.55 mV, QRS 0.04 s); S-T segment depression (0.1 mV); relatively large (in relation to R wave) negative and biphasic T wave (0.5 mV, 0.08 s). T wave changes may be due to uremia.

ECG 35

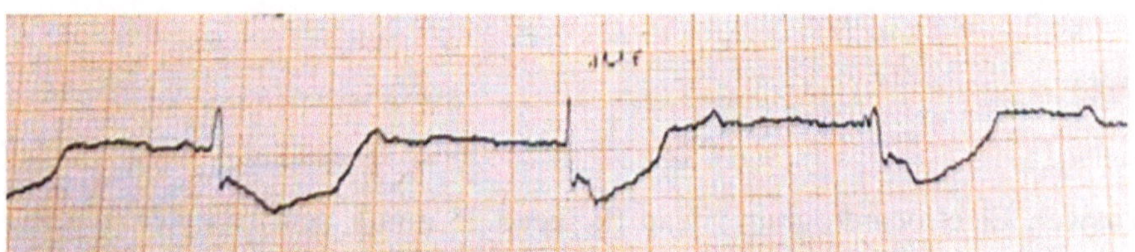

Question. It is an electrocardiogram (lead II, speed 50 mm/s, sensitivity 2) of a non-descript kitten of 35 days with shock. What are the conspicuous abnormalities in this electrocardiogram?

ECG36

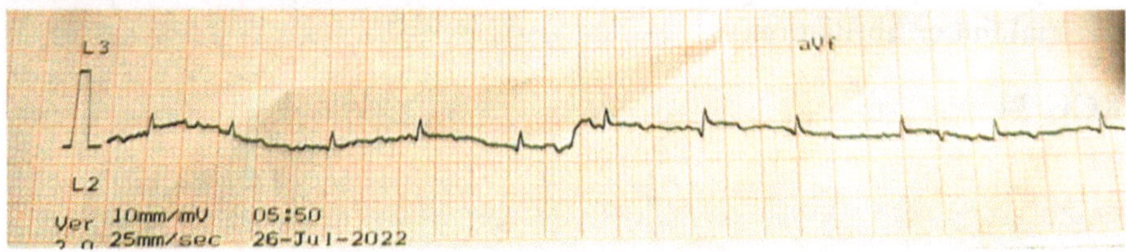

Question. It is an electrocardiogram (lead II, speed 25 mm/s, sensitivity 1) of a non-descript kitten of 50 days with anemia (Hb 5.2 g/dl, PCV 14.2%, total erythrocyte count 1.8 x 10^6/mm3),diarrhea, vomiting, anorexia, round worm infestation and hypothermia (92.0^{0}F). What is your interpretation?

ECG 35

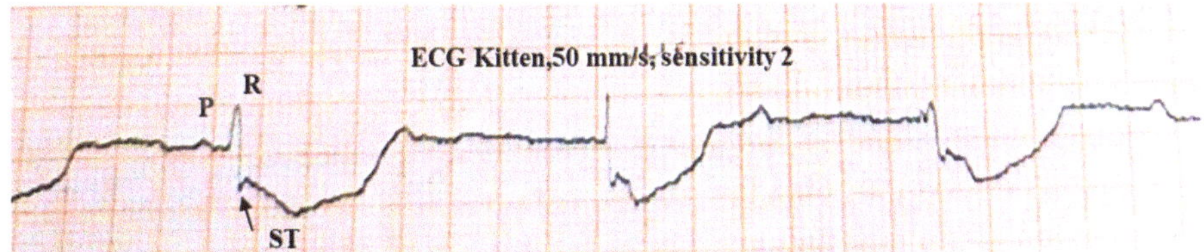

Answer .Electrocardiogram (lead II, speed 50 mm/s, sensitivity 2) of a non-descript kitten of 35 days with shock is showing bradycardia (heart rate 105 bpm), a narrow QRS, and marked ST segment depression (0.2mV).

ECG 36

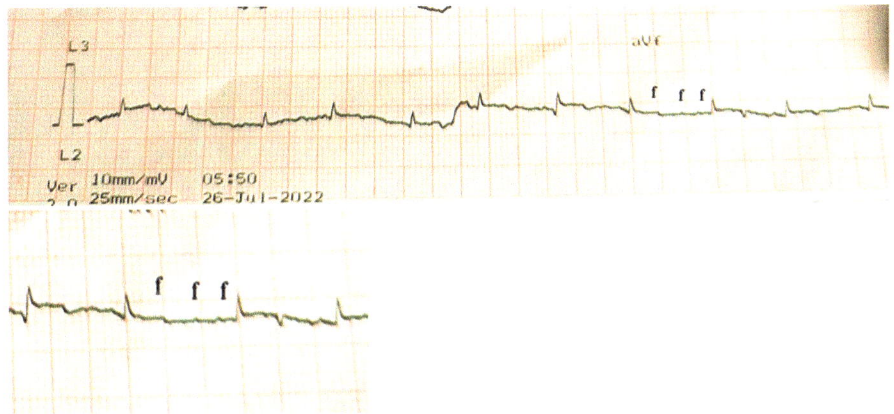

Answer. Electrocardiogram (lead II, speed 25 mm/s, sensitivity 1) of a non-descript kitten of 50 days with anemia (Hb 5.2 g/dl, PCV 14.2%, total erythrocyte count 1.8 x 10^6/mm3),diarrhea, vomiting, anorexia, round worm infestation and hypothermia (92.0 ^{0}F) is showing atrial fibrillation. The ‘P’ waves are absent and have been replaced with ‘f’ waves (fine oscillations).

ECG 37

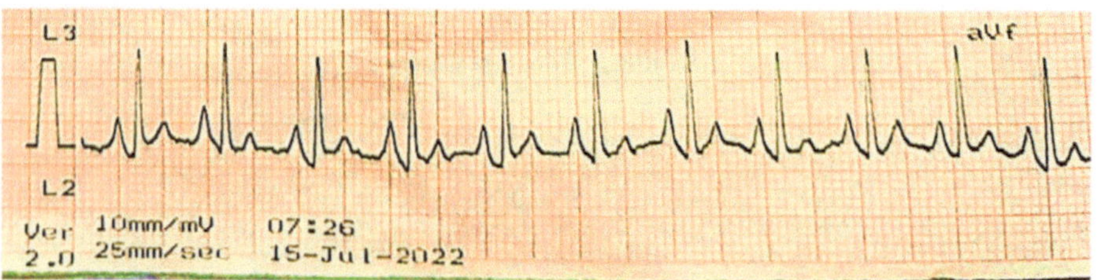

Question. It is an electrocardiogram (lead II, speed 25 mm/s, sensitivity 1) of an adult Labrador with weakness. What is your interpretation?

ECG 38

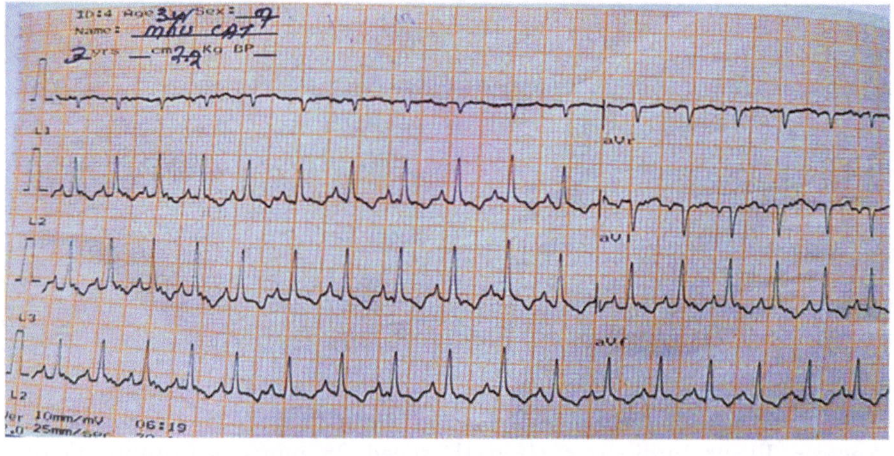

Question. It is an electrocardiogram (lead I, II, III, aVR, aVL and aVF; speed 25 mm/s, sensitivity 1) of a three year old nondescript cat with weakness and respiratory distress . What is your interpretation?

ECG37

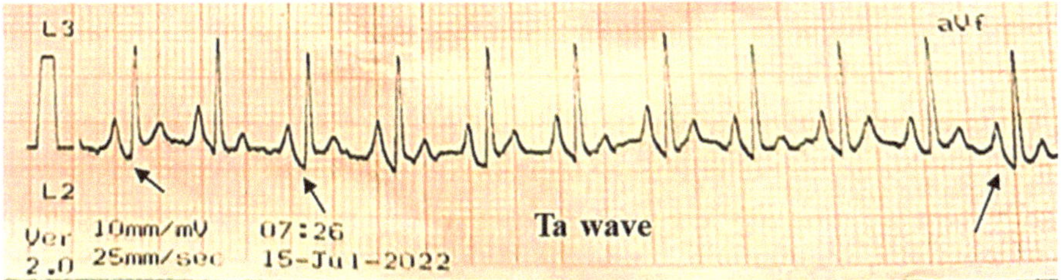

Answer. Electrocardiogram (lead II, speed 25 mm/s, sensitivity 1) of an adult Labrador, with weakness is showing sinus rhythm and Ta wave (depression of the base line following the P wave), an indication of right atrial enlargement.

ECG38

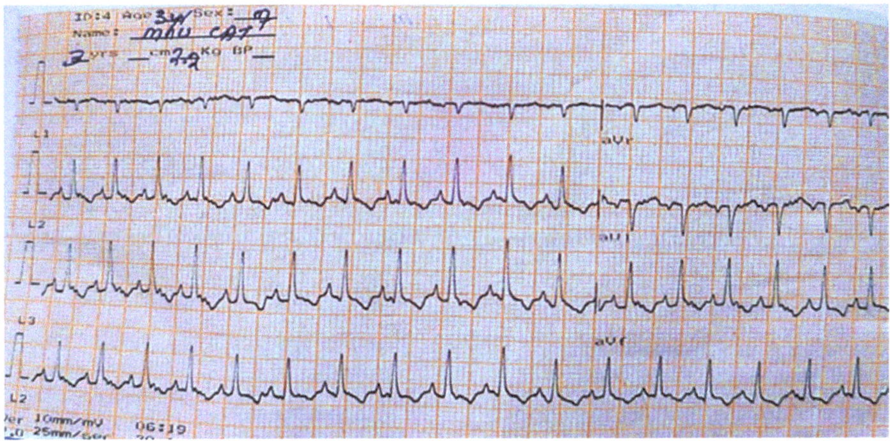

Answer. Electrocardiogram (lead I, II, III, aVR, aVL and aVF; speed 25 mm/s, sensitivity 1) of a three year old nondescript cat with weakness and respiratory distress is showing sinus rhythm (heart rate 180 bpm, R-R interval 0.33 s), normal 'P' wave (0.15-0.2 mV, 0.04 s), normal 'P-R' interval (0.1 s), slightly variable amplitude of 'R' wave (lead II 0.7 to 0.9 mV), and slightly variable 'QRS' (0.03 to 0.04 s). These changes are within range. Therefore electrocardiogram is not suggestive of any significant abnormality.

ECG 39

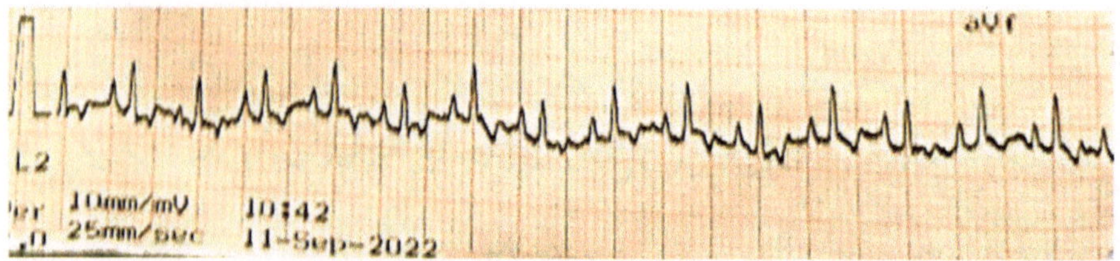

Question. It is an electrocardiogram (lead II, speed 25 mm/s, sensitivity 1) of an adult Pomeranian bitch with lymphedema. What is your interpretation?

ECG 40

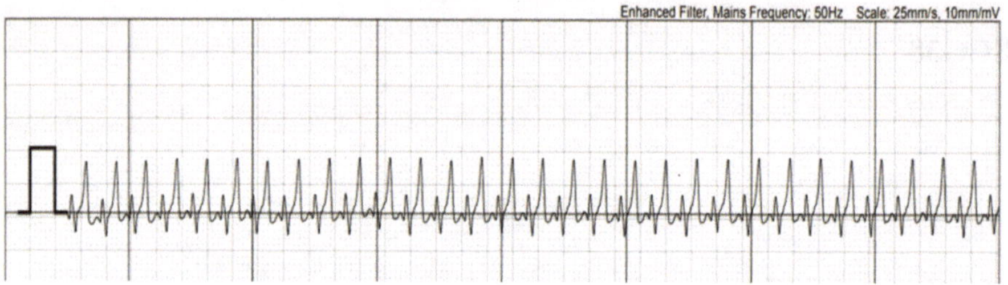

Question. It is an electrocardiogram (lead II, speed 25 mm/s, sensitivity 1) of an adult dog. Is it a normal electrocardiogram? If not. What abnormalities are there?

ECG 39

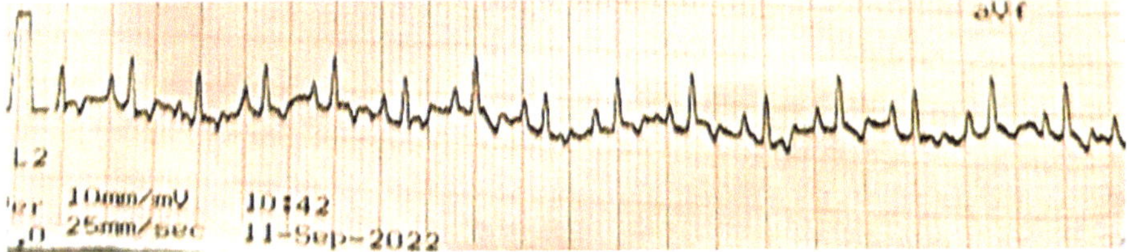

Answer. Electrocardiogram (lead II, speed 25 mm/s, sensitivity 1) of an adult Pomeranian bitch with lymphedema is showing sinus tachycardia (heart rate 200 bpm, R-R interval 0.3 s).

ECG 40

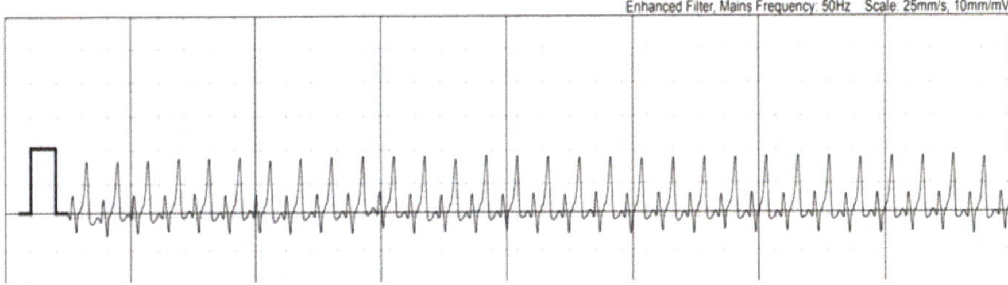

Answer. Electrocardiogram (lead II, speed 25 mm/s, sensitivity 1) of an adult dog is showing sinus tachycardia (heart rate 240 bpm, R-R interval 0.25 s), low voltage complex (R amplitude 0.3 mV) with large pointed 'T' wave (0.9 mV).

ECG 41

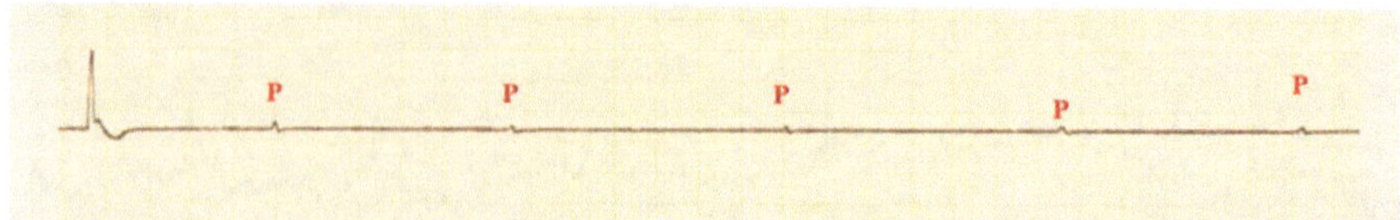

Question. It is an electrocardiogram (lead II, sensitivity 1, speed 25 mm/second) of a 5 year old male Rottweiler. What is your interpretation?

ECG 42

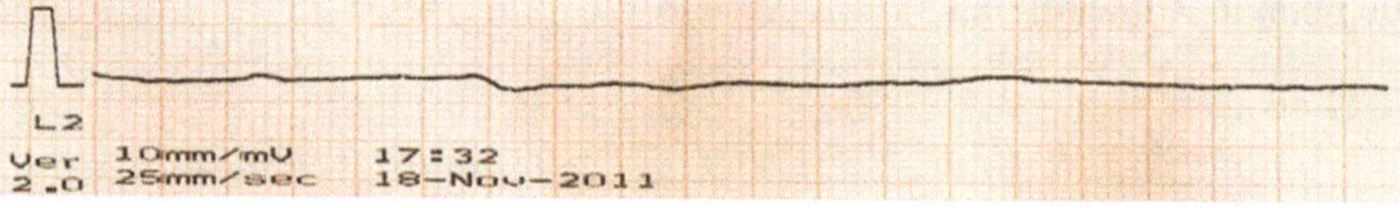

Question. It is an electrocardiogram (lead II, sensitivity 1, speed 25 mm/second) of a 7 year old male German shepherd. Interpret this electrocardiogram?

ECG 41

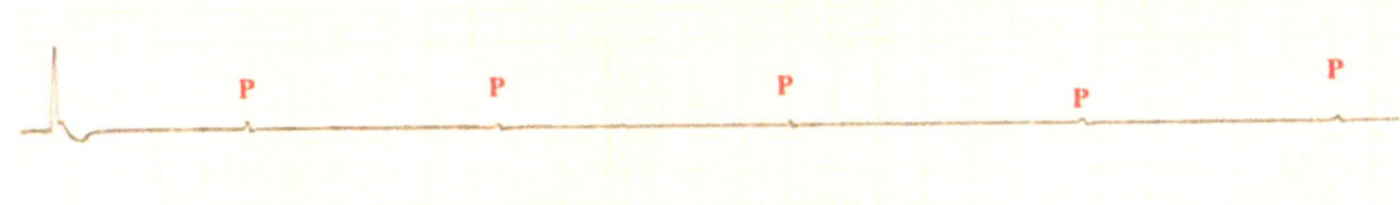

Answer. Electrocardiogram (lead II, sensitivity 1, speed 25 mm/second) of a 5 year old male Rottweiler showing ventricular asystole with severe AV Block. Ventricular activity is seen only in the beginning of the strip. Thereafter only P waves are seen without any ventricular activity. Conduction between atria and ventricles is absent. It is a case of complete heart block associated with failing ventricular pacemaker.

ECG 42

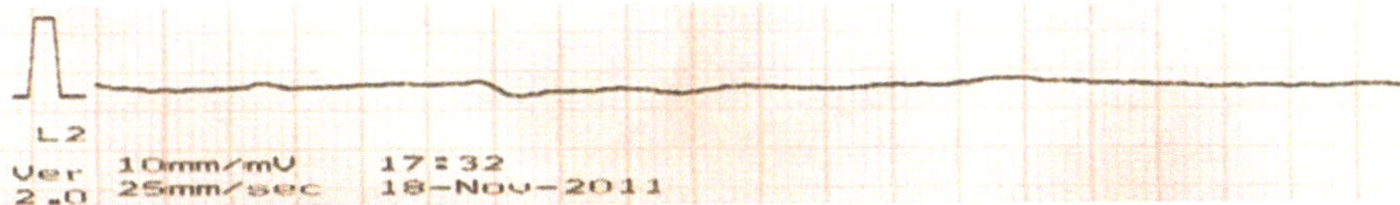

Answer. Electrocardiogram (lead II, sensitivity 1, speed 25 mm/second) of a 7 year old male German shepherd is showing no atrial and ventricular activity suggesting death.

ECG 43

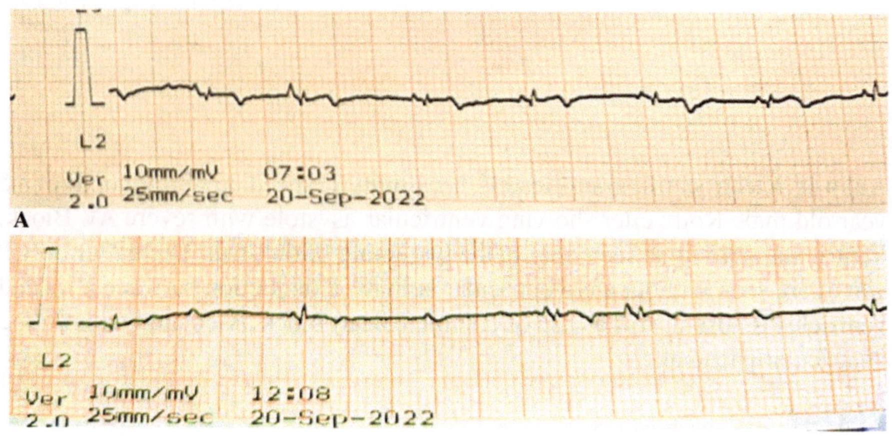

B

Question. These are two electrocardiograms (lead II, sensitivity 1, speed 25 mm/s) of a male 3 month old pocket Pomeranian with late decompensatory shock (pale mucus membranes with no capillary refill, hypotension, weak pulse, oliguria/anuria, mental depression, hypothermia (temperature 95^{0}F) , slow respiration and stupor) . What is your interpretation?

ECG 44

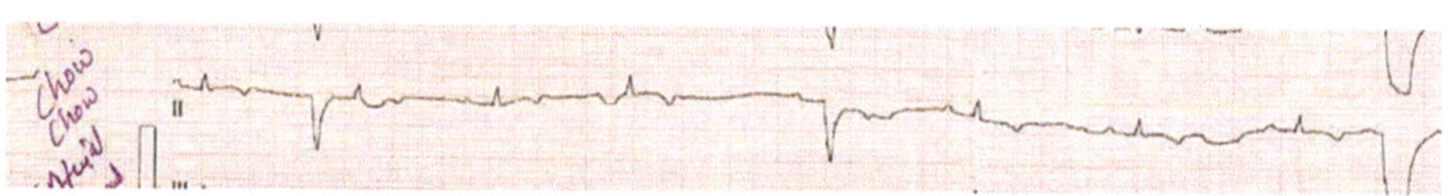

Question. It is an electrocardiograms (lead II, sensitivity 1, speed 25 mm/s) of a female 2.5 year old Chow Chow dog. What is your interpretation?

ECG 43

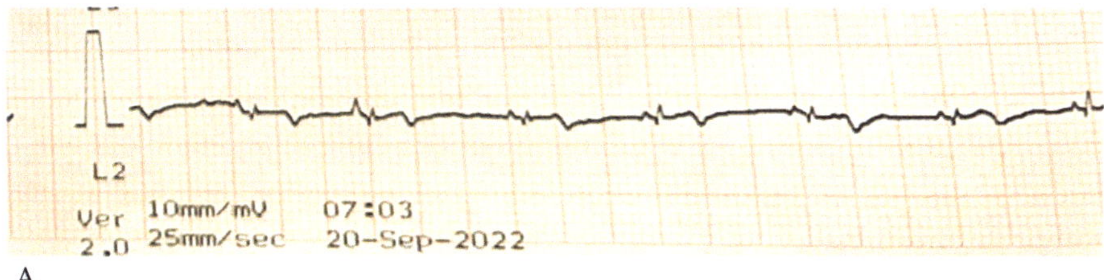

A

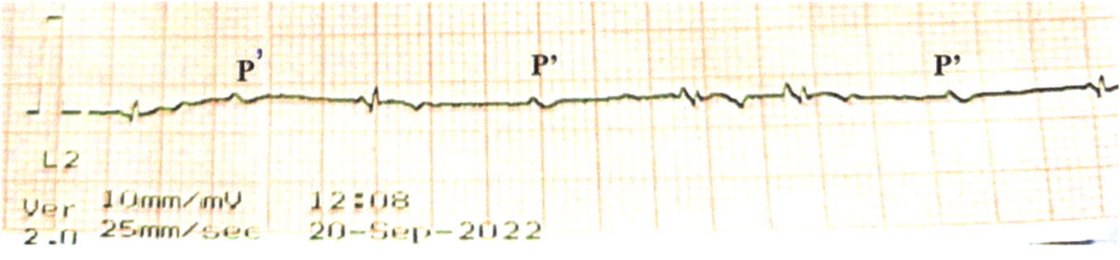

B

Answer. A. Electrocardiogram (lead II, sensitivity 1, speed 25 mm/s) of a male 3 month old pocket Pomeranian with late decompensatory shock (pale mucus membranes with no capillary refill, hypotension, weak, oliguria/anuria, mental depression, temperature 95^{0}F, slow respiration and stupor) is showing sinus bradycardia (heart rate 105 bpm, R-R interval 0.57 s). All complexes are of low amplitude because of very small heart size at this age.

B. Electrocardiogram of the same dog, taken 5 hours later, is showing development of 2nd degree AV block (intermittent disturbance of AV conduction). P' wave is not conducted. The strip shows ventricular rate of 79 / minute while atrial rate of 126 /minute.

ECG 44

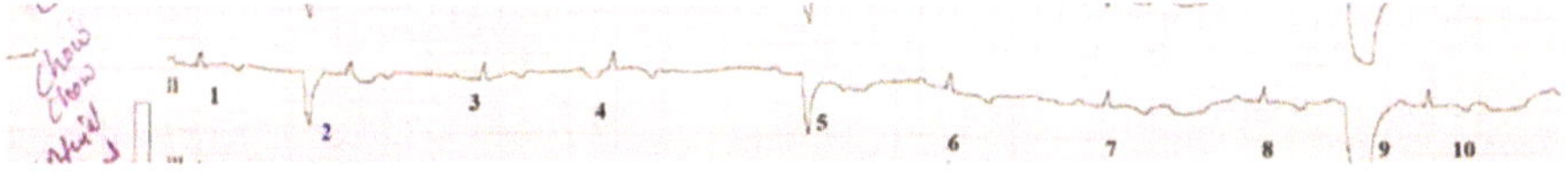

Answer. Electrocardiogram (lead II, sensitivity 1, speed 25 mm/s) of a female 2.5 year old Chow Chow dog is showing multiform ventricular premature complexes (2,5 and 9) as complexes are of variable shape and size. The other complexes (1, 3, 4,6,7,8, and 10) are sinus complexes. The rhythm is irregular due to premature and bizarre QRS complexes. VPCs are not associated with 'P' wave. The QRS deflection in VPC is negative suggesting that ectopic foci are in left ventricle.

ECG 45

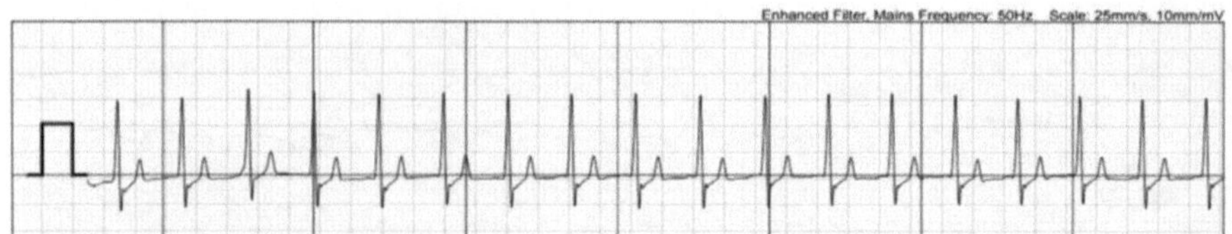

Question. It is an electrocardiogram (lead II, sensitivity 1, speed 25 mm/s) of an adult dog. What is your interpretation?

ECG 46

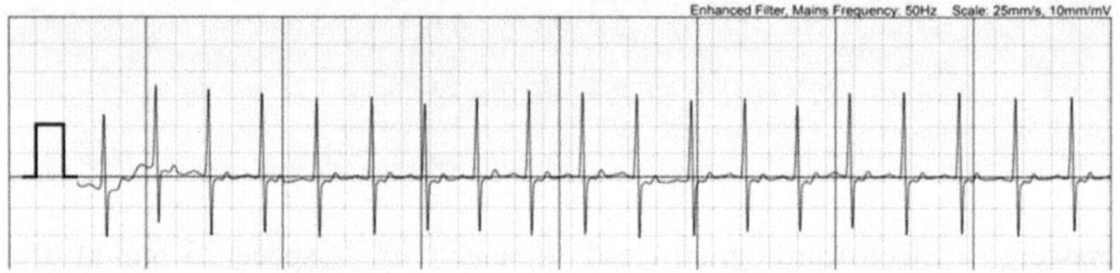

Question. It is an electrocardiogram (lead II, sensitivity 1, speed 25 mm/s) of an adult dog. What is your interpretation?

ECG 45

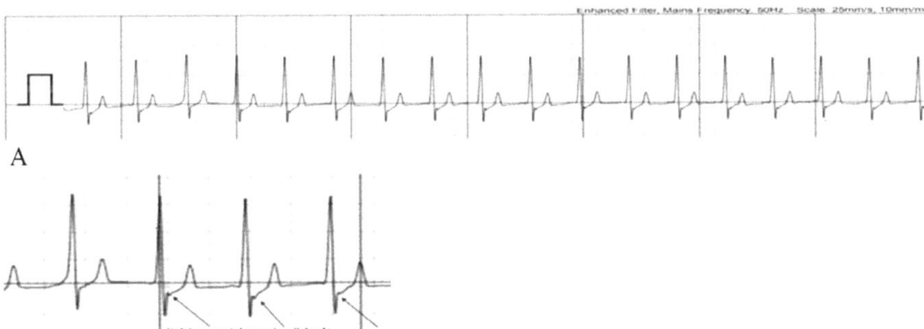

A

B

Answer. Electrocardiogram (Lead II, sensitivity 1, speed 25 mm/s) of an adult dog (A) and its cropped up portion (B) is showing ventricular heart rate of 140 bpm, fine atrial fibrillations and S-T depression of 0.3 mV.

ECG 46

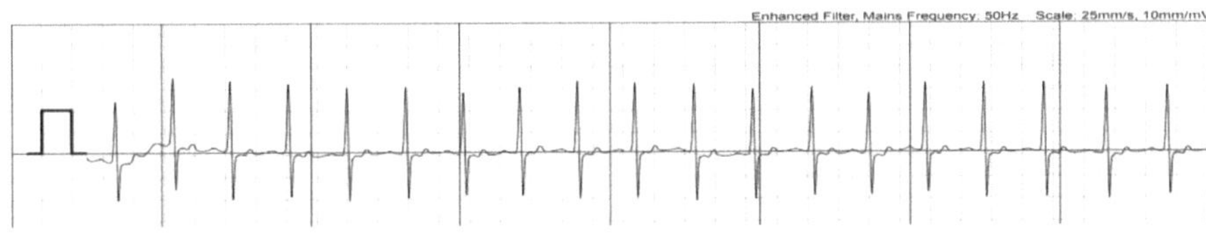

A

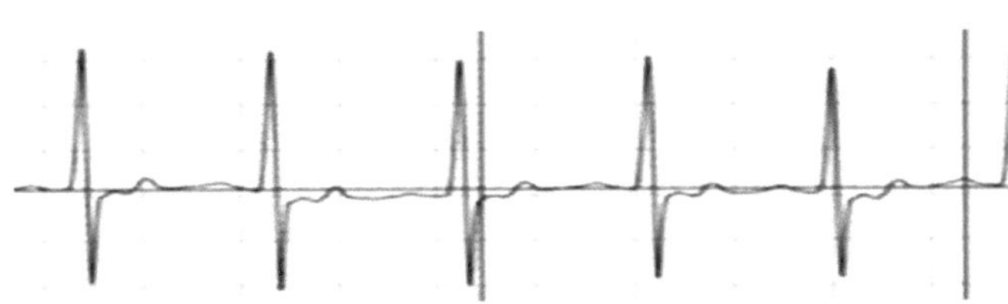

B

Answer: Electrocardiogram (lead II, sensitivity 1, speed 25 mm/s) of an adult dog is showing heart rate of 160 bpm (A) ; deep 'S' wave (0.9 to 1.0 mV), and wide 'QRS' (0.08 s) in cropped up figure (B) suggestive of right ventricle enlargement/

ECG 47

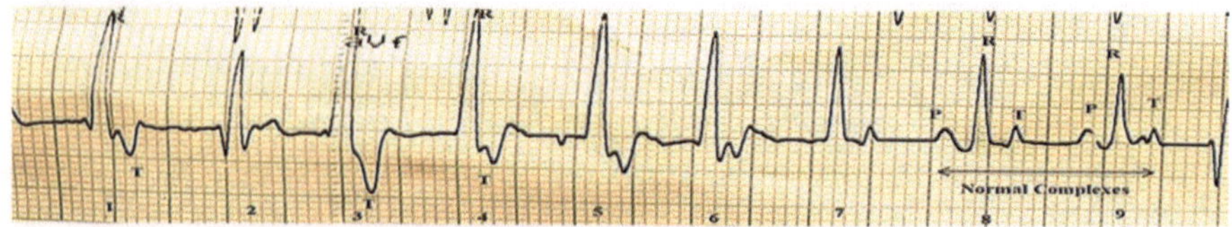

Question. It is an electrocardiogram (lead II, sensitivity 1, speed 25 mm/s) of an adult dog. What is your interpretation?

ECG 48

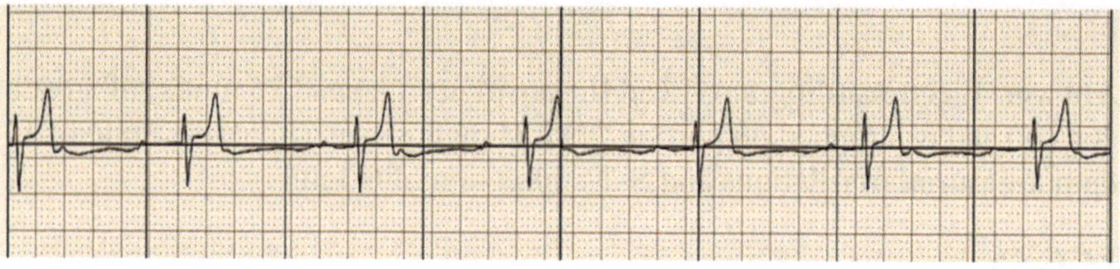

Question. It is an electrocardiogram (lead II, sensitivity 1, speed 25 mm/s) of an adult dog. What is your interpretation?

ECG 47

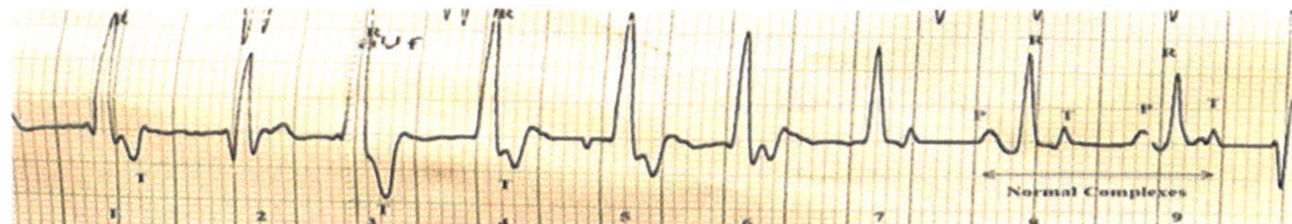

Answer .Electrocardiogram (lead II, sensitivity 1, speed 25 mm/second) of an adult dog is showing ventricular premature complexes. Heart rate is 135 bpm. Complex no. 8 and 9 are sinus complexes having 'P', 'QRS' and 'T' waves. While complex no.1,2,3 and 4 are not associated with 'P' wave and 'T' wave is negative (opposite of broad and bizarre QRS). Complex no.5 is associated with negative 'P' wave, broad and bizarre 'QRS' and negative 'T' wave. The 'QRS' of complex no .6 is having P' wave (APC) and negative 'T' wave. The complex no 7 is having very small 'P' wave broad 'QRS' and positive T .The 'QRS complex of 1,2,3,4,5,6 and 7 is broad and bizarre differing in configuration suggestive of multiform origin. Abnormal premature beat does not have 'P' wave, its QRS is bizarre and 'T' wave is opposite of QRS.

ECG 48

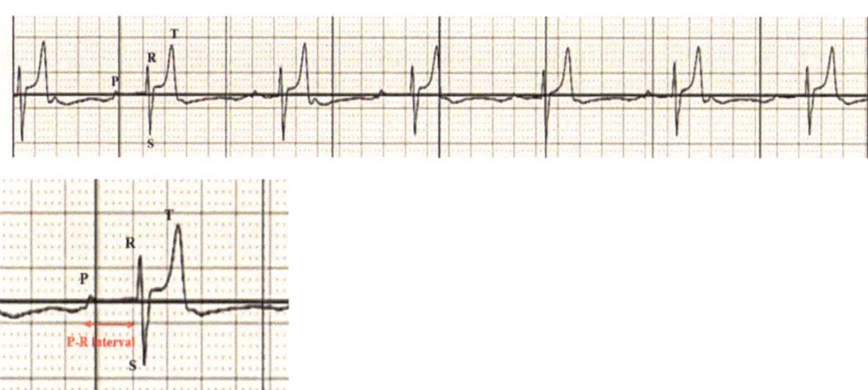

Answer . Electrocardiogram (lead II, speed 25 mm/s, sensitivity 1) of a dog showing 1st degree AV-block. The P-R interval is 0.26 to 0.28 s (> 0.13 s). It is due to delay in conduction of supraventricular impulse through AV-junction and Bundle of His.

ECG 49

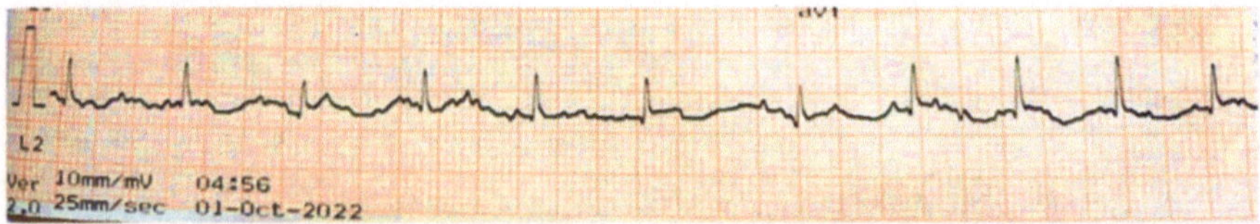

Question. It is an electrocardiogram (lead II, speed 25 mm/s, sensitivity 1) of a 5 year old male obese Labrador (50 kg weight, fat deposition on neck and thorax) with the history of syncope. cTn-I (0.12 ng/ml) and chest x-ray were unremarkable but hip x-ray was consistent with osteoarthritis. Is it a normal electrocardiogram?

ECG 50

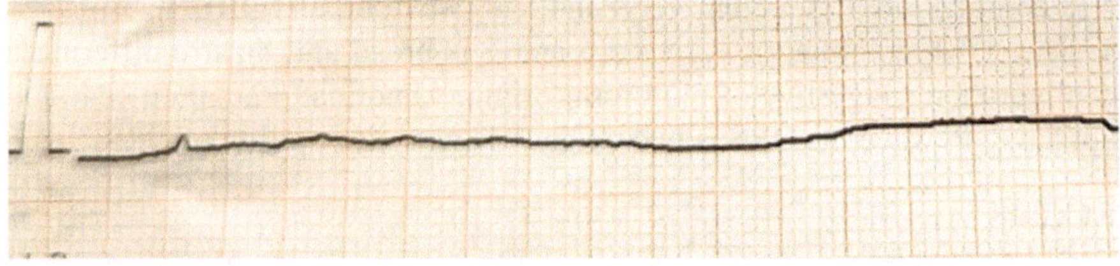

Question. Electrocardiogram (lead II, speed 25 mm/s, sensitivity 1) of an inactive turtle weighing 300g. What is your interpretation?

ECG 49

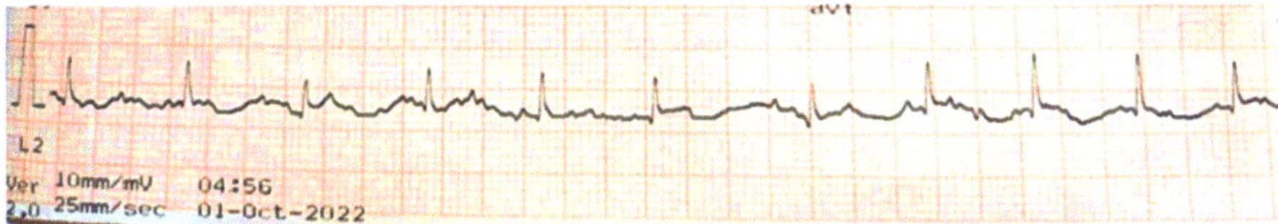

Answer. Electrocardiogram (lead II, speed 25 mm/s, sensitivity 1) of a 5 year old male obese Labrador (50 kg weight, fat deposition on neck and thorax) is showing artifacts due to erratic respiratory disturbances, heart rate of 110 bpm, and reduced voltage (0.5 mV to 0.7 mV) of 'R' wave. cTn-I (0.12 ng/dl) and chest x-ray was unremarkable but hip radiograph was consistent with osteoarthritis. It appears that reduced voltage of the 'R' was associated with obesity.

ECG 50

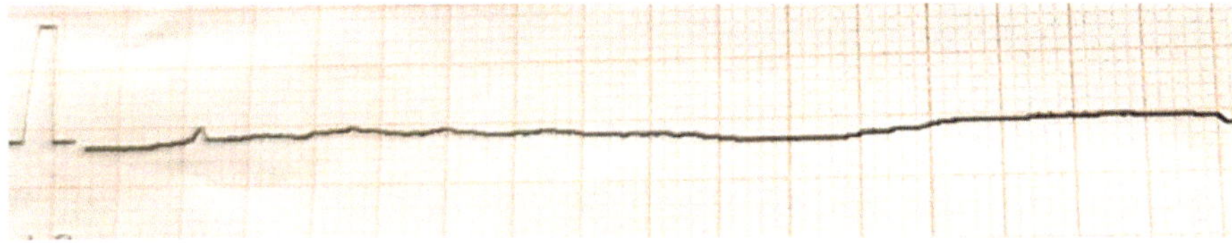

Answer. Electrocardiogram (lead II, speed 25 mm/s, sensitivity 1) of an inactive turtle weighing 300g is showing ventricular asystole. There is only one complex in the beginning of the strip. It appears that the heart made an attempt to reverse the cardiac arrest but failed.

ECG 51

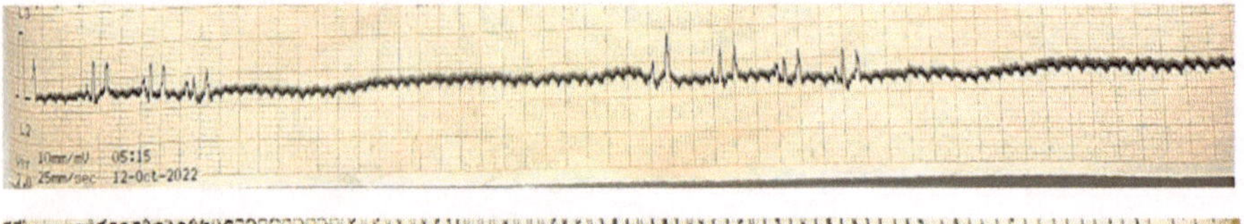

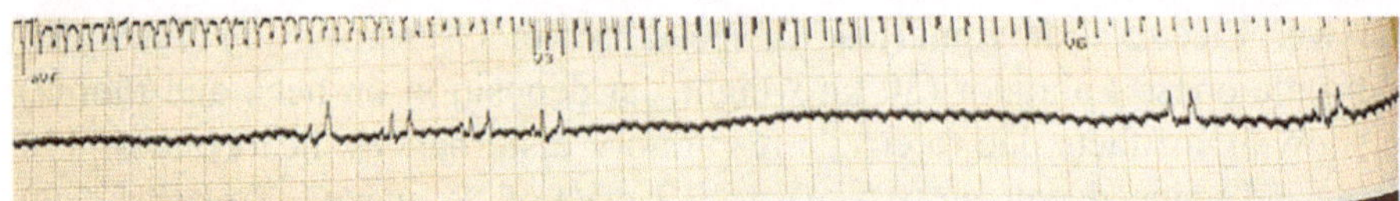

Question. It is an electrocardiogram (lead II, speed 25 mm/s, sensitivity 1) of a male adult (6 years) Lhasa Apso dog with tracheal stenosis and sudden syncope. What is your interpretation?

ECG 52

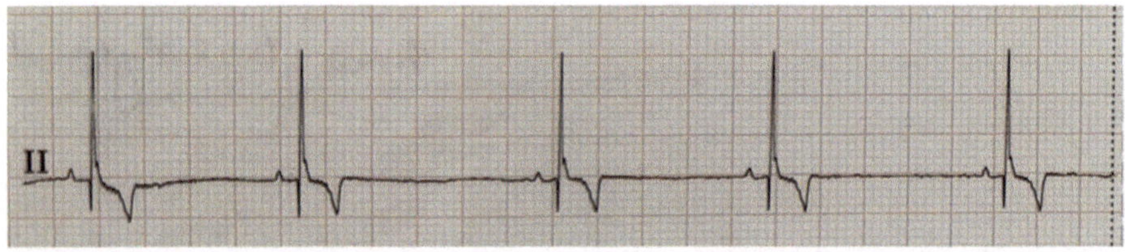

Question. It is an electrocardiogram (lead II, speed 25 mm/s, sensitivity 1) of a dog with dilated cardiomyopathy. What is your interpretation?

ECG 51

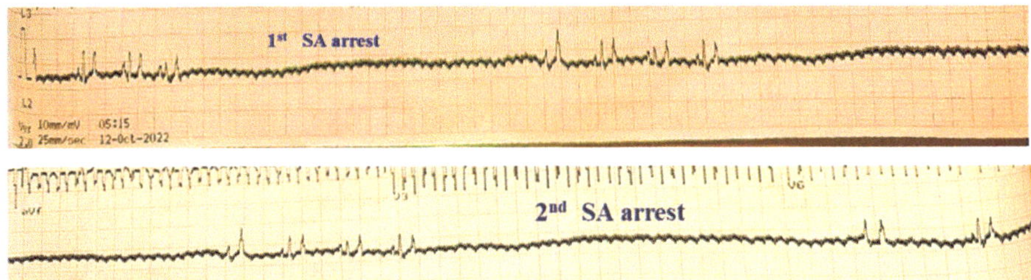

Answer. Electrocardiogram (lead II, speed 25 mm/s, sensitivity 1) of a male adult (6 years) Lhasa Apso dog with tracheal stenosis and sudden syncope is showing intermittent sinus arrest. Both arrests (marked as 1st and 2nd) are of long duration (almost 4 seconds each). The episodes of syncope were possibly due to long episodes of sinoatrial arrest. The ' P' wave is of normal configuration. QRS is also normal. R wave showing alternans. T wave is comparatively large. 60 cycle disturbances are also conspicuous in this electrocardiogram.

ECG 52

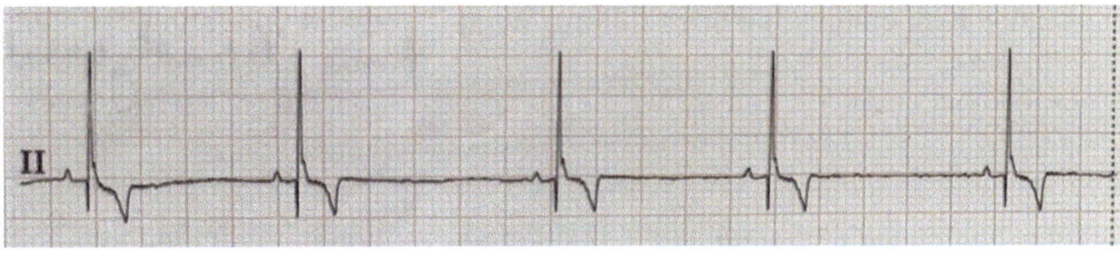

Answer. Electrocardiogram (lead II, speed 25 mm/s, sensitivity 1) of a dog with dilated cardiomyopathy is showing heart rate of 57 beats per minute and R-R interval of 0.94 to 1.14 s suggesting sinus bradycardia.

ECG 53

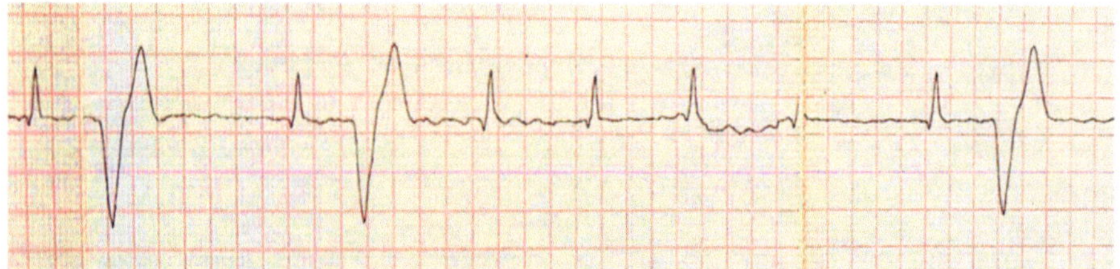

Question. It is an electrocardiogram (lead II, speed 50 mm/s, sensitivity 1) of a Rottweiler dog with dilated cardiomyopathy. What is your interpretation?

ECG 54

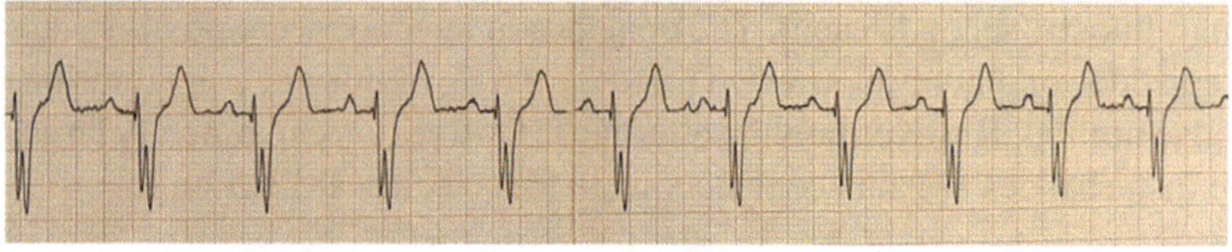

Question. It is an electrocardiogram (lead II, speed 50 mm/s, sensitivity 1) of a Labrador with congestive heart failure. What is your interpretation?

ECG 53

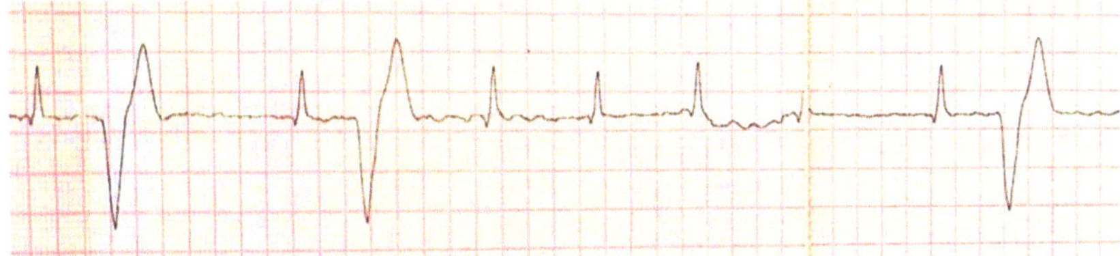

Answer. Electrocardiogram (lead II, speed 50 mm/s, sensitivity 1) of a Rottweiler dog with dilated cardiomyopathy is showing atrial fibrillations and ventricular premature complexes.

ECG 54

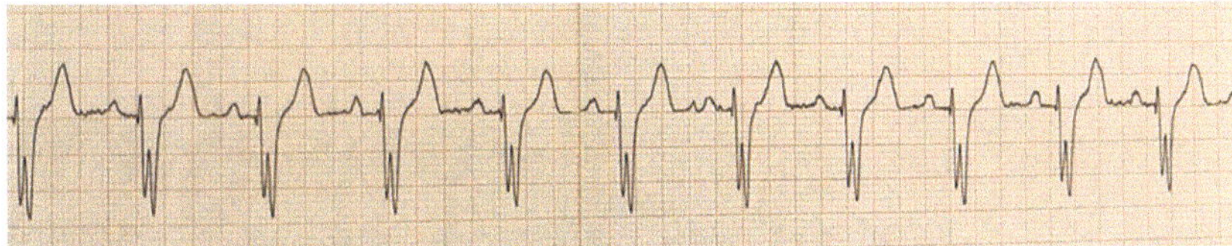

Answer. Electrocardiogram (lead II, speed 50 mm/s, sensitivity 1) of a Labrador with congestive heart failure is showing right bundle branch block. Note deep 'S' and wide 'QRS' (0.08 s).

ECG 55

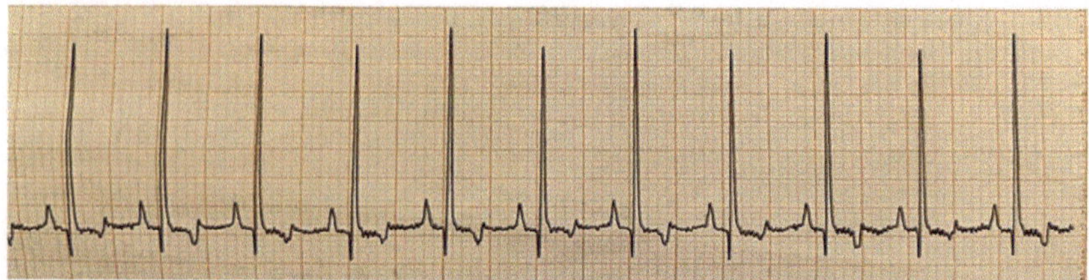

Question. It is an electrocardiogram (lead II, speed 25 mm/s, sensitivity 1) of a Labrador retriever with dilated cardiomyopathy. What is your interpretation?

ECG 56

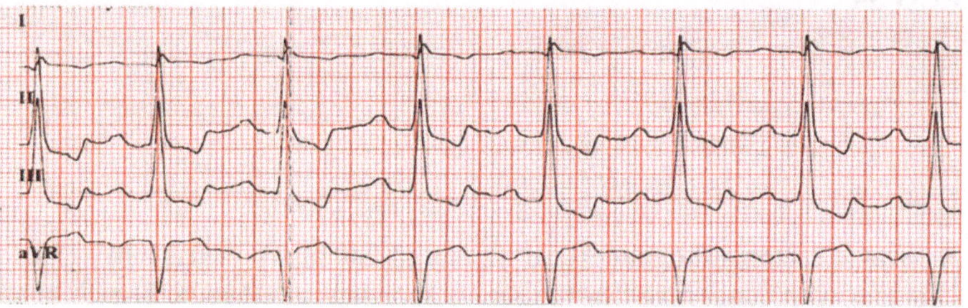

Question. It is an electrocardiogram (lead I, II, III, aVR, speed 50 mm/s, sensitivity 1) of a Labrador retriever with dilated cardiomyopathy. What is your interpretation?

ECG 55

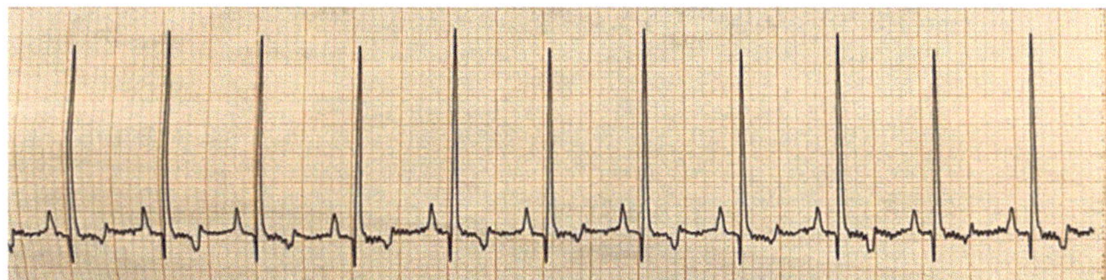

Answer. Electrocardiogram (lead II, speed 25 mm/s, sensitivity 1) of a Labrador Retriever with dilated cardiomyopathy is showing heart rate of 140 bpm, sinus rhythm (R-R interval 0.41-0.42 s), normal 'P' wave (0.4 mV. 0.04 s), normal P-R segment (0.04 s), normal P-R interval (0.08 s), small 'Q' wave (0.4 mV), variable increased amplitude of 'R' wave (3.1 to 3.5 mV), slightly broad 'QRS" (0.06 s), isoelectric S-T segment (0.06 s on base line), negative 'T' wave (0.25 mV, 0.08s) and fine muscle tremor artifacts. The electrocardiogram is suggestive of left ventricular enlargement with R alternans.

ECG 56

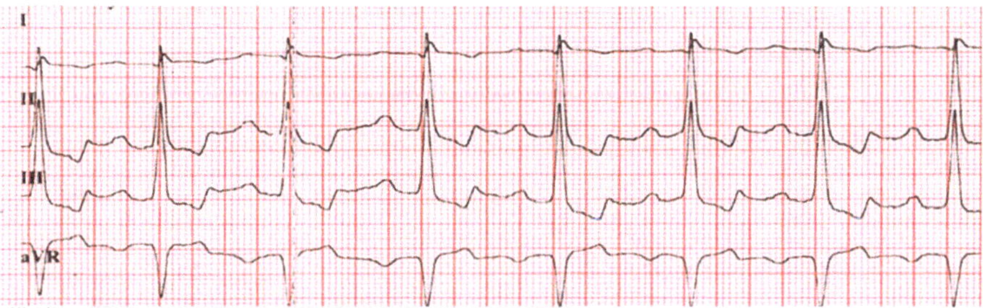

Answer. Electrocardiogram (leads I,II, III, aVR, speed 50 mm/s, sensitivity 1) of a nine year old Labrador Retriever with dilated cardiomyopathy is showing broad P (0.06 s) suggestive of left atrial enlargement (P mitrale)

ECG 57

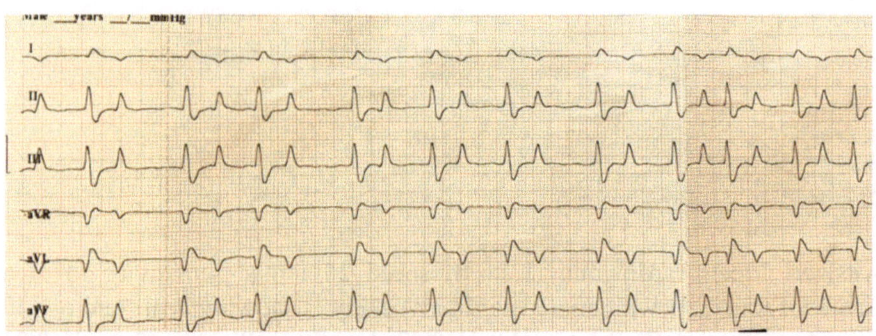

Question. It is an electrocardiogram (lead I, II, III, aVR, aVL, aVF, speed 50 mm/s, sensitivity 1) of a dog with cardio-renal syndrome . What is your interpretation?

ECG 58

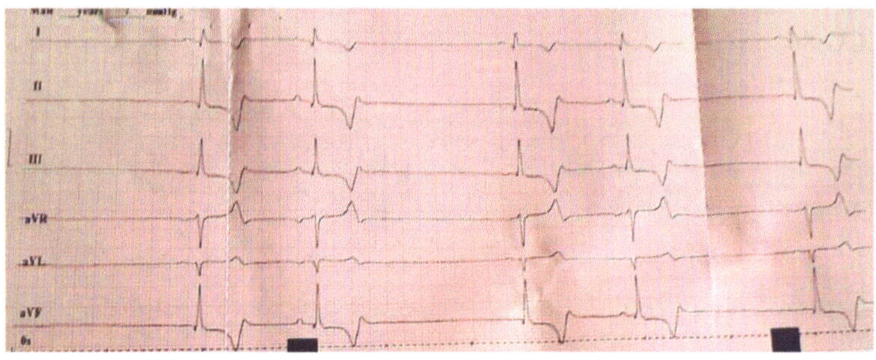

Question. It is an electrocardiogram (lead I, II, III, aVR, aVL, aVF, speed 50 mm/s, sensitivity 1) of an adult small nondescript dog. What is your interpretation?

ECG 57

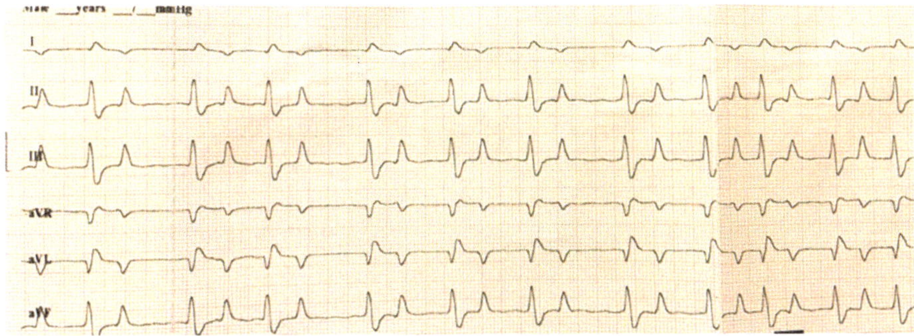

Answer. Electrocardiogram (Lead I, II, III, aVR, aVL, aVF, speed 50 mm/s, sensitivity 1) of a dog with cardio-renal syndrome is showing absence of 'P' wave, tall 'T' wave (0.4 mV) > 25% of 'R' wave (0.5 mV), indicating atrial standstill and enlarged 'T' wave.

ECG 58

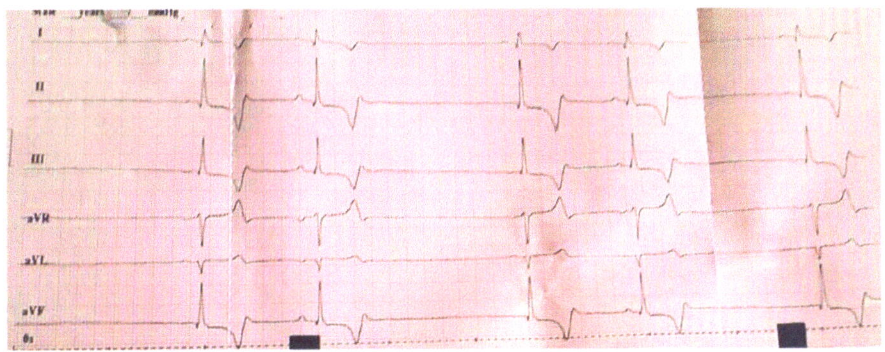

Answer. Electrocardiogram (Lead I, II, III, aVR, aVL, aVF, speed 50 mm/s, sensitivity 1) of an adult small nondescript dog is showing slow heart rate (80 bpm), and alternate ventricular escape complexes (1,3,5) without P wave following a long pause than the sinus complexes (2,4), The escape complexes (1,3,5) have not originated from SA node pacemaker but have originated from intrinsic pacemaker activity of the subsidiary lower region pacemaker located in the ventricle. Therefore these escape complexes are of ventricular origin.

ECG 59

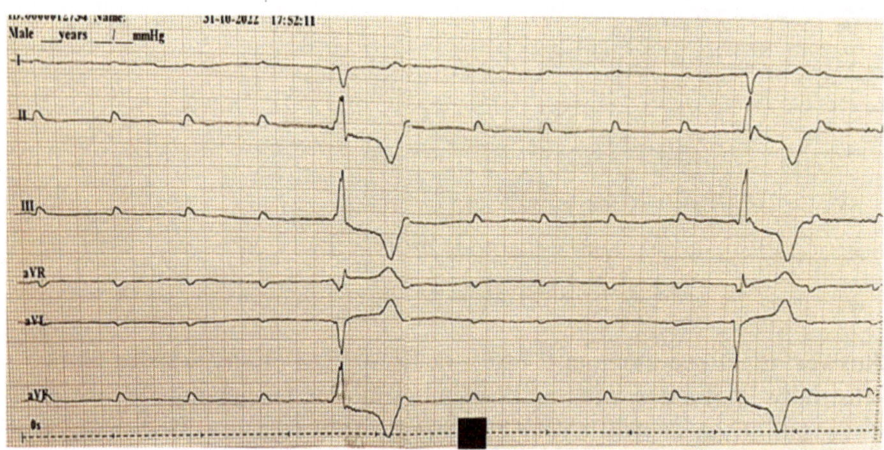

Question. It is an electrocardiogram (lead I, II, III, aVR, aVL, aVF, speed 50 mm/s, sensitivity 1) of a 10 year 6 month old pug with the history of seizures. What is your interpretation?

ECG 59

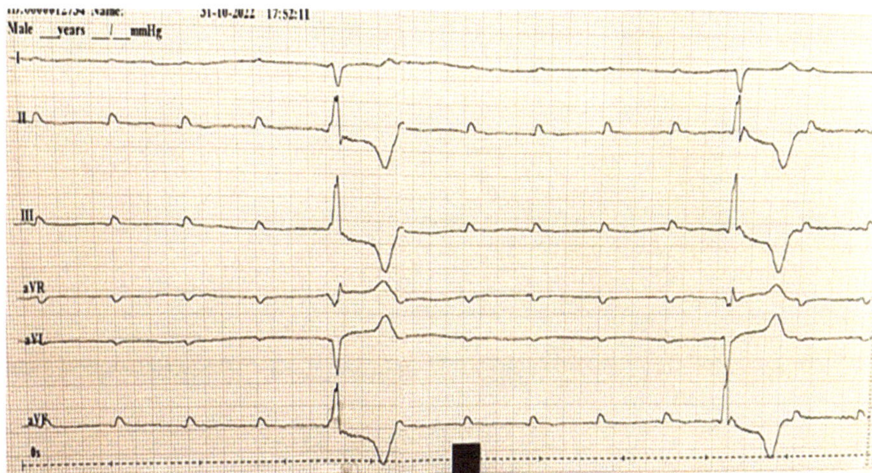

Answer. Electrocardiogram (Lead I, II, III, aVR, aVL, aVF, speed 50 mm/s, sensitivity 1) of a 10 year 6 month old pug with the history of seizures is showing complete heart block (3rd degree AV block) .The ' P' wave is occurring at a rate of 120 per minute. It (atrial activity) is independent of ventricular activity. The ventricular rate is 20 per minute. This ECG is suggestive of 3rd degree AV block,

ECG 60

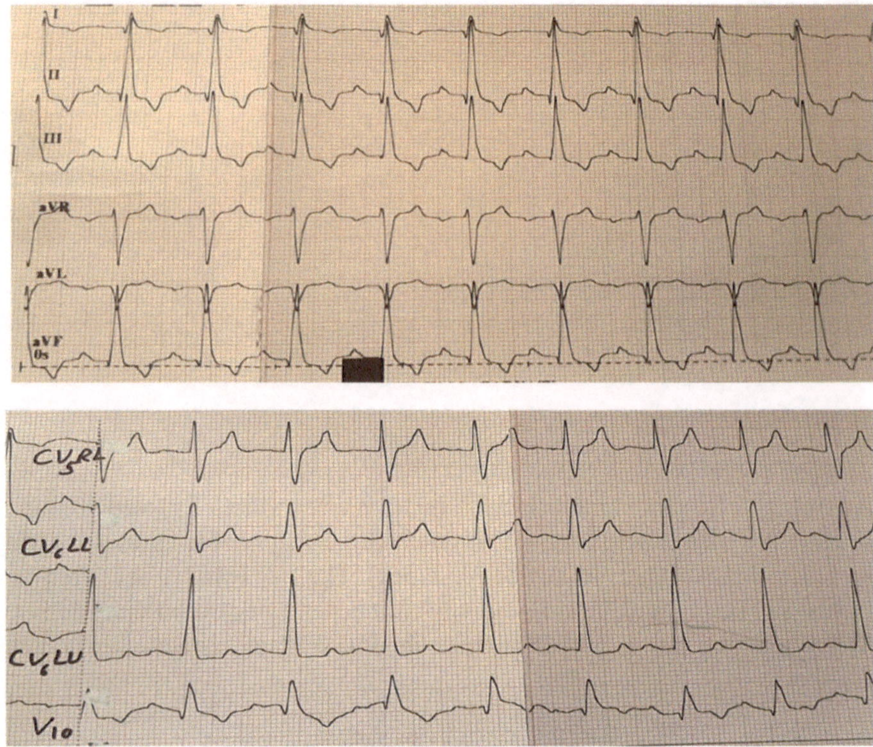

Question. It is an electrocardiogram (lead I, II, III, aVR, aVL, aVF, CV5RL, CV6LL, CV6LU ,V10, speed 50 mm/s, sensitivity 0.5) of a seven year old Labrador with signs of congestive heart failure and enlarged heart covering >82% chest cavity (X-ray). What is your interpretation?

ECG 60

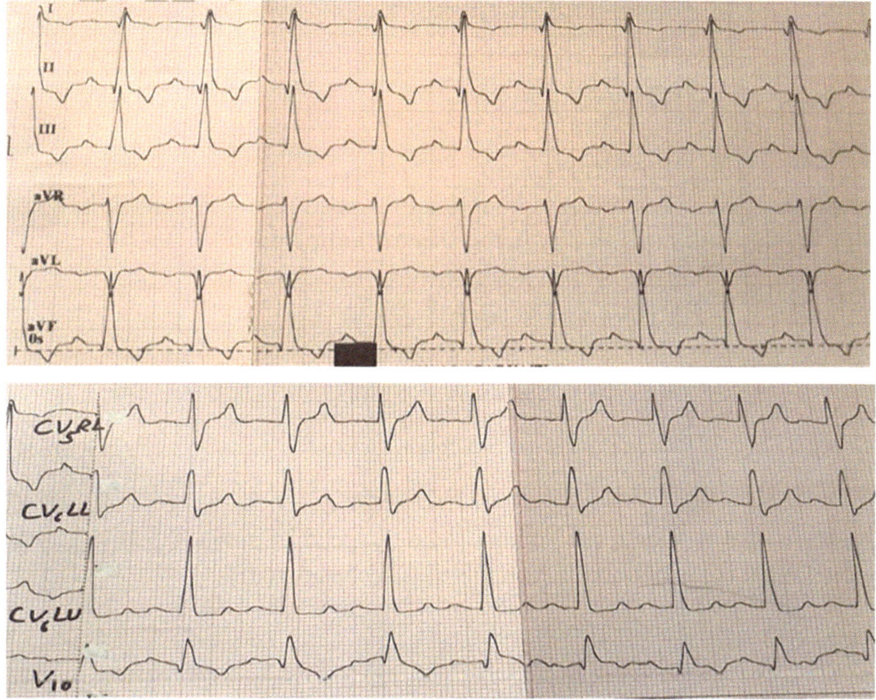

Answer. Electrocardiogram (lead I, II, III, aVR, aVL, aVF, CV5RL, CV6LL, CV6LU ,V10, speed 50 mm/s, sensitivity 0.5) of a seven year old Labrador with signs of congestive heart failure and enlarged heart covering >82% chest cavity (X-ray) is showing tachycardia (HR 177 bpm); tall R wave in Lead II (4.2 mV), III (3.1 mV), aVF (3.4 mV), and CV6 LU (4.0 mV) indicating left ventricular enlargement.

ECG 61

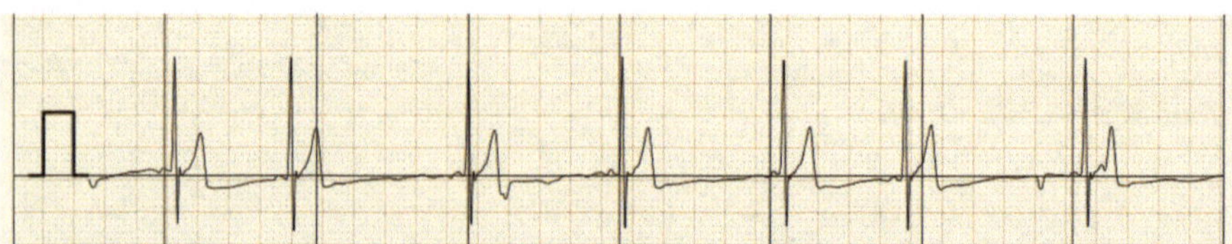

Question. It is an electrocardiogram (lead II, speed 25 mm/s, sensitivity 1) of a dog. What is the abnormality in this electrocardiogram?

ECG 62

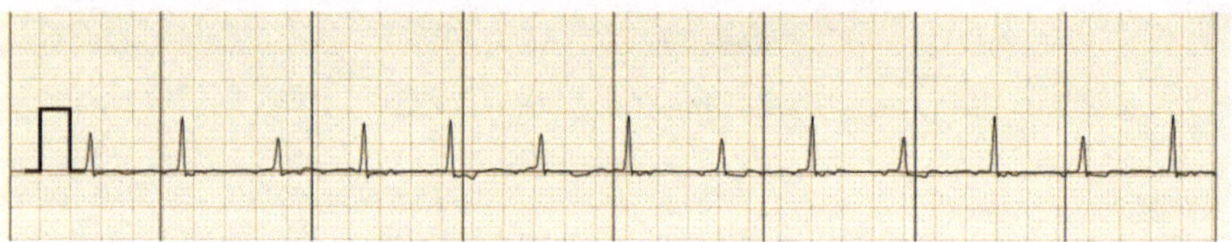

Question. It is an electrocardiogram (lead II, speed 25 mm/s, sensitivity 1) of a dog . What is the abnormality in this electrocardiogram?

ECG 61

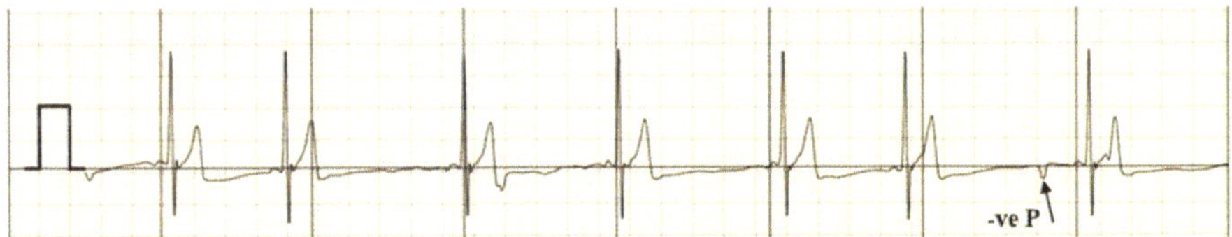

Answer. Electrocardiogram (lead II, speed 25 mm/s, sensitivity 1) of a dog is showing a -ve (negative) P wave suggestive of AV junctional premature complex.

ECG 62

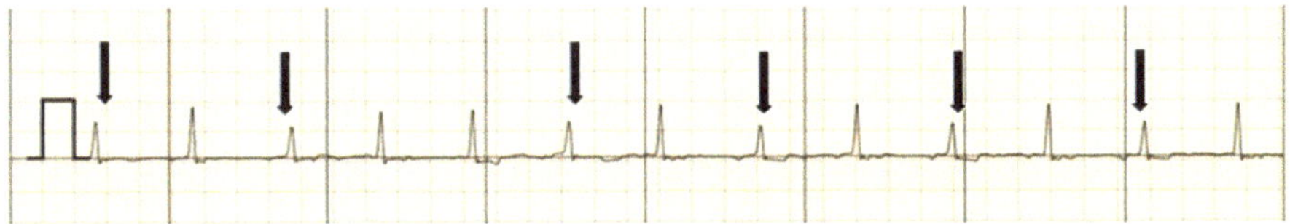

Answer. Electrocardiogram (lead II, speed 25 mm/s, sensitivity 1) of a dog is showing alteration in configuration on every other R wave (except at one place where alteration in configuration is after 2 R waves) suggestive of electrical alternans of R wave. In most of the cases it is associated with pericardial effusion.

ECG 63

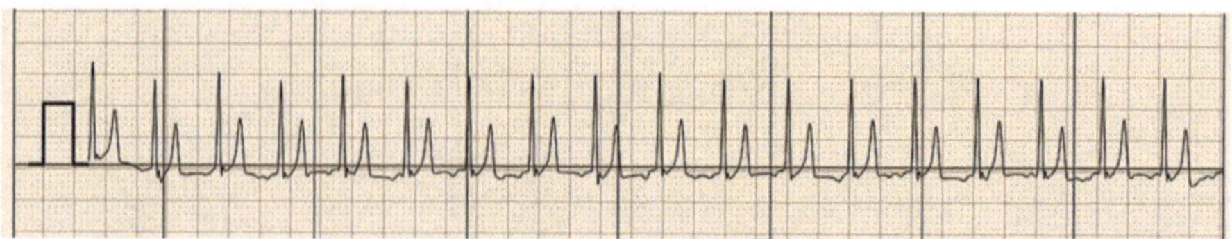

Question. It is an electrocardiogram (lead II, speed 25 mm/s, sensitivity 1) of a dog. What is your interpretation?

ECG 64

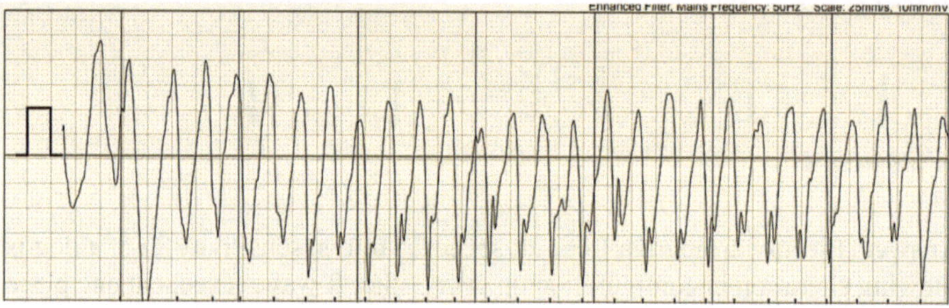

Question. It is an electrocardiogram (lead II, speed 25 mm/s, sensitivity 1) of a nine year old Cocker Spaniel with severe dyspnea at rest. What is your interpretation?

ECG 63

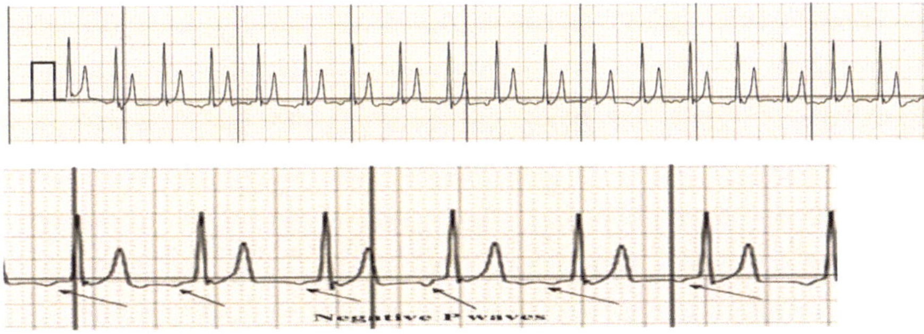

Answer. Electrocardiogram (lead II, speed 25 mm/s, sensitivity 1) of a dog is showing negative P' wave in all complexes, heart rate of 140 bpm (>60 bpm AV junctional inherent rate) regular rhythm, normal configuration of QRS complex, P'R interval is constant (0.08 s), atrioventricular conduction 1:1 suggesting supraventricular tachycardia of atrioventricular junctional (AV junctional) origin. It is also known as AV-junctional tachycardia.

ECG 64

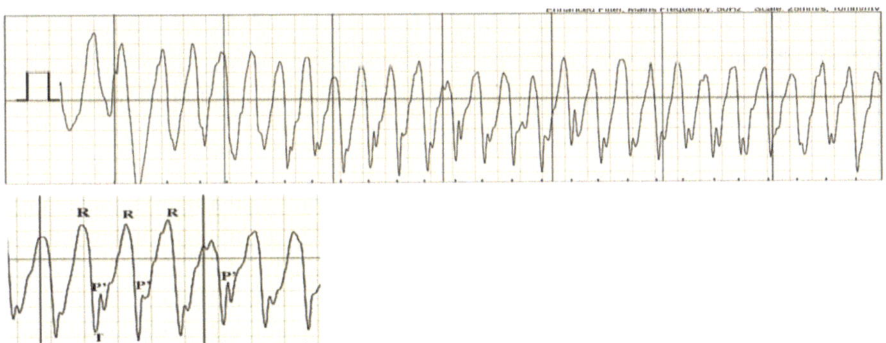

Answer. Electrocardiogram (lead II, speed 25 mm/s, sensitivity 1) of a nine year old Cocker Spaniel with severe dyspnea at rest is showing heart rate 220 bpm (>than normal heart rate), regular rhythm, positive P' wave, regular P'-P' interval, somewhat different configuration of P' wave, wide and bizarre QRS complex, constant P'-R interval, 1:1 AV conduction suggesting continuous atrial tachycardia of multifocal origin with left bundle branch block.

ECG 65

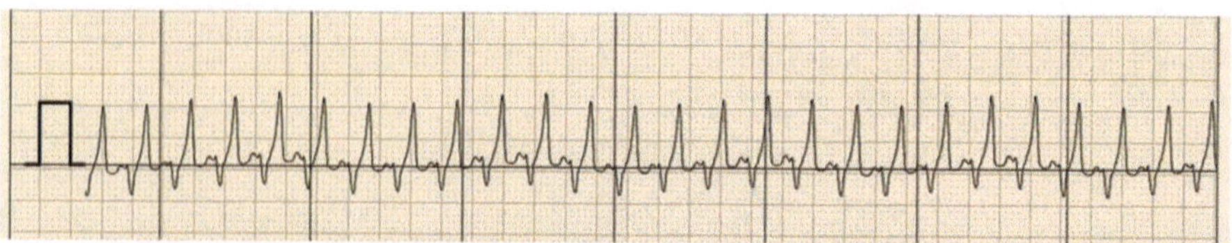

Question. It is an electrocardiogram (lead II, speed 25 mm/s, sensitivity 1) of a dog. What is your interpretation?

ECG 66

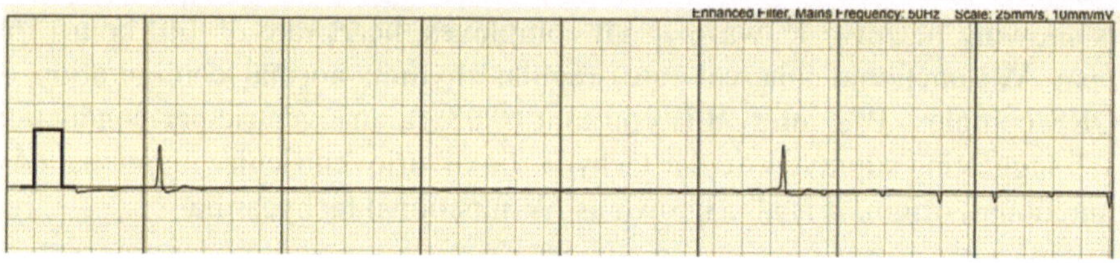

Question. It is an electrocardiogram (lead II, speed 25 mm/s, sensitivity 1) of a 12 year old Labrador presented in unconscious state. What is your interpretation?

ECG65

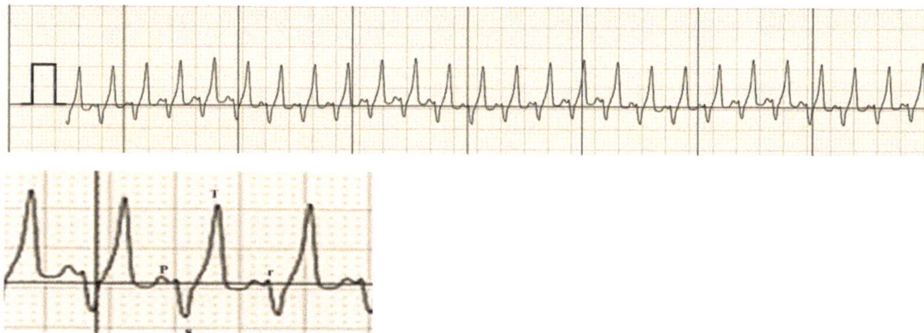

Answer. Electrocardiogram (lead II, speed 25 mm/s, sensitivity 1) of a dog is showing heart rate of 200 bpm (>than normal heart rate), regular rhythm, positive small 'P' wave (0.05 mV,0.03 s), very small 'r' wave (0.025 mV), small S wave (0.35 mV), normal duration QRS (0.05 s) and large + ve pointed 'T' wave (1.0 -1.1 mV) suggesting sinus tachycardia and tall pointed 'T' wave in relation to very small 'r' wave.

ECG 66

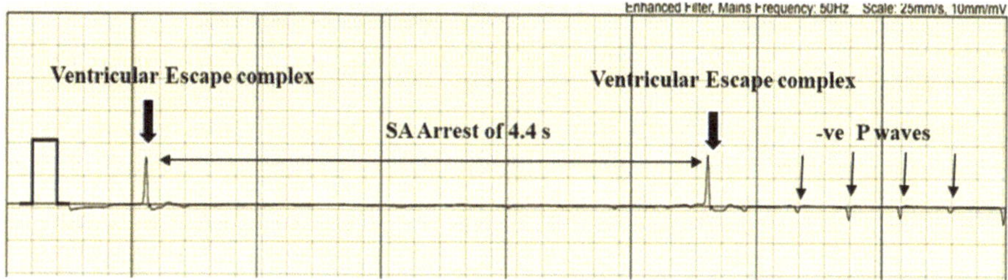

Answer. Electrocardiogram (lead II, speed 25 mm/s, sensitivity 1) of a 12 year old Labrador, presented in unconscious state, is showing ventricular asystole caused by severe sino-atrial arrest (SA arrest) of 4.4 s. No P, QRS and T complexes are seen during this period. Ventricular escape complex (no P wave in these complexes) is seen before and after the SA arrest indicating that the pace maker of the SA node stopped functioning and pace maker of lower region (the ventricle) made an attempt to rescue the heartbeat. Four AV-junctional premature complex (negative P wave) are seen after the 2nd ventricular escape complex indicating that SA node pace maker still failed to function and the pace maker at AV junction attempted to rescue the heart rhythm but failed to conduct the current further to Bundle of His to bundle branches to ventricles leading to no ventricular activity.

ECG 67

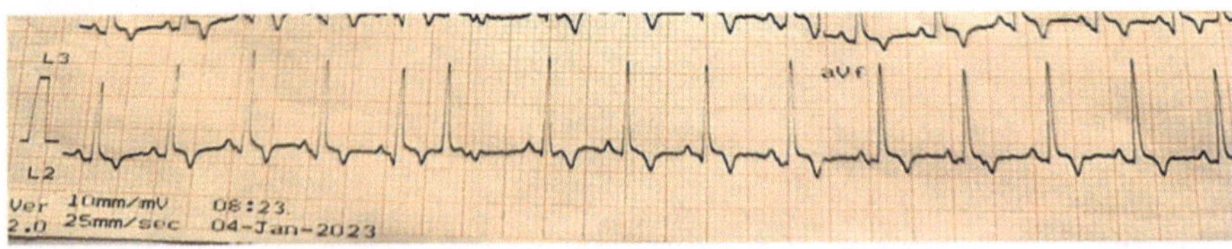

A

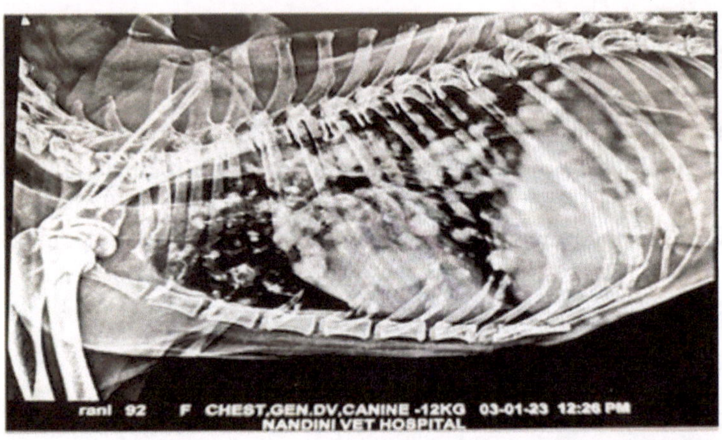

B

Question. It is an electrocardiogram (A- Lead II, speed 25 mm/s, sensitivity 1) of a 17 year old Pomeranian bitch with metastasis in lungs (B). What is your interpretation?

ECG 67

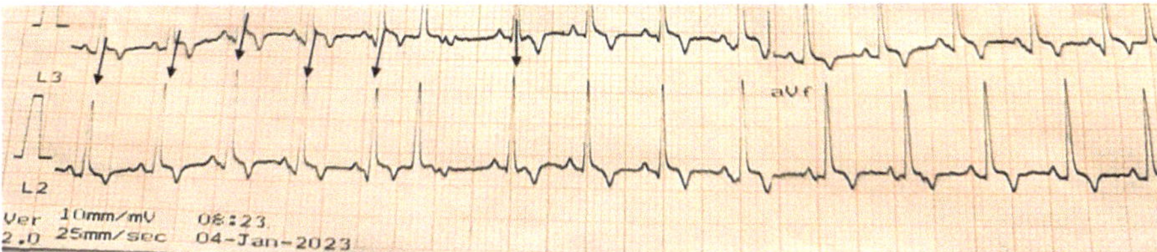

A

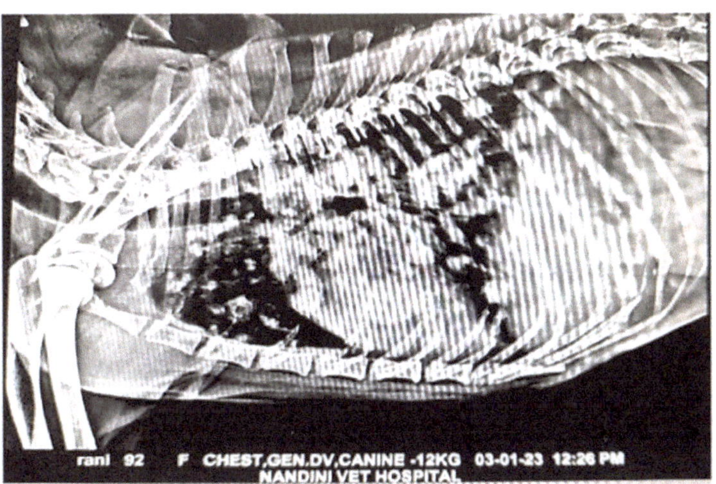

B

Answer. Electrocardiogram (A- lead II, speed 25 mm/s, sensitivity 1) of a 17 year old Pomeranian bitch with metastasis in lungs (B) is showing a heart rate of 160 bpm, 'R' alternans in all leads (amplitude of R wave is varying). The 'P' wave is related to 'QRS' of almost from the same pacemaker. Only at one place R-R interval is less than the others. Electrical alternans may be due to pericardial effusion, supraventricular tachycardia or alternating bundle branch block. In majority of cases it is due to pericardial effusion owing to neoplasia of heart base, metastatic carcinoma, right heart failure or benign idiopathic pericardial effusion. In this case electrical R alternans appears to be due to metastasis in the lungs.

Index

Q

R

S

T

V